M000250009

HEALTH AND DISEASE BEGIN IN THE COLON

Featuring: Professor Serge Jurasunas' Natural Medicine. Healthcare Strategy: Introducing Iridology, Analytic Blood Microscopy, Molecular Markers Testing and Therapeutic Microbiome and Colon Care, Detox.

A Textbook for both Laymen and Health Professionals. New Trends in Cancer Diagnostics and Early Detection.

Original translation from the Portuguese publication – copyright nº 216848/04

All rights reserved. The total or partial reproduction of the texts or images in this book through mechanical, electronic, or photocopying means without the written authorization of the author is forbidden.

Title: Health Passes Through the Intestine. Author; Serge Jurasunas

Publisher: Serge Jurasunas
English editing: Shel Stein
Cover design: Peter Anthony Design
Photographic images: Serge Jurasunas
Graphics: Serge Jurasunas, David Pesek
Formatting: Jimandzetta.com

Editor: By the Author.
Copyright 2009 no 216848/04 in Portuguese

Copyright 2016 New revised English edition
Printed in the US and UK/Europe

Print ISBN: 978-989-20-6938-8
Ebook ISBN: 978-989-20-7002-5

Health and Disease Begin in the Colon is written as a reference book with the sole objective to instruct the reader about the colon and Iridology, and to learn about how to prevent disease by suggesting Naturopathic principles for the maintenance of health. This book is solely for educational purposes and should not be construed as medical advice or as an alternative to medical checkups or hospital care. Always ask your doctor for advice before taking any detoxification regimen. Medical questions should be directed to a qualified practitioner.

Professional consultations and questions may be directed to: sergejurasunas@hotmail.com.

Please visit: www.sergejurasunas.com for more information, articles, and presentations.

Table of Contents

The Author:

Serge Jurasunas is an internationally renowned Naturopath and homeopathic medical doctor, researcher, lecturer, and writer specializing in the art of nutrition, detoxification, and Iridology.

Beginning his career in Canada in 1967, over the past four, now approaching five decades, he became involved in several directions including Live Blood Analysis, Oxidative Stress, and Oxidative Dried Blood Testing, while building a highly regarded reputation in the field of Integrative Oncology. He has travelled to over fifty countries to study and lecture on the lifestyles and health status of different cultures. In Portugal, Serge Jurasunas runs a clinic where patients come from different countries, throughout the world come seeking a solution to their disease. After nearly half a century, he contributed many new ideas, extensive new developments in complementary oncology, and developed many new nutritional and detoxification regimens and diets.

He is increasingly convinced about the importance of educating people and teaching patients, looking for the cause of illness rather than treating only apparent symptoms through medicinal drugs. He continues to hold conferences and seminars all over the world.

Thanks to his work on Iridology and other scientific publications, in 1996 he was appointed professor at Capital University of Integrative Medicine in Washington, D.C. More recently, he has just been appointed Professor of Iridology and Naturopathic Oncology at Pan American University of Natural Sciences and Medicine, and Honorary Lifetime Member of the International Institute of Iridology. He also received the Dr. Ignaz Peczely Award in recognition of his contribution to the Science of Iridology.

Professor Jurasunas further developed Iridology and furthered other health principles he learned from some of the great pioneers such as Dr. Bernard Jensen who, back in 1964, became his mentor, A. Vogel, and O. Warburg. He then studied the theories of Naturopathy with contemporary innovators like J. Tilden, B. Lust, A. Ehret, and L. Khune.

Serge Jurasunas has been honored many times and decorated for his work by Academies of Science, receiving the Silver medal of research and invention by the French Academy. He is member of over thirty professional associations and academies, including the prestigious American Academy of Anti-Aging Medicine and the New York Academy of Sciences.

"Serge Jurasunas is the author of over 150 papers from conferences and articles published over the past 15 years in The Townsend Letter Magazine (USA). In Europe he published five books including titles on Iridology, Oxidative Stress and Cancer, Lapacho, and Health Revolution." His work has been translated into 13 languages.

Chivalric Order: Serge Jurasunas is Knight Commander of the Sovereign and Military Order of St. Brigitte of Sweden, from the Order of the Temple of Jerusalem. Grand Master of the Sovereign Order of St. John of Jerusalem – Knights of Malta.

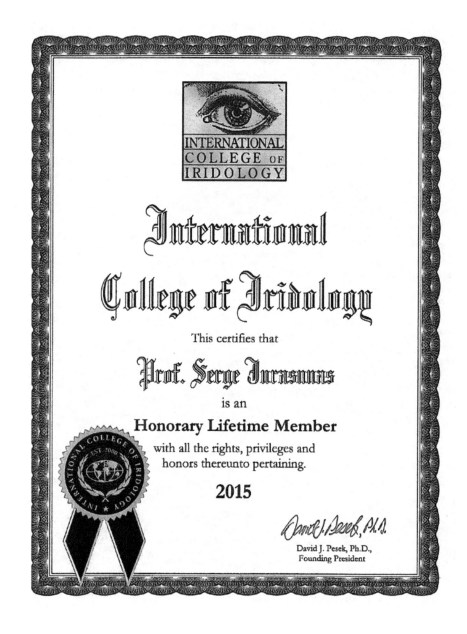

INTERNATIONAL
COLLEGE OF
IRIDOLOGY

International College of Iridology

This certifies that

Prof. Serge Jurasunas

is an

Honorary Lifetime Member

with all the rights, privileges and
honors thereunto pertaining.

2015

David J. Pesek, Ph.D.,
Founding President

The Master with His Pupil

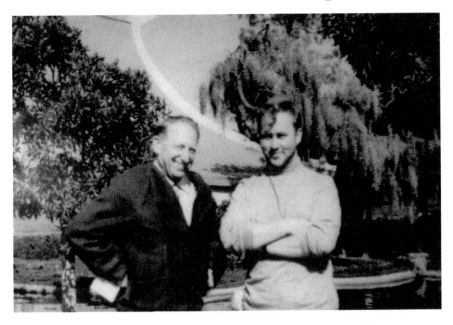

Photo of Serge Jurasunas and Bernard Jensen taken in 1962 in San Diego

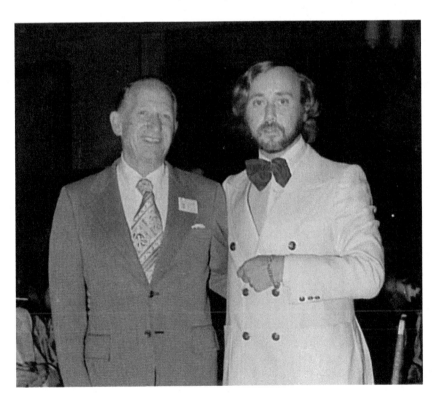

Bernard Jensen and Serge Jurasunas at the World Congress of Natural Medicine
1973 – Aix-en-Provence, France

Foreword

It is a great pleasure to write a foreword to this excellent book, *Health and Disease Begin with the Colon*. The author, Prof. Dr. Serge Jurasunas, has truly been inspired by his own life experiences and his pursuit of personal wellness. In this pursuit of wellness, at a young age Dr. Jurasunas' life path moved in the direction of helping others as he expanded his knowledge through his direct study with some of the great natural healing pioneers of the twentieth century.

Dr. Jurasunas and I met at an iridology conference in London, England in the late 1990s. We made a nice connection with each other and have been friends ever since. One of our most influential mentors was the late Dr. Bernard Jensen with whom we both had a special relationship at different times and many years before our encounter in London.

Dr. Jurasunas is one of the world's most prominent naturopathic oncologists. He is a pioneer in this field and has presented his research across the globe at numerous conferences, congresses, and symposiums. Serge has a deep and dedicated passion to helping others to transform their lives from illness to wellness. It is through this passion and a half century of clinical practice that he has created a book that is relevant today and useful for those seeking a better, healthier life. He offers to the reader well-explained, thought-provoking concepts for cleansing the organs and tissues of the human body with a primary emphasis on the large intestine or colon.

We have the ability to heal ourselves, and people today are awakening to the notion of self-responsibility. In this text, Dr. Jurasunas provides the rationale and explanations for the reader to assume the self-responsible paradigm of personal wellness.

Some of the earliest recorded practices of internal cleansing date back to the Hebrew sect, the Essenes. This sect of Judaism flourished from the second century BCE to the first century CE. They lived throughout Roman Judea. As a group, they were considered to be health conscious both spiritually and physically. They firmly believed in dietary fasting and internal cleansing. The Essenes were known to have devised a procedure, over two thousand years ago, for cleansing the colon. This technique was the forerunner of the modern day clinical procedure of colon hydrotherapy.

Until recently, medical science thought of the colon or large intestine as a mere receptacle tissue structure of the body. It was believed to be a storage tube for digested food material and metabolic waste waiting to be evacuated out of the body transiting the rectum and anus. Today, the colon is said to be our second brain due to the neurotransmitters it produces.

Dr. Jurasunas draws on his clinical practice experience to educate the reader to the present-day knowledge of the colon with his wealth of information on this structure of the gastrointestinal tract that is so vital to our overall health and wellbeing, physically, emotionally, and mentally.

In the second half of the twentieth century a growing awareness of the importance of diet, nutrition, and internal hygiene was beginning to emerge. By the early 1970s, this awareness was gaining momentum. People were starting to take nutritional supplements and eat foods that were whole and free of chemicals. Today, these foods are referred to as "organic." All living things that have a metabolism are actually organic, as compared to rocks which are inorganic. However, the term "organic" has also been designated to mean all natural and free of industrial chemicals.

While this phenomenon was blossoming, conventional thought in the allopathic medical model held firm that an individual's diet, nutrition, and internal hygiene had little or no relationship to his or her physical health and that we could receive all the vitamins and minerals we require by simply eating over-processed, industrial, chemical-laden meats, grains, and dairy products. A particular State Board of Psychology that I was compelled to be a member of took a blanket position that diet, nutrition, and body toxicity had no relationship to an individual's mental and/or emotional health, even in light of research evidence at the time to the contrary. This was as recently as the early 1990s.

Dr. Jurasunas has dedicated decades of his life to studying and observing the correlation between diet and nutrition, constipation, and breast cancer. He has seen a strong link between these three factors. Over the past several years he has been working with the molecular markers related to cancer. One such marker is the P53 tumor suppressor, the guardian against cancer. More than 50% of all cancers are linked to a mutation of the P53 gene.

Most of us have had the experience of a friend or family member who has been diagnosed with cancer. And far too many people have succumbed to this dreadful, preventable disease. With the onslaught of environmental toxins, our health and immunity are constantly under siege. Internal tissue cleansing or organ detoxification is necessary to give the body a fighting chance to ward off disease and build a healthy immune system. Dr. Jurasunas drives this point home in this informative book about the critical importance of cleansing the colon as the starting point on the physical level.

Today there is tremendous, worldwide interest in human health and disease prevention. Healthy aging is of utmost interest to people who are conscious about their wellbeing. I am happy to say that over the past several years the allopathic medical model has begun to adopt limited forms of natural therapies, along with some diet, nutritional and detoxification practices, albeit motivated by profit-loss. Billions of dollars are willingly spent, out-of-pocket, annually by people seeking natural forms of healthcare either to prevent disease or to heal themselves.

As natural, traditional, and age-old remedies and therapies began to receive limited acceptance by mainstream medicine, they were referred to as "alternative therapies." Later the reference was changed to "complimentary medicine." Now, progressive physicians have begun to experience and realize the power in natural healing modalities, the current term most commonly used is "integrative medicine." This is a combination of both allopathic and naturopathic practices, and perhaps, is the best of both worlds.

The human body has many ways to give us information about its levels of function and overall health. Some techniques are ancient, such as pulse diagnosis, fingernail analysis, observation of the tongue, and iris analysis. Other, more modern techniques include various evaluations of the blood, whether it be a dried sample or a live cell. One of these more progressive techniques is known as the Oxidative Dried Blood Test. This evaluation examines the fibrin web structure and morphological changes under a microscope using multiphase contrast. Through this procedure, other information can indicate potential issues such as allergies, bowel toxicity, and levels of inflammation, heavy metal toxicity, and hormonal imbalances. Another procedure discussed in this text is the Live Blood Analysis and how it is used to evaluate potential conditions such as oxidative stress, risk of brain stroke, as well as toxins resulting from lowered liver and kidney function. Serge also integrates the ancient technique of Tongue Diagnosis that provides further information about the health of the digestive, hepatic, renal, and respiratory systems. It also includes the heart and spleen. The aforementioned are but three of the many tools of analysis Dr. Jurasunas employs to help guide his patients to wellness.

The medical paradigm of the quick fix and the suppression of symptoms of dis-ease does not correct the recurring problem, nor does it prevent degenerative disease. Thus, there is an inevitable disenchantment with the current, allopathic, medical business. The natural healthcare seeker is experiencing positive results where the way of toxic pharmaceutical drugs (not actually medicine) and the surgeon's scalpel are, in most cases, ineffective at curing the problem.

Over the past forty years that I have practiced natural healthcare, I have seen a significant trend in the population toward people assuming personal responsibility and developing an attitude of self-reliance for their own levels of health. As a clinician and natural health educator, this is very gratifying for me. People are realizing that the doctor does not do the healing (not even the natural healthcare doctor) and that, ultimately, it is up to them in their consciousness and their relationship with the creative source of all, God.

In those early years of my practice, the mainstream thinking was that the spiritual, mental, emotional, and physical aspects of our human nature are uniquely separate. Today, scientific research has proven, overwhelmingly, the interconnectedness of these aspects. There has even been research that shows the positive effects of prayer in one's healing process. Western Civilization is beginning to wake up to a new way of thinking and being.

Our bodies contain genetic information in the DNA. Most people understand that our physical traits are inherited. Some examples are blue eyes, medium build, brown hair, bold chin, etc. What most people do not know is that we also inherit thought and emotional patterns from our ancestors that can go back several generations, just like the physical traits.

Predispositions to degenerative diseases that run in the family are understood to be genetically transferred and can be further induced by the ways we eat, drink, feel, think, live, and love. Personality traits are also present in the genetic material we have received from our ancestors. Individuals who have one or more of the following: deep-seated anger, low self-esteem, survival issues, relationship difficulties, grief and sadness, or depression, to name a few, may have genetics that predispose them to these conditions. Keep in mind that we may also inherit conditions and traits that we consider positive or constructive, such as determination, strong self-esteem, or forgiving and loving easily.

Beyond genetics, we know today that we also have epigenetics. The term "epigenetics" refers to heritable changes in gene expression (active versus inactive genes). Epigenetic change is a regular and natural occurrence and can also be influenced by many factors including environment, lifestyle, thoughts, feelings, behaviors and more. In simple terms, we are capable of influencing the expression of the genetics we are born with. We can keep the P53 gene and other aspects of our immune system healthy and functioning. This is a constant process throughout our lives which can happen unconsciously or consciously. One of my favorite mottos that I emphasize in my practice and seminar teaching is, "Good Health is Your Choice!"™ This is scientifically true.

The science and practice of Iridology is not new. The oldest records uncovered thus far have shown that a form of iris interpretation was used in Central Asia (Mesopotamia) as far back as 1000 BC, nearly three thousand years ago, in the Chaldean civilization. In the Bible, St. Luke writes that Christ said, "The lamp of your body is the eye. When your eyes are sound, you have light for the whole body, but when your eyes are bad, you are in darkness."

Conscious or unconscious genetic patterns of physical, emotional and mental traits, both constructive and destructive, can be seen in the irises (colored portion) of the eyes through the use of the science and practice of iridology. This particular system of iris analysis is called Holistic Iridology®.

From the physiological standpoint, the eyes are connected and continuous with the brain's dura mater through the fibrous sheath of the optic nerves. The eyes are connected directly with the sympathetic nervous system and spinal cord. The optic tract extends to the thalamus area of the brain. This creates a close association with the hypothalamus, pituitary, and pineal glands. These endocrine glands within the brain are major control and processing centers for the entire body. Because of this anatomy and physiology, the eyes are in direct contact with the biochemical, hormonal, structural and metabolic processes of the body via the nerves, blood vessels, lymph and connective tissue. It is estimated that the brain processes 400 billion bits of information every second and that only two thousand bits of this information reaches a person's conscious awareness. This information is recorded in the various structures of the eye, i.e. iris, retina, sclera, cornea, pupil and conjunctiva. Thus, it can be said that the eyes are reflexes or windows into the bioenergetics of the physical body and a person's feelings and thoughts.

Through his tireless efforts with clinical practice and research, Serge has discovered markers in the irises that correlate to disease conditions in the body. One of these contributions relates to breast cancer. You will learn more about Iridology in Part V.

The information interpreted from the eyes helps reveal the root causes of a person's conditions. By getting to these root causes and eliminating them, it is possible to effect true healing rather than just suppression of symptoms. Imagine that you have a beautiful flower garden and it has weeds growing amongst the colorful and fragrant blossoms. Would you tend to your garden by merely cutting the weeds off at the ground? Of course not, they would return only to be stronger. You would pull them out by their roots to eliminate them, giving your beautiful flowers a better opportunity to grow. This analogy holds true for the healing process within you. It is necessary to get to the root causes of dis-ease and disease, most of which begin in the colon.

Each and every one of us has the innate ability to be healthy. Quantum physics tells us that we truly create our own reality second by second, a reality of infinite possibilities. Our spirit and consciousness sustain thoughts, from which arise emotions, which in turn affect the physical body on a cellular level. Simply put, all of this information flows through the body, as neuropeptides and hormones via the nervous system, the cerebrospinal fluid, the blood, and lymphatic circulatory systems, as well as the subtle energy systems.

All healing begins on the spiritual level first, then into the mental and emotional levels, and finally into the physical body. This is the true nature of the healing process. You have the God-given power to change your life on all levels. "Remember…Good Health is Your Choice!"™

I recommend this book as a guide to anyone who is seeking natural healthcare information and choosing wellness through the process of detoxification. Read, learn, and enjoy.

David J. Pesek, Ph.D.
January 2016

Preface

Earlier in my life I felt a particular interest for the healing power of nature and the Naturopathic system to prevent and treat disease. Back in the year 1962, recently emigrating from France and living in Los Angeles, I had the opportunity to meet Dr. Bernard Jensen, one of the greatest pioneers in Iridology, and had an iris examination in his office where he suggested I change my dietary style and take some supplementation. Later on, Dr. Jensen invited me to come along with him to Hidden Valley Health Ranch in Escondido where I could immediately observe how patients were treated with natural food, diet, organic vegetable juice, chiropractic, detox, and colon irrigation, which was something new for me.

It could not have been more opportune for me to observe with my own eyes, during the several occasions that I stayed there, how patients with different types of disease would improve and get better without taking any pharmaceutical drugs. This personal training from Dr. Jensen, especially being directly in contact with patients, talking to them, asking questions, and observing how they were improving, was certainly the main reason for me to decide to pursue the same road and choose this as my profession. From this contact where Dr. Jensen was also teaching patients what to do to improve their lifestyle, definitely showed me that also I would need to teach people a better way of life, to eat better food, and how to change their mind and their spirit. This is what I followed for the past fifty years.

After graduating in Naturopathy, and later on in Homeopathic medicine, I started learning about other methods, other sciences, other medicines and theories, all of which took place over the past five decades, but of course Iridology remained to me of major interest, especially how the iris reveals your genetic stature, which I found incredible. My interest in treating disease drove me toward study, research, and the clinical application of new approaches to treat the disease of cancer. During the last several years I have been involved with molecular markers and molecular medicine. I am however still convinced that colon cleansing is still important, even for cancer patients, since years ago I learned about the cancer therapy method of Dr. Max Gerson who was using enema therapy for his patients. Later on I made the correlation between pre-cancerous signs visible in iris and molecular markers testing, mainly the P53 tumor suppressor gene, with additional details to follow in this book.

In 1978 I opened my first clinic in Lisbon, then in 1983 a much larger one outside of the city with more space, where I could have more treatment rooms, including ones for colon hydrotherapy. I have treated thousands of patients from all over the world with all types of diseases, but always had a particular interest in the field of Naturopathic Oncology. I have spent much time teaching people, taught so many doctors, and traveled to many countries around the world to lecture, but also to learn about other methods and diagnostics. For this reason, I introduced Live Blood Analysis and the oxidative dried blood test that I pioneered, which really give me a better opportunity to better understand the role of natural food, diet, and detoxification over junk food. You observe before and then you observe after how the patient has done with a diet, or even a detox, how incredible is the change in blood status! Then you observe how medical doctors are not able to show interest or to observe since it is a way to learn and to grow. This is why I decided to introduce these two blood tests in this new English version of my book in Chapter III, so the reader will readily see the difference between clean blood and intoxicated blood, not even mentioning the change in free radical activity.

To begin with, in Chapters I and II, I discuss the gut system and the microbiome; in Chapter III, about all the intestinal problems including constipation and the link between breast cancer and constipation. In Chapter IV we have a large section about auto-intoxication and its consequences, which is one of the main pillars of my theory associated with disease. Chapter V is very important as it contains some approaches to Iridology from an embryonic standpoint, the intestine as our second brain, about our intestinal immune system, and a major explanation about the science of Iridology and how it can reflect genetic reflex disease, which is one important theory of Naturopathy. Finally, in Chapter VI, we focus on a detoxification program, dietary approach, the nutritional value of food, and different techniques such as colon hydrotherapy and other bowel management methods for those people who wish to cleanse their body.

Over the years I could observe in my patients the benefit of detoxification, no matter what the disease or just as a preventive measure. We can even approach disease from solely a molecular standpoint and proclaim that disease is just a problem associated with only four letters of the alphabet of our genome, such as ATCG and mutation of one of these letters, but we are still missing the total body and how to approach the disease and the patient. In fact, intoxication of the colon leads to intoxication of the blood and the body; a leaky gut increases the penetration of bacteria and Candida in the blood that can in turn intoxicate cells and even induce a P53 mutation that leads to cancer.

Therefore, without a doubt, diet, detoxification, colon cleansing, and liver detox remain an important approach to improving health condition. Each time I have a patient in my clinic, no matter what the disease, I first check through Iridology the main elimination channels which are the colon, kidney, lungs, skin, liver, and lymphatic system, along with a Live Blood Analysis observation through a special microscope which may show how much the blood is intoxicated. You can also be sure that the patient has a bad bowel function. Being a specialist in Naturopathic Oncology and molecular markers, we also cannot forget we can target cancer cells in several simultaneous directions with a molecular approach, while also not forgetting the emunctory organs and detoxifying the body, all of which in turn synergistically increases immune defense.

Finally, we have to remember one thing. Our health status depends on what we eat, how we absorb food, and how much foreign waste and toxins are eliminated. Healthy cells make healthy tissues, healthy tissues make healthy organs, and healthy organs make a healthy body. This can only be achieved through a diet of natural food, oxygen, and exercise for the sake of the body's own detoxification and clean blood. It cannot be any other way. For this reason I decided to write this book to present my clinical and experimental observations about how our digestive system functions, about some new facts and discoveries, about our intestinal system, and how it can be associated with disease, reflex disease, and how we can treat our bodies better through detoxification and in return improve our health status.

As an underlying foundation, I teach that Iridology is the most important method to visualize the whole body, especially the organs that carry on the duty to detoxify then expulse waste matter and keep the body in harmony, even without the perspective of disease. The last chapter shows interesting iris clinical cases, although I finally decided to include some real patient cases to demonstrate how we can really treat disease with a natural approach and keep some patients healthy for many years to come.

Introduction

In his extraordinary work published in 1944, *Man, the Unknown*, by Dr. Alexis Carrel, Nobel Prize winner for Medicine, we may read the following quotation:

"Our ignorance is naturally very strange. It is the result of the extreme abundance and confusion of concepts that mankind has amassed about itself and apportioned into an almost infinite number of segments allocated to the study of our body by science."

The division of the human body by placing each of its organs into a separate compartment, encouraged medicine to create for each organ or system, a specialty followed by intensive study into each of the organ's mechanisms, supposedly independent from each other. For each one, specific medicines supposed to control the abnormal or damaged mechanisms were developed.

In this way the specializations of cardiology, neurology, stomatology, dermatology, and psychiatry came about giving birth to medical specialists and their long list of drugs, which according to Dr. Alexis Carrel was one of the major medical mistakes. Notwithstanding the enormous amount of progress we have seen, we must remember that these organs depend upon one another, where the study of embryology can confirm this theory.

We must also remember that these organs also depend on the quality of the food we eat, the water we drink, and the air we breathe. They depend on good digestion and the assimilation of food. Make no mistake, the human body has a unique organizational system. It digests and transforms food, assimilates it, and with the help of oxygen, transforms it into cellular energy. It then expels toxic waste from the transformation and assimilation of food passing through the intestine. The food we ingest, be it meat, fish, or carrots do not enter the organism with a specific label of meat or fish, but simply as food molecules transformed into amino acids, lipids, and carbohydrates.

An entire infrastructure is necessary in order for this transformation to take place, an organization we take for granted, especially in the stressful context of modern society. Eating cannot be directed only toward satisfying one's taste and filling the stomach rather than fulfilling a biological need to activate and to maintain all the organism's functions. Today we have started to see food as much more important in our daily life since it can be seen as our medicine, as proclaimed by Hippocrates 2,500 years ago. Recently, a well-known French oncologist, Professor Henri Joyeux, published the sixth edition of his popular book, *Changing Your Diet - Prevention of Cancer*, where he claims that food is our medicine. What progress! What changed concerning the real value of food that we ourselves have proclaimed during the past decades? We are the pioneers in this field, not always the medical doctor or oncologists, but we the Naturopaths and Integrative Practitioners.

I also think an essential factor has been overlooked. This is the terrain, which insures and maintains a healthy body organism. The intestine and the colon have the special tasks of absorbing food, expelling, detoxifying, and cleaning. Naturally, we must keep in mind that the colon is only one of two factors linked to a more complex process of detoxification through five other systems: the skin, kidney, liver, lung, and lymphatic system.

The colon and the intestine have long been regarded as very important for our health and to prevent against intoxication. Some references go back as far as 1886 with the French doctor, C.H. Bouchard, Professor of Pathology in Paris who wrote a book about auto-intoxication and the colon. In 1916, Dr. G. Guelpa, M.D., wrote a book about constipation as the cause of disease. Another successful book was published in the USA in 1922 by Dr. Arnold Ehret, *The Definite Cure of Chronic Constipation* and also, *Mucusless Diet Healing System*, which at the time sold 150,000 copies and was republished twelve times. During the years from 1965 to1967, when I was furthering my studies in Naturopathy and nutrition, I was lucky to have bought these books that opened my mind about the importance of the colon and detoxification, although it was Dr. Bernard Jensen who first taught me about some of these principles. Today these early authors may very likely be unknown, but they were among the pioneers who stressed the importance of detoxification of the colon in the health system.

John Tilden, M.D., the "Father of Natural Hygiene" in the USA, well-known in the Naturopathic field, wrote a book, *Toxemia: The True Interpretation of the Cause of Disease* (1926), which was also part of my research. According to his theories, most health problems and illness are caused by colon intoxication.

I also cited Dr. Max Gerson, a famous Austrian medical doctor who immigrated to the United States, who was the first to understand the importance of intestinal detoxification in the treatment of cancer. His work, entitled *A Cancer Therapy – The Result of Fifty Cases*, greatly influenced my studies in this field. I also knew his daughter, Charlotte Gerson, very well. She came to see me in Lisbon to discuss cancer and how to best treat this disease. At the time it was published (1948), it had enormous repercussions in the United States and was the subject of various sessions in the American Congress.

Nor can I overlook our much-missed professor, genius of Naturopathy, nutrition, and Iridology, Dr. Bernard Jensen. He was my great professor and guide in the Art of Healing through nature-cure, nutrition and detoxification. Thanks to him, I learned how an intoxicated colon can influence an individual's health and well-being. How chronic constipation can intoxicate the body leading to auto-intoxication of the colon, organic imbalance and diseases. How constipation can lead to illness, auto-intoxication of the colon, and organic imbalance. Unfortunately, for the past 90 years, constipation and its accompanying problems seemed to be of little interest to the medical system that only focuses on local pathology. Understanding of their origin, has not been widely accepted, and doesn't solve the underlying problem.

In this book we will learn how the intestine can cause numerous illnesses and various symptoms, which are medically complex to explain. We will also understand that in order to treat any illness, we must first consider the colon, the intestine and the microbiome.

Food, diet, and detoxification are fundamental elements essential in the improvement of intestinal functions. It is the most natural way of maintaining health, or in case of illness, a return to health.

In order to treat pain one must be aware of its cause and origin. Treating the symptoms of an organ without understanding their origin is incomplete.

Some time ago, I was contacted by a young girl who suffered from virulent acne. After two years of unsuccessful dermatological treatments, being tired of using medicines and creams, she asked her dermatologist if a special diet might be useful in her case. He answered that food had nothing to do with her skin or with her problem. An answer like this seems to ignore the fact that the skin is a reflection of the intestine and what we eat.

This young lady wanted to gain a better understanding and do something different for her problem, as the treatment she had been on had not given any results. It is here that the function of a doctor is important; he must teach the patient to understand and improve their state of health in order to balance it. Should this not be the aim of current as well as future medicine? Should this not be the real meaning of the word Doctor? (The word "doctor" comes from the Latin word *docere*, which means "to teach").

People need education in the field of health, and more importance should be given, with more time dedicated to education rather than to prescribing medicines.

Even after nearly a half century of practice, I am increasingly convinced of the importance of explaining the role a healthy colon plays in the prevention of disease and teaching healthy living concepts while educating people to look for the cause of illness rather than apparent symptoms.

It is a good way of getting rid of the chronic illnesses that afflict 80% of the population. In spite of the major advances in medicine, supported by statistics and reported in the media, cancer, which was #8 on the list of causes of mortality in 1900, is now #2. Cardiovascular disorders have gone from #4 to #1.

Our body has been working just the same way since Hippocrates put forth his treatises. In order to live, we need food produced by nature, which will then be transformed, assimilated, and expelled. If food is badly digested, it stagnates in our intestines often causing severe disorders. We become sick, without knowing why. We may age rapidly, without realizing why.

If we analyze this situation we can see that our society spends a lot of time and money trying to treat diseases or best keeping patients taking toxic medications for lifetime and neglect other healthy direction to avoid or decrease the percentage of disease. Hospitals, clinics, and doctor's waiting rooms are full of patients with symptoms, which doctors hardly manage to keep up with or hardly understand.

We are all aware of the fact that we need to change our life style, our bad habits, our dietary style, and the way we treat illness. The habit of eating bad foods has become dramatic in USA. Obesity now seems to be a normal condition. Did you know that the average American annually consumes sixty-four dozen doughnuts, over fifty gallons of soda pop, nearly two hundred pounds of refined sugar, and over four pounds of food additives and preservatives? Surely this is not the food created for humans to be healthy.

It is important to cut back on our financial donations to institutions and associations which only manage illnesses. Alternatively, we ought to invest in better institutions which study health.

With this in mind, I have written this book in simple and easily understood terms, supported by scientific evidence to arouse the interest of health professionals. I will also discuss some important foundations gained from my practice of Iridology. Had it not been for Iridology, I would never have accumulated so much experience or understood the cause of so many illnesses, especially the importance of the colon and the way it influences organic disorders.

Today, more than ever, our body needs more attention and more respect, just the same as our planet. We polluted our environment as well as our bodies and seem not to realize that we are also destroying ourselves. The most important thing is not some miracle cure or what the newspapers say; the important thing lies in what we can learn and do for ourselves.

Special thanks go to my wife Lucie, who has been very helpful being the first to support my work, especially to review the book in Portuguese as well as for her advice. This English translation and update would not have been possible without the editorial help of Shel Stein from Florida, himself an adept of health, nutrition, detox, and an admirer of Dr. Jensen's work. Also special thanks to my secretary Ana Cristina, who spent so much time with this book, especially with the correction, and her valuable contribution in working with the various figures and illustrations included in this book.

Serge Jurasunas

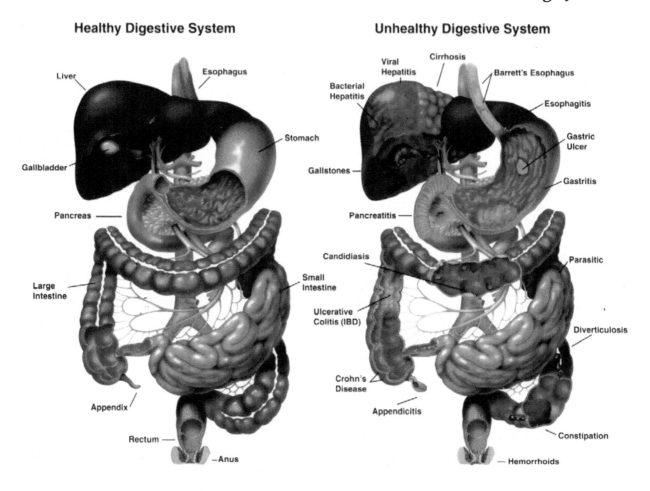

The Digestive System

Quotations:

A wise man should consider that health is the greatest of human blessings and learn how, by his own thought, to derive benefit from his illness. Everyone has a doctor in him or her, but many people are not aware about this and prefer to rely on medical care where for many people, they become drug dependent. The natural healing force is one of the great powers within our body, in each and every one of us, and contributes greatly in getting well and recovery from disease.

Our food should be our medicine. Our medicine should be our food. But to eat when you are sick is to feed your sickness.

—Hippocrates

If we could give every individual the right amount of nourishment and exercise, not too little and not too much, we would have found the safest way to Health.

—Hippocrates

Sometimes medical drugs may lessen pains but do not own any healing virtue to bring back health from disease.

—Serge Jurasunas, 2006

Part I

Embryology
Anatomy of the Intestine
Intestinal Functions
Digestion and Assimilation

Embryology

Without intending to first give a lecture on embryology, it is however necessary to impart some basic knowledge on the role the intestinal system from an embryological perspective. This knowledge will lead us to a better understanding of the importance of the intestinal system in maintaining health and above all in relation to the colon and the other organs that make up our body. We have always had an idea of this relationship, but what I am going to present follows the theories on the specialization of organs according to conventional medicine.

First of all, I would like to consider the first element in the treatment of a disease: the cause. In Western medicine the body is merely reduced to a box divided into compartments, ignoring that one certainly affects the other, which gives rise to medical specialties and total misunderstanding of the real conception of our organism.

Each day we are faced with miracles which often seem hard to explain simply because we do not understand or we forget about the mystery and the power which created life. Life is something more transcendental than the creation of a medication to which beneficial qualities are attributed. Whether we consider a tree, an egg in a nest, or the miracles of the human body, where is the force from which they originated?

Apparently, everything derives from nothing, but in reality everything is triggered by a complicated force that is beyond our imagination.

In the beginning there is simply a fertilized egg, a mixture of twenty-three chromosomes from the father and twenty-three chromosomes from the mother. When these two halves unite creating a fertilized egg, the chromosomes join together to create a combination of hereditary traits from the father and from the mother that at the same time contain the hereditary traits of their predecessors. Each organ, each System, will develop in accordance with the hereditary conditions, good or bad, transported and transmitted by the parents, grandparents, and great-grandparents.

The more aggression an organism suffers, the greater the possibility of creating new organisms, which are increasingly more frail and prone to disease.

The chromosomes are made up of thousands of genes that represent our genetic inheritance, or our hereditary traits, and are found within each cell. It is our greatest wealth.

Each cell contains forty-six human chromosomes, between 10,000 to 30,000 genes, and 3 billion DNA subunits (the base: ATCG), which seems difficult to believe especially when we consider that this is all contained in the nucleus of a cell which is microscopic and invisible to the naked eye. The genes are made up of DNA and each DNA nucleus contains the basis of the genetic program which is responsible for the color of our eyes, our hair, our organs, and hence our health. Our genes hold the information necessary for the formation and maintenance of our cells.

DNA sequences are read like the letters of the alphabet, but four letters are enough to program the diversity of the living being, represented in the double helixes of DNA.

DNA Structure

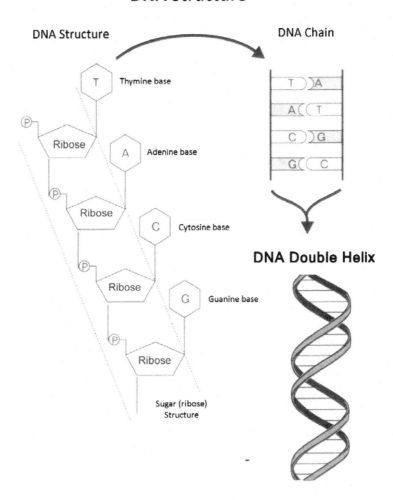

Structure of DNA Chain
Thymine base
Adenine base
Cytosine base
Guanine base

Double Helixes of DNA
Sugar (ribose) Structure

A – Adenine   T - Thymine
G - Guanine C - Cytosine

As we can see in the double helixes in the table, there is coordination in the frequencies of amino acids. **A** goes with **T** and **C** with **G**. Free radicals are unstable and toxic molecules caused by stress, sun exposure, radiation, tobacco, etc., and can cause cellular imbalance.

A lengthy exposure to these toxic factors causes anomalies, rupture, or mutation in the pair base which can cause pathologies such as cancer.

Thankfully, DNA contains repair agents, certain enzymes and polymers that intervene upon these damaged segments. Protected and apparently in good health we can, however, have certain hereditary weaknesses and be vulnerable to different pathologies. But let us return to the

3

embryo. In the beginning there is just a mass of cells, and the development of the human body starts to form between the second and the eighth week.

It is also during this phase that each germinal layer follows its own process of differentiation in order to create the different tissues and specific organs. In this way, by the end of this phase, all the systems have been established and will have taken their own particular form. All the elements of the human body—the organs, the defense systems, the sixty billion cells, as well as the extraordinary computer we call the brain—derive from one single cell. All the organs of the human body are formed from three germinal layers of tissue, which in turn derive from this original cell, which are:

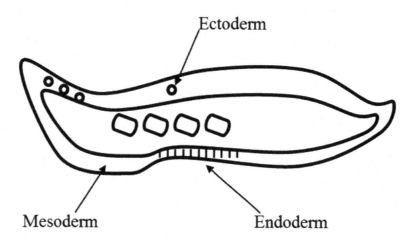

-Endoderm

-Mesoderm

-Ectoderm

The *endoderm* – gives origin to the gastrointestinal system, liver, pancreas, gall bladder, urogenital system, prostate, eardrum, and the auditory canal.

The *mesoderm* – is the origin of muscles, connective tissues, bones, cartilage, joints, heart, cardiovascular and lymphatic systems, kidneys, gonad epithelium, reproductive system, teeth, cortex and adrenal glands, spleen, blood cells, lymphatic, and blood vessels.

The *ectoderm* – gives origin to the central and peripheral nervous systems, sensory organs, subcutaneous glands, iris musculature, lens of the eye, mammary glands, and skin/epidermis.

In this stage of embryonic development we observe that there is an existing relationship between certain organs that also exists between the layers of the germinal tissues.

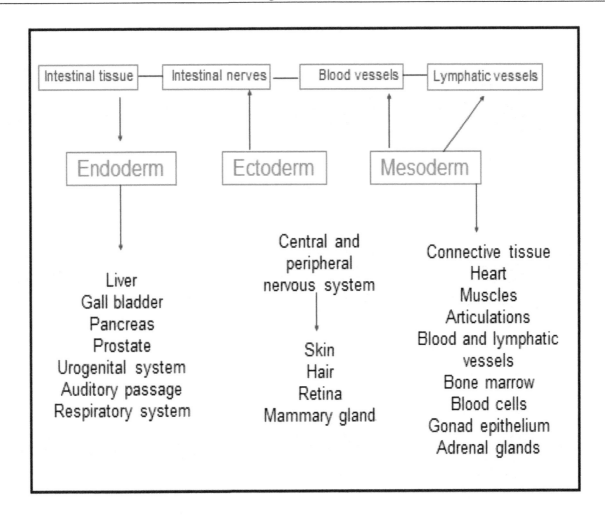

This way, and according to our table, we can see that the blood or lymphatic systems existing within an organ are not formed by the same layer or tissues which gave origin to the organ. For example, not all the organs are developed from the same embryonic tissue. Do you think that the intestinal tube is developed under the same germinal layers as the nervous system, the connective tissue, blood, and lymph? Actually not, while the intestinal system is formed by the endoderm layer of tissue, the nervous system is formed by ectodermic tissue, and the blood vessels are in turn formed by the mesoderm.

It becomes easier to understand how different embryonic and post-natal organs are related to the intestines. For example, how and where certain organs derive from the embryonic tissue of the ectoderm. The above figure clearly demonstrates this theory.

We can also observe that two important systems, the skin and the nervous system, have a common origin: the ectoderm.

Therefore it is comprehensible that there is a direct relationship between the skin and the nervous system, which both are subject to endogenous and exogenous attacks, such as the skin from pollution and endogenous toxins, oxidized lipids, and the nervous system from toxins, bacteria, and social events. In case of any skin disease that suddenly appears and worsens or becomes more critical, we have to consider internal disorders, the microbiome, and toxemia, but also what is affecting the nervous system.

Often in case of skin disease we have to start with the nervous system, and this is true in the case of psoriasis. More recently I had a case of a twenty-three-year-old man with severe psoriasis who was so nervous that I told him that he had to change something in his life and build a better nervous system if he wanted to improve.

I also give an example of a case of a mother whose son was diagnosed with tuberculosis, without any visible signs pointing to the problem. Suddenly, the woman started itching between her fingers. Although she had resorted to various types of treatment, the alleviation and disappearance of the problem only took place when her son's illness stabilized and he was on the way to recovery.

Therefore it is necessary to pay more attention to the nervous system and have a direct approach in case of skin disease. According to my experience, supplementation such as vitamin B complex, taurine, magnesium, GABA, lecithin, herbal preparation with hops, crataegus, passion flower, chamomile, and valerian is excellent, and if necessary, some homeopathic preparations for the nervous system such as Nerve Heel from Heel Laboratory may be useful. In a severe case, why not utilize therapy from live cells! "Hypothalamus" i.m. is quite efficient to balance nervous disorders, anxiety etc. This therapy is very efficient in case of skin disease associated with chronic nerve dysfunction. Of course detoxification is important, but often we realize that you will have to treat the nervous system as well. As one medical doctor stressed speaking about skin disease, don't forget the skin and the nervous system are cousins by embryonic origin.

On so many occasions during my lifetime of practice I faced such problems and always obtained excellent results treating both at the same time. More recently a nineteen-year-old girl came in for consultation with her mother for a very severe skin problem with large red plaques all over the body and legs, frequent scratching and, of course, she was very nervous with anxiety, always worrying about her studies. The mother consulted the best dermatologists, including the top one in Portugal, who prescribed about the same treatment of cortisone, antibiotics, and ointment, but nothing else without success. After fifteen days under my treatment, she started to improve from her scratching, and after two months, she was free of the disease. In her case I had to approach her nervous system beside the regular, normal treatment to boost her liver, colon, kidney and diet. My idea was to try some injectable live cells. I.M. basically hypothalamus for at least to obtain an immediate result from scratching, and it worked.

In this marvelous embryonic development of our organs, we observe a relationship (Arc Reflex) existing between certain organs, once this relation has been established between the layers of the germinal tissues.

Relationships of this type exist between the tissues of the breast, colon, and nervous system. Through Iridology one can observe what we call an "arc reflex," which, in the case of breast pathology, associates the colon and the nervous system. I have performed hundreds of iris observations of breast cancer pathology and breast tumors that have shown evidence of this relationship. It needs careful observation and interpretation. One can see an arc reflex, which, often in case of breast pathology, I observed an association with the colon and the nervous system: the collarette. It is also evident that our health status greatly depends on the hereditary condition of our gut system. This being true for many people, but we don't like to pay attention. In the embryo, the gut is formed like a tube and starts at one end, the foregut, and goes to the other end, the hindgut. One end begins with the mouth and the other terminates with the anus. The gut becomes the center of life as soon as the brain and other organs are formed. The primitive gut nourishes all the organs in the embryo. But did you also know that the gut or intestine is the first soft tissue organ formed in the embryo? In the embryo, cells become rapidly differentiated, but they need nutrients and oxygen, not only for the cells themselves, but for the mitochondria as well. As soon as we are born, the digestive system supplies the nutrients, which is a fundamental process for the making of new tissue, new cells, good blood and activating the function of our immune cells. Not mentioning the microbiome that is now well-known plays a crucial role in many defense mechanisms.

When the entire organism is formed, food and nutrients are fundamental to all our body's processes, the making of new tissue, new cells, good blood and activating the function of our immune cells.

After the intestine, the nervous system also plays an important role in the formation of the organs of the embryo. Indeed, while the intestine is developing, the spinal cord, called the "notochord," has little branches that go almost everywhere in the body but especially to completely surround and innervate the colon. These nerves are linked to the sympathetic and parasympathetic nervous system and consequently with our entire organism. Unfortunately, we continue to dissociate from the interrelationship between our organs, and treat the organs separately, forgetting the whole, often with severe consequences and an increase in neurological disorders.

The topography in the chapter dedicated to Iridology gives us a better understanding of the relationship between the colon and the other organs, as well as the knowledge of how and from which organs the human body is formed.

It is easy to understand that some people may have localized hereditary weakness in certain areas of the colon. On the other hand, the colon plays a key role in the health of our body since every organ, gland and tissue depend on what the intestine is absorbing and expulsing, but also from an embryological perspective. For example there is a relationship between the liver, lungs, pancreas, prostate and the colon since they derive from the same embryological tissue, the endoderm. The study of embryology is currently answering these questions as well as confirming additional factors, about which, little is known.

Conventional medicine treats pain locally and forgets about the body as a whole. This is the problem. By comparing the patient to a box, the neurologist's specialized compartment of interest is the nervous system. Hence the problem will be treated with anxiolytic or antidepressants drugs, not free from side effects, forgetting about the bad influence of toxins and bacteria circulating in blood, while more recently the intestine is now seen as our second brain.

In this way, we may also damage our nervous system and make it worse, particularly for those people who already have a weak nervous system and poor hereditary status. Many suicides around the world are now seen as caused by the medical drug Prozac. This all depends on hereditary factors
which can take up to the fourth generation in order to know if a fetus will have normal or abnormal genes, or even for a baby to be born with a good or bad intestinal system.

Unfortunately, the Cartesian medical system lists all newborns as healthy as there is no visible deficiency. Without concern for hereditary factors or any organic weakness medicine, doctors will prescribe the same vaccines, medicines, antibiotics etc. for every case. Recently a young twenty-three-year-old female asked me for help with nutrition as a result of having nearly her entire intestinal tract removed. She had more than one hundred cysts scattered throughout her intestine. I asked myself: Did this woman have a good intestinal system when she was born? From an embryological point of view, in what condition was the tissue that caused a case like this one? How many years did it take for the one hundred cysts to develop? How is it possible for a person not to feel anything and to have been considered to be in perfect health?

Obviously, in the embryonic stage she must have already had some bad tissue and intestinal cells, a bad nervous system or other deficiencies. During the ensuing years, the cysts slowly formed all over, especially in the weakest areas, because of bad eating habits and lack of intestinal hygiene.

In this case, we have more than one basic element that shows us how important it would have been to know our hereditary constitution in order to prevent certain illnesses. But, above all, we now know and we have seen more clearly how our gastrointestinal system plays a major role in maintaining health, and in many cases, how it can influence the entire organism.

Anatomy of the Intestine

The digestive system can be compared to a twenty-three-foot long passage that goes through the body, like a major boulevard, extending from the mouth to the anus. It is along this gastrointestinal tract that food goes through the various transformative stages of digestion where it will be ground, prepared for assimilation and then assimilated by the organism.

The non-assimilated food is expelled as a component part of the remains from our body's elimination. It so happens that the function of elimination is just as important as the process of assimilation. It is not so strange that our *health depends on these two stages.*

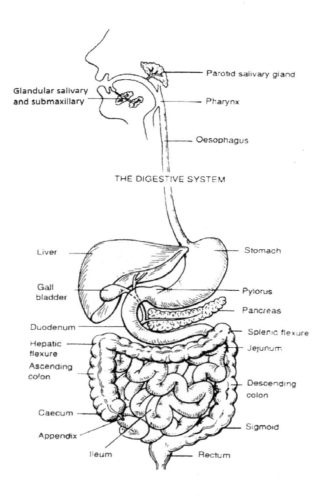

Intestinal Anatomy

Mouth – the chewing and salivating organ, which uses teeth and salivary glands to perform its function.

Pharynx – an area between the digestive and respiratory tracts. It is the organ for swallowing and propelling food from the mouth to the stomach.

Stomach – the tumescence of the digestive tract situated in the upper part of the abdomen, to the left of the liver, which it covers slightly. In aspect, it is like a 10-inch sack shaped like a capital J. The superior orifice, which connects the stomach to the esophagus, is

9

situated not far from the heart, from which it gets the name "cardia." The end orifice, the "pylorus" connects with the small intestine.

Intestine – made up of two sections: the small and the large intestine. The first wraps around itself in a molding formed by the second. The small intestine begins in the pylorus and ends in the large intestine or colon.

The small intestine can be divided into two sections: the duodenum, which forms a C like curve, coiled around the upper part of the pancreas. It measures about ten inches and receives secretions from the liver and the pancreas. The jejunum measures approximately sixteen feet and forms fifteen or sixteen curves—coils—of different lengths. They are highly flexible and coil around each other.

The small intestine contains the intestinal glands, which secrete a rich mucous that constitutes the intestinal juice.

The large intestine, or colon, is separated from the small intestine by the ileocecal valve, which prevents reflux of the contents of the colon (a phenomenon which may occur).

The large intestine measures about five feet and is divided into five parts:

1st - The cecum, a small sac two inches long and three inches wide, situated in the join between the intestine and the colon and extending to a small tube, the appendix, which seems to have an immune function.

2nd - The ascending colon, which extends along the right side of the abdomen in front of the liver where it makes a 90-degree bend.

3rd - The transverse colon curves slightly, passes under the umbilical, and heads towards the left flank where it begins the second 90-degree curve.

4th - The descending colon continues along the left flank before the iliac crest where it bends towards the center.

5th - The sigmoid colon, which ends in the rectum, is situated in the hollow of the inlet; leads to the outside through the anus.

The stomach, the small and large intestine are surrounded by the peritoneum, a thin membrane which forms a sac with no openings, made up of two leaf-like layers that run one on top of the other. The peritoneum contains numerous blood and lymphatic vessels and in cases of obesity can contain significant amounts of fat.

Living beings, as soon as the fetus begins to develop, have a very complex anatomical system, which we have just mentioned and I will repeat. Its principal role is receiving food, transforming it, assimilating it and expelling it. The reason is simple, due to the fact that the organism contains more than forty trillion cells, tissues, endocrine glands, bones, hair, teeth, blood and immune cells, various systems etc., for which it must continually provide vital elements for the needs of this miniature universe. There is another less-known function that depends on this system.

Mitochondria, known as our power house, are small, sub-cellular organelles that play a crucial role in our body by utilizing oxygen and break down foods into small molecules of electrons to generate high amounts of chemical energy called Adenosine Triphosphate or ATP, essential to powering all our cell's biochemical reactions, as well as for the functioning of the entire body. Recent evidence and experimental studies demonstrate the functions of mitochondria in the regulation of the DNA genome, relate to a cell's differentiation, even apoptosis. Decreasing ATP energy production today is linked with many symptoms and chronic/degenerative diseases ranging from Chronic Fatigue Syndrome (CFS), to Fibromyalgia and Parkinson's, as well as cancer.

The main function of this process is to receive food that is first digested and transformed, then assimilated by the body while the remaining wastes are expelled. Our cells are dependent on our nutrition, oxygen and clean blood, which is dependent on our emunctory organs and detoxification process, and especially the colon and liver, which in turn is dependent on our detoxification process and especially the colon. We have to remember that healthy cells give rise to a healthy body.

Intestinal Functions

Before explaining all the different functions of the gastrointestinal system, we are going to talk about the harmful factors, capable of disturbing good intestinal function. I would like to explain how important it is for every one of us to acquire and maintain a minimum of knowledge about the intestinal functions.

Today science actually confirms that our health status largely depends on the quality and variety of food we eat. While sixty years ago, eating was not considered as important for our health, natural food was not even considered as a preventive factor against cancer. We can eat for pleasure, which is still common today, or for a physiological need triggered by hunger, i.e.: "I am hungry" or "I need to eat." This can be for any kind of food. But you should know that eating, while being a necessity, is first a biological act, which is actually quite complex.

We now know our digestive system is not adapted to industrial-processed foods, as I will explain further on in the book and even to incorrect combinations of heavy foods that overtax the digestive system. Today's industrial and processed foods contain transformed food structures, inadequate if not ill-suited for our genome. Combining proteins with one or two carbohydrate(s), or other heavy foods, is totally incorrect, overtaxing our digestive system.

We have come to the point at which the human gastrointestinal system is suffering from deteriorating conditions from hereditary predisposition, industrial foods, social or physical stress, an excess of pharmaceutical drugs and is under constant attack. If we are unable to gain this basic knowledge ourselves, to receive adequate information and education from our medical doctors, we must at least have some priority and should learn about what we should eat. We should also learn how we can reduce the stressful conditions which affect our body and the intestinal system. We need to learn how to naturally activate our intestinal function so we can keep it healthy.

Sitting at a table in order to eat is not as important as ingesting, digesting, absorbing and expelling. For these we must rely on a well-functioning gastrointestinal system. In order for our organism to function well, we need to have a good intestinal structure. We need to get the best natural food as possible so the intestine can transform and absorb the nutrients and expel the waste matter. This is what we can expect to keep us healthy.

We now know our digestive system is not adapted to artificially processed food or to incorrect combinations of heavy foods. The stress of modern life, hereditary factors and bad eating habits, all have a very negative influence on the digestive and elimination organs in spite of their toughness and ability to adapt.

We have come to the point at which the human gastrointestinal system is under constant attack. If, on one hand, we are able to understand the functions of this digestive system, then on the other, it is absolutely essential to understand the difference between bad and good food.

I recently received a visit from a young, single girl suffering from serious hepatic and digestive problems. Amongst other symptoms, she vomited, complained of strong intestinal pain, nervousness, and insomnia. After various medical consultations, the cause of her problem remaining undetected. She was referred to a psychiatrist for an evaluation. This happens in at least 50% of hospital emergencies.

After thirty days on a dietary regime, with antioxidants and supplements for her nervous system, the symptoms began to attenuate and then disappeared. In spite of these results, she was scared the problem might reoccur. I then tried to tell her how we could prevent these kinds of problems through the understanding about our health, what to eat, how to understand the biological function of the gastrointestinal system and the need to detox ourselves.

One other case is a fourteen-year-old girl who suffered from constipation, abdominal pains, pains in the bone, nervousness, dizziness and chronic fatigue, but eating a very bad diet of red meat, white rice, spaghetti, potatoes and no vegetables or fruit intake. Her medical doctor paid little attention to her food habits and state of constipation. Actually, this is what the mother told me: "Our physician never told me about changing the diet of my daughter." He only prescribed analgesic pills and some drugs for the nervous system. For a fourteen-year-old girl, we can probably do better!

This type of knowledge is best acquired by reading books concerning our health, especially those written about health and nutrition which are important to learn about our body's needs, about the value of nutrients and about how to feed our cells. Books written by Dr. Bernard Jensen, and especially Dr. Catherine Kousmine, a Swiss medical doctor, are to me a must to acquire for some proper, basic knowledge. Attending lectures is also another good suggestion to learn about health principles, and this includes colon health, may I say. Today we have more opportunities than ever to learn about our body's system and healthful condition, especially through the Internet.

It is important to understand intestinal physiology, or even better digestive functions, which begin in the mouth and end in the colon with the eventual elimination of feces. This way, we can understand that our marvelous system of organs can, in spite of everything, suffer damage and become altered.

Intestinal Physiology (Functions)

Food digestion begins in the mouth with chewing and salivating, where care must be taken, especially with thorough mastication of carbohydrates.

The act of chewing depends on the cortex, the region of the brain controlled by the parasympathetic nervous system. Obviously people who swallow food quickly without chewing have a problem with the brain and the nervous system. It is very important to chew food properly first by crushing it, and then moisten it through salivation from our three pairs of salivary glands. Under stress and anxiety, the production of saliva, which is usually, in an adult, a liter and a half in twenty-four hours, becomes diminished and can disturb proper digestion.

The objective of digestion is to break down food from its main nutrients (carbohydrates, proteins, lipids) into more simple chemical substances, which can be absorbed into the blood stream to be used by the cells in the organism.

After being chewed and saturated with saliva, the food will form into a ball, which will be propelled in to the stomach after being swallowed.

The stomach secretes an average of two liters of gastric juices per day; these contain hydrochloric acid and two enzymes called chymosin and pepsin. Hydrochloric acid is highly concentrated. Its purpose is to decompose the mass of food, but it also has antiseptic properties for destroying the bacteria ingested with food.

It is essential to have a good level of hydrochloric acid, not only to break down proteins, but also to preserve the balance between sodium and calcium in our body. Hyper-secretion of hydrochloric acid chemically transforms the sodium within the intestinal walls.

With time, the destruction of sodium causes an imbalance in the production of hydrochloric acid resulting in difficulty in digesting protein. According to some American researchers, the reduction in hydrochloric acid is one of the first factors leading to premature aging in human beings.

Digestion in the stomach ends with the creation of a kind of semi-fluid acidic mush called chyme, which slowly drains into the duodenum due to the mobility of the stomach.

The stomach also creates a mixture, which combines our food with the gastric juices. This is one of the reasons why one must not remain sedentary after having eaten. A nice 20- or 30-minute walk after meals, especially after dinner, stimulates our intestinal muscles and enzyme secretion for better digestion and quicker absorption. All the taxi drivers who have consulted me suffer from gastrointestinal problems, particularly of the stomach.

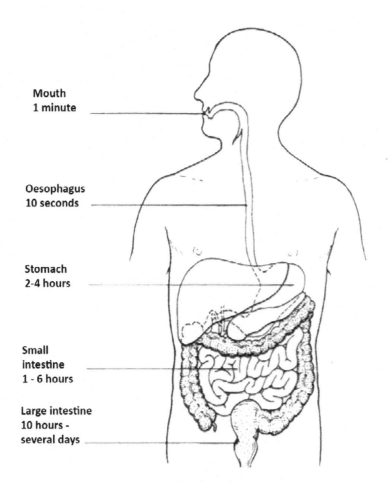

Mouth
1 minute

Oesophagus
10 seconds

Stomach
2-4 hours

Small
intestine
1 - 6 hours

Large intestine
10 hours -
several days

**The Digestive system. The diagram illustrates the average time that
food spends in each part of the digestive system.**

*The time the mass of food remains in the stomach and its expulsion varies according to
meals between three and ten hours. Meat alone takes about three to four hours to be
completely digested. A mixture of fat meat, fried foods, and fermented cheeses can take
more than five to ten hours to digest (while further taxing our digestive system).*

This is why so many people arise in the morning with coated tongues, belching out flavors
reminiscent of the previous meal. Obviously the repast from the day before was not entirely
digested.

Finally, the mass of food is pushed towards the duodenum in small quantities every twenty
seconds. At this stage, the chyme is extremely acidic as it contains a high concentration of
hydrochloric acid and enzymes, which help digest the large protein molecules.

In fact, it is necessary to prepare and facilitate the new process that begins in the intestine.
Fortunately, the small intestine secretes bicarbonate, an alkaline substance needed to neutralize
the acid in the stomach. In the first phase, proteins are transformed into amino acids in the
stomach in order to undergo further transformation in the intestine. Animal proteins are more
difficult to break down and digest compared with sub-animal or plant protein. An excess of
animal protein and bad mastication can cause even more strain on the entire digestive system.
Hence, many amino acids transform into toxic amines that poison the body and increases aging of
the organism. Industrialized processed foods, excessive alcohol and stress may also damage the
micro-villi impairing the good absorption of food.

In the small intestine, all nutritive elements are reduced to microscopic size, after having lost their initial identity. Absorption at this level depends greatly on the quality of digestion and the breakdown of food, with the helpful participation of specific bacteria and finally on the intestinal micro-villi where food is absorbed into the blood circulation. Industrially processed commercial foods, excess of alcohol, and food additives may damage the micro-villi impairing the good absorption of food. Dr. Jensen used to tell me, "Eating food is one thing, but the absorption is another, and many people are not knowledgeable on this subject."

Some substances, like fibers, are neither transformed nor absorbed but they play a very important role in the intestinal tract.

The duodenum is another very active part of the intestine. It receives the influx of bile, which has an important role in the digestion of fat. Biliary salts have a similar action to that of a detergent capable of perfectly emulsifying these small drops of fat. The biliary salts produced by the liver help dissolve the fatty acids from fats in order to facilitate their absorption at the level of the intestinal mucosa.

One of the causes of colon cancer is a diet rich in fat and a reduction in the secretion of biliary salts, which ensures a greater concentration of lipids in the colon.

The presence of bile is equally important at the intestinal level for the absorption of the liposoluble vitamins A, D, E and K, present in fats such as butter or cream. Drinking only skim milk deprives the organism of these important vitamins, not to mention selenium. Bile also helps the absorption of cholesterol, which poses the question of whether the means used to control cholesterol are correct, or not?

In truth, bile has many functions within our intestinal system. One of them concerns the protection of intestinal mucosa ensuring the fluidity of mucus it secretes. It also helps elimination and regulates the intestinal flora combating pollution of certain bacteria.

The bile is concentrated in the gall bladder and is expelled during digestion with an average of one liter every twenty-four hours.

The pancreas is another important organ that participates in the process of digestion. For example, before the chyme enters the duodenum, it is mixed with pancreatic secretions. In general terms, these are enzymes that separate proteins, carbohydrates and fat. We can find similar enzymes in the intestinal juices, such as the amylase and trypsin, which act on the proteins. Pancreatic juices also help the absorption of vitamin B12 allowing the fixation of its intrinsic factor on the intestinal mucosa. The intrinsic factor is a protein produced by the stomach, the presence of which is essential for the absorption of this vitamin. The pancreatic juice also has an important function in limiting the absorption of iron. Indeed, an excess of iron in the blood depresses the immune system and can favor the multiplication of cancerous cells. Later it was discovered that iron increases the level of oxidative stress in reacting with the free radicals of oxygen.

When chyme is precisely mixed and split, it is then ready to be absorbed through the blood stream. Carbohydrates transform into glucose (which increases our glycemic level). Lipids are now in the form of fatty acids and glycerol. The proteins are finally reduced into their constitutive amino acids. In brief, after they lose their individuality and original specificity, they are no longer molecules of fish or meat but simply amino acids and nothing more.

Here is a small note to say that fatty acids are not absorbed in the same way as proteins or carbohydrates. Their absorption is slower and depends on their chemical structure, whether made up of long chains or medium chains. In both cases the particles of fatty acids are absorbed by villosities.

However, long chains of amino acids are split into forms of triglycerides and are then absorbed in the form of miniscule particles, better known as chylomicrons, which penetrate the lymphatic system. The chylomicrons are transported by the lymphatic system, which allows them to enter into the blood circulation through a vein found in the neck called the superior vena cava.

The medium chains of fatty acids represent 10% to 20% of all fat. They are absorbed directly through the portal vein without passing through the lymphatic system. Both types of fatty acids end their journey by passing through the liver where they are metabolized and transformed into energy.

Digestion and Elimination in the Large Intestine

The intestine absorbs nutrients as the remaining residue is pushed into the cecum, the first part of the large intestine. The role of the large intestine consists mainly of the formation and elimination of what we call fecal matter. This occurs as the result of some chemical phenomena, which are no longer caused by enzymes, as in the small intestine, the stomach or the mouth but rather by certain microorganisms.

Toxic waste material, or feces, is still in a fluid state when it enters the large intestine, which measures more or less 5.3 feet. The straight part, called the ascending colon, contains the remains of used food and cellulose. The former can still be reabsorbed, while cellulose (fiber) is partially broken down through the action of bacteria, eventually to be expelled as fecal matter. The colon, in contrast to the small intestine, does not work based upon chemical phenomenon, or the action of enzymes but instead with microorganisms.

In the intestine the chyme is mixed and immediately pushed towards the large intestine by the rhythmic movement of the intestinal muscles called peristalsis. This mixture, along with circular and longitudinal movements, is used to transform the larger particles into smaller ones and, above all, to expose the surfaces of the chyme as much as possible to the digestive enzymes. Then, movement helps the chyme continue to the colon where it will be expelled.

Let us examine how the organism works in eliminating the remains when food is absorbed. Do not think that fecal matter forms by itself, suddenly or without complex mechanisms. The mechanism of formation of fecal matter is incredibly precise. First of all, a certain percentage of water (86%), must be reabsorbed so that the feces have a normal consistency. With 88% of reabsorbed water, the feces become too solid; with 82% they are too watery. This mechanism is almost as precise as a Swiss watch.

The feces, which have been formed, still contain badly or partially chewed fragments of food which escape the digestive processes, carrying toxins, microbes, and dead cells in the magnitude of 30 trillion to 100 trillion every twenty-four hours.

The colon, as opposed to the intestine, does not work by chemical phenomenon or by the action of enzymes, but thankfully by the (interaction of) microorganisms.

The flora of the colon changes at an incredible rate compared to that of the small intestine. Aerobic Bacteria that travel into the large intestine require oxygen. Anaerobic flora present in the colon, have processes by which microorganisms biodegrade fecal material, converting these materials in the absence of oxygen. In the presence of nondigested food and accumulated feces, anaerobic bacteria multiply very quickly, create some bad fermentation, gases, and toxic substances which pollute the colon. Even worse, they can even penetrate into blood circulation. The flora in the colon, in relation to those in the small intestine, are not the same, and quite different. Bacteria present in the colon are no longer aerobic but mainly anaerobic and are not able to survive in an oxygen atmosphere.

The correct acid balance of the intestine can be maintained with the help of appropriate foods such as kefir, cider vinegar, acidophilus, apple juice and whey. This kind of food, on the other hand, also helps the colon not to be overly alkaline, so as to discourage putrefaction and the development of harmful bacteria.

It is therefore of key importance to understand the difference between the small intestine and colon. This way, the intestinal flora must be encouraged as much as possible, maintaining a low level of anaerobic bacteria, which might settle there. They can only exist when there are putrefactions where they multiply. It is much better to maintain the correct acid balance of the intestine with the help of appropriate food. On the other hand, the colon should not be too alkaline, so as to not encourage the development of harmful bacteria.

Usually between one year and a few months after birth, many children no longer are given maternal milk and are often fed with cow's milk from birth. Maternal milk gives the baby acid feces and cow's milk causes alkaline feces. This is when such problems as intestinal disorders, constipation, diarrhea and infections arise.

A good diet must be the pillar of intestinal integrity. Certain foods are essential for good intestinal function and bowel elimination. For example, fibers play a very important role in the entire intestinal system. Fibers are food for the good bacteria of the colon and they assist in digestion, producing fermentation, and maintaining the acidity of the feces.

This is not their only task. Fibers also have the power to accelerate intestinal transit. Denis P. Burkitt, a famous English surgeon, distinguished himself for his research in the dietetic of fibers. He proved the relationship between a fiber-rich diet and the duration of intestinal transit. Dr. Burkitt observed various African populations, in particular their eating habits, and the effect on the colon.

After having observed thousands of Africans, and then the English, and their eating habits, he compared the time of duration of the digestive transit and the average weight of the feces.

On one hand, the rural Africans have a diet rich in fresh fruit, vegetables, and roughly ground cereals. The bran only partially removed from the cereal is still present in the food. It absorbs the water in the intestine, increases the volume of the matter in the colon and is totally eliminated much faster. In this way, the colon is always clean and in good, healthy condition.

He also observed that refined foods such as flour, sugar, or other carbohydrates were not available to the Africans who were part of this study.

Today, the situation is slightly different, with intercontinental travel, tourism and the introduction of commercial foods in Africa. This explains how the door to illness was opened.

On the other hand, in Western countries we mostly consume refined carbohydrates. We eat an excess of meat and animal by-products and forget about fruit and vegetables. There is a greater retention of feces in the colon, toxic wastes and bacteria. Therefore, according to Dr. Burkitt's comparisons, the weight of the feces of a rural African is between 300g and 500g a day, and those of Englishmen weigh 110g on average.

Insufficient and thin fecal matter implies that there is retention of feces and other toxic waste, including dead microbes, bacteria, undigested and unabsorbed food. Modern medicine seems not to worry about the higher incidence of colon diseases and symptoms, which include appendicitis, gall stones, hemorrhoids, colon cancer, irritable bowel syndrome, inflammation, diarrhea and constipation, all of which are linked to our eating habits. Over 100 million North Americans suffer from intermittent forms of intestinal disease that cost, medically speaking, twenty billion dollars or more per year.

This mass of food can remain in the small intestine from four to six hours, according to the person and their eating habits. The chyme stays in the large intestine from ten to twelve hours and sometimes even several days. The total time for a normal transit is more or less eighteen hours from a meal to its total elimination, while a period of forty-eight hours increases the risk of intestinal disorders and of colon cancer. In modern countries and in Portugal, the time for a total elimination of a meal is particularly long. Often the patients tell me that they experience difficulty. This means that feces are not fully eliminated and accumulate.

About 50% is retained after two days, and after five days, feces contain 90% of the residue of that same meal. Incredible! The colon sometimes retains five to nine meals considering that we eat three times a day. Nobody considers this important, and even the gastroenterologists give little thought to this fact which is actually easily understood. In the book we will present several examples of patients with chronic constipation and a bowel function every three or seven days.

At the end of the transit, fecal matter accumulates in the sigmoid colon (80% of colon cancer occurs here), where the peristalsis pushes it towards the rectum. The bloating caused by this matter on the organ makes elimination necessary. So, if feces are small in quantity and of a hard texture, they are not sufficient in volume to expand the rectum. Sometimes they remain stuck the rectum causing inflammation, and even anal fistulas, with intense pain. Elderly people on an incorrect diet can retain bad food, non-digested, in their intestinal tract for up to fifteen days or more before being absorbed or eliminated. This is why they accumulate more toxins and often are ill. The consequences are evident in circulatory disorders in the lower limbs, dilated abdomens, and the general fatigue they often experience.

Anyone of us can perform an experiment to calculate the duration of our intestinal transit by mixing a colorant into our food. For example, you can eat a dish of red beetroot with your diner and make a note of time you have your meal. Take note of time of the meal when the beetroot was eaten. Pay attention and then note the hour in which the feces come out red. This way, one can tell the duration of their intestinal transit.

After all these considerations, one must be keenly aware of the importance of a healthy colon: good intestinal function in accordance with a better and balanced food diet.

Some people will be uneasy about how little attention they have paid to their intestinal system and their dietary style, and not many are aware that wrong food may really harm and damage our intestine (sometimes these improperly digested materials remain stuck to rectum), but of course, there is always time to correct the past errors.

Digestion and Assimilation

Our health not only depends on what we eat but also on how we digest and later assimilate food. That is, the way in which our digestive tract manages to benefit from it. For a long time we thought that our notions of digestion and assimilation were only secondary to the theory that man's needs are expressed in calories. Hence, only food measured in calories, and not by its qualities or digestive effects, was considered important.

Today, many people suffer from digestive and intestinal problems but are happy to take some medicines, digestive salts or antacids to diminish the accumulation of intestinal gasses, but they continue eating the same foods.

It is true that man can adapt to foods composed of very different quantities and qualities.

It is true that our digestive system can adapt to bad food without digestive disorders or disease. Each individual is different, and some people have a very good digestive enzyme system and can abuse food for years before they feel some problems or even are suddenly diagnosed with a cancer of the colon or pancreas. Digestibility of food, a first requirement for the benefit of the organism, greatly depends on the conditions of the digestive tract. It is true that eating habits vary in different countries. In different regions of Portugal, the inhabitants seem to get used to them, but a regional staple diet can cause indigestion in a person who is new to a different region.

All this implies a highly complex genetic mechanism necessary for the digestion and assimilation of food composed of three families of nutrients: fats (lipids), sugar (glucose) and proteins which combine with the mineral salts, vitamins and water, which we also need. As we will see, digestion involves a particularly important enzymatic mechanism.

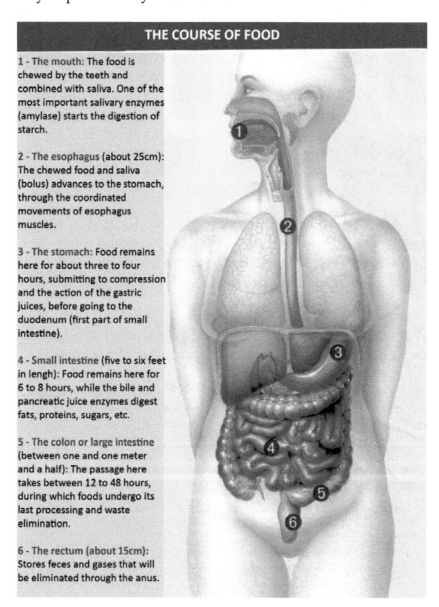

THE COURSE OF FOOD

1 - The mouth: The food is chewed by the teeth and combined with saliva. One of the most important salivary enzymes (amylase) starts the digestion of starch.

2 - The esophagus (about 25cm): The chewed food and saliva (bolus) advances to the stomach, through the coordinated movements of esophagus muscles.

3 - The stomach: Food remains here for about three to four hours, submitting to compression and the action of the gastric juices, before going to the duodenum (first part of small intestine).

4 - Small intestine (five to six feet in lengh): Food remains here for 6 to 8 hours, while the bile and pancreatic juice enzymes digest fats, proteins, sugars, etc.

5 - The colon or large intestine (between one and one meter and a half): The passage here takes between 12 to 48 hours, during which foods undergo its last processing and waste elimination.

6 - The rectum (about 15cm): Stores feces and gases that will be eliminated through the anus.

1) The mouth: Food is chewed by teeth and mixed with saliva. One of the most important enzymes present in saliva (amylase) begins by digesting yeast.

2) The esophagus (about ten inches): Food chewed and saturated with saliva (food mass) continues towards the stomach through the coordinated movements of the esophagus.

3) The stomach: Food remains here for about three to four hours undergoing compression under the action of gastric juices before proceeding towards the duodenum (initial part of the small intestine).

4) The small intestine (between fifteen and eighteen feet in length): Food is held here for six to eight hours while the bile and the enzymes in the pancreatic juices digest fats, proteins and sugars.

5) The colon or large intestine (about three and a half to four and a half feet): The journey through here lasts between twelve to forty-eight hours, during which food undergoes its last transformation and the remnants are excreted.

6) The rectum (about five inches): Stores the feces and gasses, which are eliminated through the anus.

The organism has various ways of dealing with large molecules of nutrients which cannot be used by the organism. These are reduced before passing through the blood. The molecules and proteins that enter the blood stream and were not properly broken down, digested and assimilated, unbalance the immune and the nervous systems.

The process of digestion begins in the mouth where food is ground by means of salivary mastication.

This process prepares our food for intestinal digestion. During mastication, food undergoes the action of ptyalin, a ferment that acts on yeast transforming it into smaller molecules (dextrin). We have said that, indirectly, chewing triggers the secretion of digestive juices in the rest of the digestive system. Food, which has already been transformed into a mush, is then swallowed and enters the stomach and mixed with the gastric juices formed by the secretions of the gastric mucus.

This juice contains hydrochloric acid and a myriad of digestive enzymes. For example, the stomach secretes pepsin, which reduces food proteins into smaller complexes called peptones, in order to be dissected in the intestine into elementary particles or amino acids which enter the blood stream and from which human proteins are reconstructed. At this stage, the intestine and the pancreas secrete digestive ferments used to degrade proteins, amino acids and fat. These are namely amylase, trypsin and lipase.

The stomach has the role of a reservoir, as it processes the food through the action of the gastric juices, and then slowly allows it to pass through to the small intestine. In humans, food quickly leaves the stomach after ingestion. Liquids only take about to one or two seconds, but a complete elimination of a meal takes place over a period that varies between three to ten hours, according the individual, their digestive capabilities and the type of food.

Glucides or carbohydrates pass through to the duodenum very quickly; proteins, on the whole, pass after two or three hours, while lipids or fats remain in the stomach a lot longer. Their presence in the food ingested, such as fried food, slows digestion. This causes an imbalance in the harmony between the speed of digestion and the movement of food through the digestive tract, which can also cause gastrointestinal and nutritional problems. Furthermore, eating a lot or eating fast, eating under stress or under strong emotions diminishes and often blocks the emptying of the stomach contents into the duodenum.

Just like the small intestine, the stomach is also richly innervated with filaments of sympathetic and parasympathetic nerves linked to the brain. Information is transmitted both ways and is eminently capable of causing gastrointestinal disturbances.

Food undergoes the most important of transformations once in the small intestine, in particular in the duodenum. Under the combined action of the pancreatic juices, the bile, and the intestinal juices, food substances will be absorbed where as those which are not (often because the quantity is excessive) will be eliminated. The excess of food contributes to increasing the secretion of the enzymes amylase and trypsin. With age, there is much waste and the secretions become increasingly more difficult causing a great number of digestive disorders.

Excessive animal proteins and bad mastication are responsible for the accumulation of poorly digested proteins in the intestinal canal, which become toxic.

Hence, many amino acids transform into toxic amines that poison the body and may trigger chronic and degenerative diseases such as cancer and increase aging process in our body:

Intestinal Putrefaction

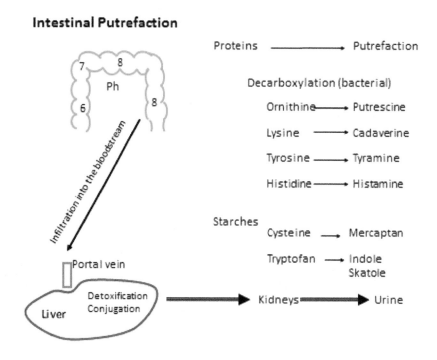

In these cases, we can help the body to detoxify by taking some proteolytic enzymes (such as Inflazyme Forte from AB.) which help to absorb non-digested proteins and to dissolve clusters of fats, necrotic tissue circulating in the blood and help the digestion of heavy food. Otherwise, a mixture of papaya or pineapple enzymes that also contain papain and bromelain is also good. Aloe Vera offers excellent results especially when associated with papain and pau d'arco. As the stomach and the small intestine move, their mobility aids the action of the juices, ensuring the progression of the contents of the small intestine towards the large intestine. The average length of transit in the small intestine is about four hours, from the moment the stomach passes on its contents.

When a person is very hungry, the stomach quickly transfers its content into the duodenum. If one is not hungry, it rids itself from its content in about two to three hours after having eaten. This shows that from the physiological point of view, it is better to space meals (four to six hours apart), and above all, not to pick in-between meals. Apparently, the pylorus will not allow the passage of food to the duodenum until the organism really needs food. The pancreas is an organ with a double function: it is a digestive gland that secretes pancreatic juices into the duodenum, but it is also an endocrine gland that passes insulin directly into the capillary blood vessels. When there is an excess of sugar in the blood, the pancreas produces insulin in order to rebalance the sugar level. Thanks to insulin production, the cellular membranes increase their permeability so that sugar can be absorbed by the cells.

The duodenum is a very active center because, besides the pancreatic juice, it receives bile that plays a very important role in digesting fat due to biliary salts, which allow the emulsification of drops of fat. Biliary salts help solute the fatty acids derived from ingested fat, making it easier to be absorbed at the level of the intestinal mucus.

If fat is not emulsified, it will circulate into the blood in the form of large molecules, and in the presence of oxygen, will oxidize if the level of antioxidants like vitamin C, and above all vitamin E, are low in the blood plasma. If we ingest saturated fats, it will be difficult to absorb them and they become rancid very quickly. This results in various pathologies including cholesterol and cardiovascular illnesses, and also arthrosis (joint degeneration) and breast cancer.

At the intestinal mucus level, the presence of bile is essential for absorption of the liposoluble vitamins A, D, E and K that are present in lipids.

Eliminating all fats without considering the needs of the organism, as many people (incorrectly do) in order to fight cholesterol, causes a poor absorption of liposoluble vitamins. The consequences can be tragic, causing an almost total deficiency of vitamins A and E.

In the same way, bile helps the absorption of cholesterol. It protects the intestinal mucosa by facilitating the fluidity of the mucus it secretes. It increases peristalsis in the small intestine, assisting intestinal function and lubricating the colon walls. People who suffer from constipation must think about activating the gallbladder. Bile increases the efficacy of pancreatic fermentations. The biliary secretion is approximately one liter a day while the volume of liquids of the digestive juices amount to about six liters daily, that is, two liters per meal. Finally, the small intestine itself secretes a juice, which complements the action of the pancreatic juice and the bile, in order to allow digestion and absorption of ingested food.

Food Absorption

The absorption of nutrients takes place within the digestive tract, which goes from the mouth to the colon.

Usually, it is thought that the passage of food through the mouth and the esophagus happens too fast for absorption to have any importance at this level. However, there is absorption, especially in the sublingual area of the mouth. This characteristic is often taken advantage of in the ingestion of certain medicines or nutrients, which will therefore not be attacked by the digestive juices.

The blood vessels that are in contact with the mucus of the mouth and the tongue launch directly into the external jugular vein draining the blood from the head and from the neck. This prevents the immediate passage through the liver and allows for extremely rapid absorption. For example, some medicines in the form of small pills used in the treatment of chest angina are placed under the tongue and stop pain after just a few minutes. The same occurs with supplements administered under the tongue.

There is another danger connected with sugar. There are children who eat sweets all day, chocolates, which melt in the mouth and chewing gum masticated for hours on end. These children prepare themselves for obesity and diabetes, but little importance is given to this fact.

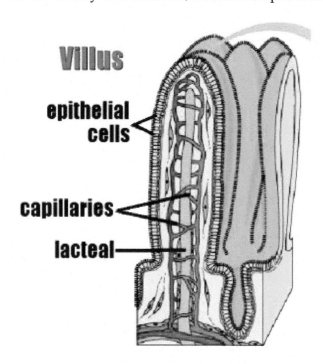

In the image we can see a cut in the small intestine showing the villosities. Each villus is like a small factory with its own network of fine capillaries and blood vessels capable of receiving and transmitting nutrients ready for distribution.

In the small intestine, the food mass is absorbed by its walls. These are covered by about 10 to 20 million valves and villi. The villi are in direct contact with the blood stream and lymph, allowing the nutritive substances to be directly absorbed into the blood and transported to the liver where they are transformed and stored, while others are sent to the lymph where they join the blood stream after having passed through the lungs.

Each villus plays the role of a small factory in the final process of the absorption of food. They all have their own network of tiny capillaries and lymphatic vessels, which are ready to enter the blood stream. These villi are similar to thousands of absorbing hairs, around which bacteria, appropriate laboratories, transform the food mass into actual vitamins.

We must also understand that eating is more than assimilating and absorbing. It is also something else, something more important.

Now one of the recent problems is what we call "leaky gut syndrome," which can allow harmful organisms such as fungi, parasites, bacteria, toxins and non-digested food to enter the blood circulation, due to increased intestinal permeability. The Live Blood Analysis observation is one good method for a practitioner to check the blood of patients via a microscope, to monitor and observe the intestinal bacteria dancing between blood cells. One other big problem with leaky gut is an impaired ability to absorb nutrients which is a key function of a healthy gut. People become malnourished because food isn't properly absorbed and assimilated. Partially digested food entering into to the blood circulation, activates an immune response and may initiate an auto-immune cascade and disease since immune cells start to attack their own tissues. We will discuss this situation in more depth further into this book. Industrial food, oxidative stress, inflammation, and EFA deficiency may also be associated with leaky gut. Inflammation can also be caused by medical drug prescriptions in large amounts.

Leaky gut syndrome means an increased intestinal permeability, opening the door to bacteria and partially digested food particles into the blood circulation.

Damaged Villosities

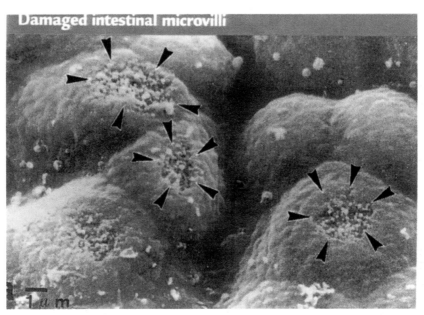

Damaged intestinal microvilli

The mucosa can also be attacked by unwanted bacteria or by harmful food that triggers certain inflammatory states; cases which now have become even more frequent.

Normal intestinal villi

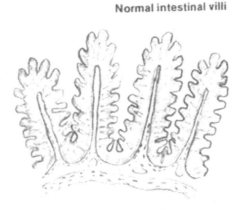

Intestinal villi affected by celiac disease

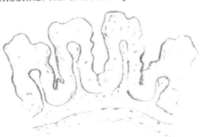

Normal intestinal villosity, intestinal villosity affected by celiac disease and partly on the quality and condition of the intestinal mucosa.

Inflammation can also be caused, not only by industrial food, but with pharmaceutical drugs taken in large quantity or on a permanent basis, not usual these days. Many pharmaceutical drugs are taken to treat diseases, where today especially we can speak of "over prescribing of drugs." I have seen patients coming to my clinic, especially aged people, but also those who were middle-aged, taking up to ten to sixteen different drugs per day, which may induce strong side effects and in the long run may cause severe damage to the intestinal mucosa, not to mention the liver, causing new disorders, including cognitive disorders, which may be linked with mortality. This factor produces serious conditions like allergies as well as drug interactions and side effects.

A chronic inflammation of the intestinal walls can, after many years and other factors, cause an alteration of the mucosa, which then lets unchanged and harmful substances into the blood. For example, when white sugar is consumed on a large scale, that exceeds the available capacity that the intertase (an enzyme of the intestinal juice) has to transform it into easily assimilated glucose and fructose, it can cause headaches and allergies and itching when entering the blood stream. Animal proteins, as well as some vegetable proteins, are the most likely to pass through the intestinal mucosa. It is necessary to understand that before proteins are absorbed, they must completely lose their identity. They cannot be cheese, beef, egg or soy, but simply amino acids that form new proteins in the body once they have been absorbed.

Today this factor is responsible for a variety of serious symptoms and disorders like allergies, hives, nervousness, and even auto immune disease. Over time and in certain individuals, depending on their genetic status, it can trigger degenerative disease such as multiple sclerosis.

This is why detoxification is a prime factor in Naturopathic medicine. As you have seen, eating is not such a simple act! Nobody knows the reaction to a meal when placed in the mouth.

Absorption in the small intestine is primordial; it partly depends on the quality of digestion (food ingested must be well chewed) and partly on the healthy intestinal mucosa and their villi. For example, if the passage through the small intestine is very rapid because the food was poorly transformed, then there is no time for final digestion and assimilation to take place. Partially digested food can penetrate the intestinal mucosa, but other non-digested food enters the large intestine where it becomes food for putrefying bacteria. Generally these bacteria increase the process of putrefaction developing more toxicity, feeding on food residues and producing an excess of gasses.

When they are overfed, they proliferate, become aggressive, increase the putrefaction process and excrete more toxic matter. They trigger abnormal fermentation, diarrhea and other physical symptoms. Some growing bacteria and toxins can reenter into the small intestine, which becomes toxic, and these toxins can even pass through the intestinal barrier, travelling throughout the blood circulation and even be responsible for weakness.

On the other hand, one must not forget that there is something called the "intestinal ecosystem" (or microbiome). There are more than five hundred species of bacteria and an equal amount of fungi that colonize the microbiome. We have said that there are microbes that live in the layers of the intestinal mucosa and there has, as yet, been no serious research on their behavior. We know that there is a good aerobe micro-flora necessary for the transformation of vitamins and other biological processes and hostile anaerobe micro-flora that is strictly controlled by the aerobe bacteria, which stop their proliferation. Little importance has been given to the intestinal ecosystem, associated with our health; however over the past few years, science is now discovering how important our intestinal microbiome is for maintaining health and preventing disease.

Once the process of assimilation has ended, the chyme (mass of food) reaches the end of its journey. The organism has selected the elements it needs to maintain its energy, regenerate and finally eliminate the undesirable substances. The residue enters the large intestine in a liquid form. The straight part of the intestine is called ascending colon, which contains food and cellulose remains. The first can still be absorbed. Cellulose under the action of bacteria is partially broken down into glucose, which then can also be absorbed. The large intestine is rich in micro-organisms that synthesize a good number of vitamins useful for the organism (vitamins B and K). Water and some of the bile are recovered while going through the transverse colon and then the descending colon.

The remaining residues are concentrated in the sigmoid (above of the rectum), used as a reservoir for feces that will then be expelled. This area is particularly dangerous because it accumulates many acidic feces, which stagnate for long periods and cause severe putrefactions where the growth of bacteria may be liable to activate carcinogenic factors and mutagenic substances. Bacteria, which develop and grow in the presence of food lacking fiber, produce the putrefactions: i.e. meat, eggs, milk, cheese, white flour, sugar and fat.

Proteins and fat, as well as excess food which escape digestion and assimilation, are attacked by the colon's bacteria, and instead of participating in the construction of the body, they cause diseases and illnesses. Overeating obstructs the organism, causing daily and permanent sources of intoxication. A diet rich in fiber is important to increase the amount of water in the colon, and for the feces to be more solid. Eating fiber-rich food helps move the contents of the large intestine more quickly and to absorb water, softening stools so that they pass easier. Fibers also help to reduce the blood cholesterol level, accelerate elimination, and reduce the risk of cardiovascular illnesses, of gallstones and colon cancer.

Why not ask ourselves these simple questions: Why do hospitals and the general public seem to ignore these important subjects concerning intestinal function and hygiene? What about the quality of food, above all, when it directly concerns patients hospitalized and affected with intestinal disorders or even colon cancer?

Conclusions:

- Eat a balanced diet, not too much and not too little, and vary your food.
- Eat slowly and calmly.
- Chew food properly in order to activate the digestive mechanisms.
- Avoid bloating the stomach with large quantities and mixture of food. A one-dish meal is a simple way to eat and not overtax the digestive system.
- Light exercise (walking) after meals facilitates digestion, but heavy physical activity makes digestion difficult.
- Drink one to two liters of pure water a day, especially between meals.

Part II

The Intestinal Ecosystem
The Intestinal Immune System
Elimination Organs

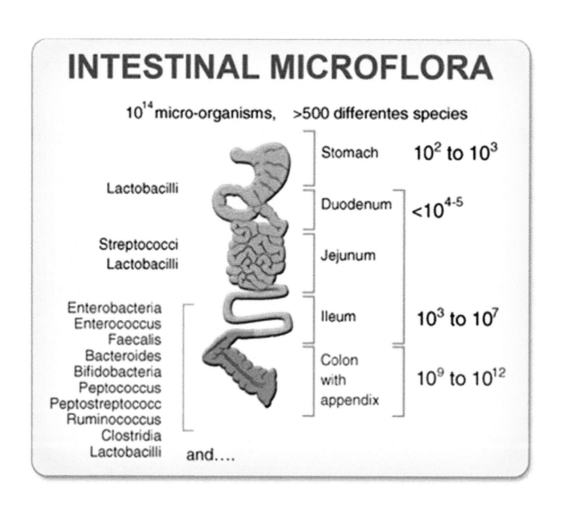

The Intestinal Ecosystem

When we talk about preserving nature, we talk about an ecological balance of the ecosystem destined to maintain an environment favorable to life. We try to create a line of defense and a balance between the benefits of nature and pollution.

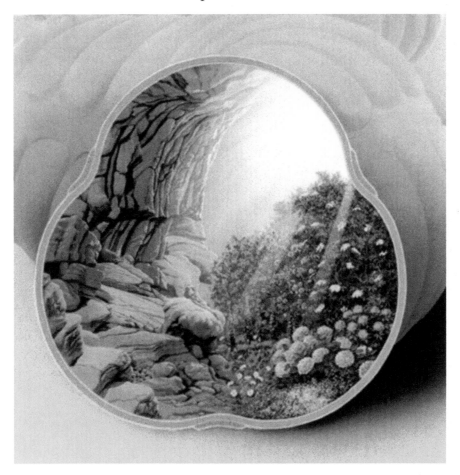

The intestinal micro-flora is similar to nature's ecosystem. Our intestinal ecosystem health needs the same elements as in earth or vice-versa. In an alkaline earth, the aerobic bacteria die, same as in the human intestines.

On close analysis we notice that nature's ecosystem and our intestinal system are perfectly identical. To begin with, the microbial floras found in the ground and the intestinal flora, are considered a real defense barrier, and are essential for various biochemical processes.

I remind you that the microbial flora of fertile soil is particularly rich. In two and a half acres of land there are about 1,104 pounds of bacteria, 552 pounds of fungus, and more or less 220 pounds of worms. Healthy soil is essential for agriculture as it is full of life and is quite complex. We will prove that our intestine has a similar role. It must be so in order for humans to be healthy and resistant. When I was at Hidden Valley Health Ranch with Dr. Bernard Jensen, I saw how they gave much attention to the quality of soil to have organic vegetables growth of high nutritional value. Dr. Jensen was a pioneer in raising bed worms for use in top soil, with horse manure, composting, and dolomite. But worms were important to balance the soils eco-system. It is incredible that we are only now discovering about our body's

29

mechanisms of balance and defense, when conventional medicine boasts about having all the secrets of the human body in hand. Research concentrates on the mechanisms of the immune cells without considering that there could be other even more subtle mechanisms. However, more recently it is true that science has shown a growing interest for the intestinal micro-flora that could be seen as the guardian of our health. The concept of healthy intestinal flora being essential to human health originated from the work of Russian microbiologist Elie Metchnikoff (1845-1916), a disciple of Pasteur, who elaborated his theory on longevity in relation to intestinal micro-flora.

Today, we know that a healthy aerobe intestinal flora plays an essential role, not only against infections but against chronic diseases such as diabetes, rheumatoid arthritis, and functions to balance cholesterol and to reinforce our immune defense. Some variety of bacteria that belong to the group of Gram+, once entering into the blood circulation, reaches the lymphatic ganglions and stimulates the production of some white cells named pTh17. This cell acts as a new immune defense in our body fighting against cancer cells. We need to pay more attention to this intestinal ecosystem through quality food and not abusing medical drugs, especially antibiotics that destroy this sensitive flora.

An anaerobe intestinal flora can cause various chronic illnesses, even respiratory illnesses, not forgetting about unpleasant digestive disorders. The intestine is colonized by good bacteria, which increase enormously in the terminal part of the colon, just as the bacteria linked to the process of putrefaction.

The digestive tract contains about 100 trillion bacteria that weigh about three pounds that renew themselves two to three times a day. Today the microbiome is recognized as central to keep our body healthy, acting as a barrier against many diseases. Bacteria participate in the maturation of our immune defense system and are important to produce many vitamins from transformed food such as vitamins B6, Biotin, B1, B2, B6, B12, folic acid, and vitamin K. According to certain precursors, such as Dr. John Harvey Kellog from the United States, good bacteria are conserved in the clean colon and build a barrier against harmful bacteria. A good balance between the two types of bacteria minimizes the possibility of putrefaction, gas, and fermentation. According to Dr. Kellog, the correct balance in a healthy colon is about 85% good bacteria and 15% bad bacteria. We may ask ourselves where these bacteria come from because a child, in the fetal stage, is completely protected. Well, on the one hand, the child colonizes its intestinal bacteria from the mother at the moment of birth, and thereafter the rest depends on breast feeding from which the child builds its good intestinal flora, but surely not from processed formula feeding.

Today young children are over-prescribed antibiotics while their intestinal flora has yet not matured and their immune system is weaker. Consequences to their health condition can be serious in the future, and today there is an alert to medical doctors to prescribe fewer antibiotics.

Distribution of Bacteria in the Human Intestine

Unfortunately, currently the balance in most people has reverted to 15% good bacteria and 85% bad bacteria. This difference tending to a greater multiplication of bad bacteria shows bad eating habits.

Caffeine, over-cooked foods, white sugar, and white bread favor the development of harmful bacteria which live without oxygen (anaerobe). It is important to know that good intestinal bacteria also have another task: producing almost all the hydrosoluble vitamins, except for vitamin C. Some of the important vitamins include vitamin B1, vitamin B2, pantothenic acid, vitamin B3, nicotinic acid, vitamin B12, and folic acid. Note the production of vitamin K by the intestinal bacteria.

It is incredible, if not truly miraculous; we have a real pharmaceutical laboratory in our intestine, which is vital to our health and well-being. Most of the time we take our body for granted, almost without noticing, as if our digestive tract works on auto-pilot. We should value, maintain, and not harm this natural gift that, even today, we still have a tendency to abuse. Our organism's nutritional needs not only depend on the quality of the food we eat, but also on our intestine's bacterial flora. Again we should learn more about our body's conception, how it functions. We should then determine the best food alternatives in order to preserve and maintain our good health.

The fat metabolism and the level of cholesterol are just another two factors related to the bacterial flora. Today for example, we have the tendency to abuse the use of antibiotics, thereby greatly reducing the normal bacterial population of the small intestine, which will only regain its balance very slowly. In time, this becomes dangerous for an adult. Now just imagine what happens in a baby! It is a mortal blow, as its intestinal flora is not yet balanced. Antibiotics are not the only medicines guilty of harming the microbial flora. Certain analgesics, for example, are also very destructive. It has been proven that fibers are necessary to improve the intestinal transit and combat constipation. Old theories are now reemerging showing that fibers are good for preventing colon cancer.

The English surgeon Dr. Denis P. Burkitt, who carried out an in-depth study on the role of fibers in relation to colon illnesses, stated that fiber is the food for normal colon bacteria. They are the ones responsible for fermenting fibers and producing and maintaining acidity of the feces. Fibers also promote a certain acidity in the colon, preventing it from becoming too alkaline, which also favors cancer.

While multiplying, friendly bacteria use the proteins from food, which have not been digested by the small intestine. By using the bulk of the non-digested amino acids in their own metabolism, bacteria limit their production of ammonia, which is a toxic substance, especially for the brain and nerves.

The role of fibers is not limited only to these functions. They increase the volume of the feces, dilute the toxic substances that can exist in the colon and accelerate intestinal transit thereby diminishing the contact time with the mucosa of the colon. This way, the fat deriving from food is eliminated more rapidly through the feces. Otherwise it would remain in the colon and easily enter the organism. Intestinal bacteria control the digestion and absorption of fat preventing its accumulation in the organism.

The intestine and the colon can be compared to a main boulevard that runs through our body, guarding us against harmful bacteria and toxins for our defense and protection. The intestine plays a protective role and is the guardian angel of our well-being. Therefore, it needs correct, specific, and special food.

I have often stated that man is both hardy and fragile. We are internally colonized by billions of friendly bacteria, and in smaller quantity, by harmful bacteria. We must try our hardest to conserve the 85-15% balance between good bacteria and bad or anaerobe bacteria. With the introduction of commercial and unnatural foods, we alter the balance, opening doors to all kinds of illnesses. The list of disorders and diseases associated with the contamination of our intestine is long and becomes increasingly longer. Infections are one of the first consequences.

Unfortunately, all the effort to combat these conditions is concentrated in antibiotic therapy with increasingly alarming results that cause an even greater imbalance of the intestinal flora.

There is a more natural and effective way to increase immune cell activity and prevent cases of infection, sinusitis, and bronchitis. In our clinic I like to use in particular a treatment called microtherapy or "intestinal vaccination," using autolysates of human bacteria in the form of drops. It is a natural treatment developed in Germany, called Symbioflor, that renews the micro-flora, activates macrophages and acts on the intestinal immune system, stimulating antibodies, B and T Lymphocytes, suppresses pathogens and penetrates the organism through the lymphatic system. There are three different mixtures, and one is adapted to cancer, particularly colon cancer. Results are often very quick while in any case it also increases bowel movement. I have recommended Symbioflor (Pro- Symbioflor and Symbioflor 1 and 2) for more than twenty years to stimulate the immunity, for infantile respiratory disorders, asthma, allergies, and constipation. At the same time, it is very important to understand the value of nutrition in order to supply the body with the necessary nutrients, vitamins, fibers, and enzymes. One must not forget that probiotics are so important in strengthening the immune system and balancing the intestinal flora.

Intestinal Eco-System

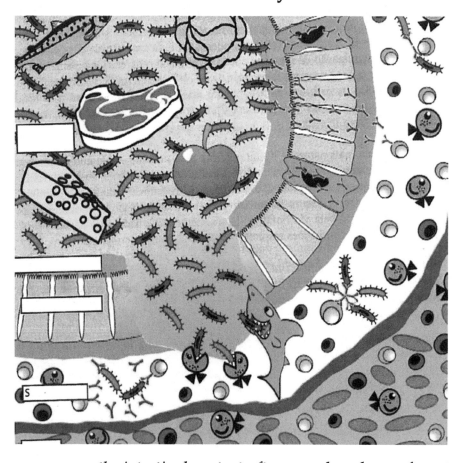

In this image we can see the intestinal content after a meal made up of meat, fish, cheese, cabbage, and apples. The mixture of food is a source of putrefaction and proliferation of harmful bacteria (in red and blue in the intestine) capable of passing through the intestine and entering the blood stream. Initially the immune system and the bacteria are there to protect us against this invasion, which can cause allergic, cutaneous, arthritic, and rheumatoid diseases. The intestinal mucous can be damaged by bad bacteria or irritated by industrial food, which induces inflammatory processes frequent in our society.

The Intestinal Immune System

There is an important factor which must be explained and which patients hardly know about, i.e. the intestinal immune system.

In truth, we all know that immune cells are produced by the bone marrow. On the other hand, we still ignore some new research regarding another important source of immune cell production: the intestine.

The small intestine contains an area called the Peyer's Patch in which the mucosa contain immune cells and antibodies which are our defense against infection and inflammation both in the intestine and our body. For instance, mucosal dendritic cells interact with specialized capillaries that allow antigens to move from the blood then to lymph nodes and will increase our immune defense. Other antigens are directly processed by intestinal dendritic cells to induce the production of a type of T cell that controls intestinal inflammation. Mucosa dendritic cells of the small intestine primarily monitor intestinal content both to suppress inflammatory reaction against food and to protect against invading pathogens.

And yet, many of the infections, recurrences, allergies, and respiratory disorders, among others, are a consequence of the absence of immunoglobulin produced by the intestine's lymphoid tissues. Do not be surprised to find that the intestine produces 70 to 80% of our immune cells, essentially T lymphocytes, B lymphocytes, macrophages, and dendritic cells. Evidence shows that these cells have a basic role to play against intruders, which enter the intestine. The cellular layers lining the intestine create a barrier between the inside and the outside of the organism. Through food and water we swallow a large number of microbes and bacteria, which are fortunately destroyed by the immune system.

Unfortunately, it all seems to be ignored with the use and abuse of antibiotics which indeed do not resolve the recurring problems of infections, allergies, respiratory disorders, or intestinal inflammation which is a consequence of a poor intestinal immune defense and the absence of immunoglobulin produced by the intestine's lymphoid tissues.

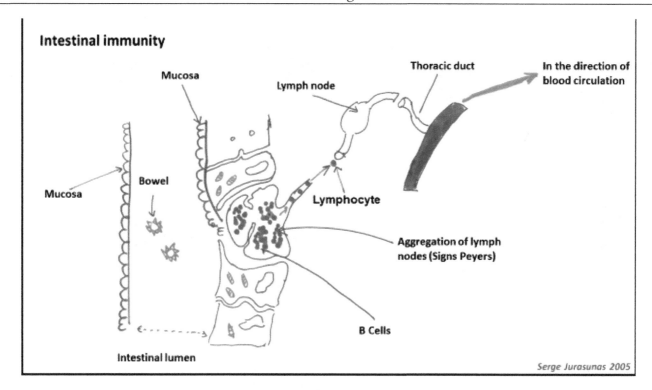

Intestinal Immunity

The image shows the intestines lymphatic tissues and the local Peyer's Patches that produce immune cells.

We must not forget that the surface of the intestinal mucosa is substantial, ranging from 10,600 and 14,130 cubic feet, according to the individual. The large intestine is the about the same in size as a tennis court. This enormous surface is permanently in contact with modern food, toxins, and microbes. Increasingly we are more often faced with low quality food, often served at restaurants, which are not very scrupulous and lacking in hygiene, as well as in malls with an atmosphere filled with microbes and pollution imbedded in the food. Fortunately, we are primarily protected against these invaders by the intestinal immune system, but this does not occur in every case. Let us consider the local intestinal protection. The immune cells migrate from the intestine through the thoracic duct into the lymphatic stream to the mucosa of the bronchials and the lungs, with the aim of protecting and combating infections.

The integrity of this system is essential in maintaining our immune system against infections. Apparently, this concept is still ignored above all, in cases of infection as doctors limit themselves to prescribing antibiotics or promoting vaccines. To date, the cases of infections in winter have not diminished, but on the contrary they have increased in a disturbing way.

According to recent studies published in the United States, one in four hundred people are deficient in immunoglobulin A, which shows an immune deficiency. Now, in Portugal the situation must be similar if not more serious, promoted by an excessive use of medicines and antibiotics by a health care system that has become increasingly industrial, and much less effective in actually treating disease. Adolescents currently are given excess medication, leading to a reduction in immune defenses and sooner or later, this translates into a lack of defense and a greater susceptibility to infections. Already in France during 1984, certain doctors considered that three to five antibiotic treatments taken by adolescents during one winter could be highly injurious to their future health.

Today, up to ten treatments are used on some children during winter. It is thoughtlessness without regards for the health of children, which mainly blocks up their immune defense. Preventative medicine should be used to reinforce the immune system in order to offer and promote better health, offering greater attention through a better diet, dietary support, and decreasing oxidative stress. This protection in cases of severe diseases, such as cancer, even passes through the intestine's immune defenses via the micro-flora and colonies of aerobe bacteria.

Without overemphasizing the importance of the intestinal defense system, we must, however, concede that it is important and is enclosed in a complex system, which has been ignored up to now. Instead of giving our immune system greater attention through a better diet, dietary support, and decreasing oxidative stress, we rely on vaccination and antibiotics which now, according to a recent report dated April 30, 2014, antibiotic resistance has become tragic in more than 144 countries, because of the these bacteria and a weak immune defense system. Instead we keep carrying on attacking it with excessive medical prescriptions, polluted foods, and bad life style. We have effectually eliminated the efficacy of the immune defense mechanism and detoxification process. This is probably the greatest aggression medicine has done to repress a genetically built immune defense.

More recent research from the Institute Gustave–Roussy (Villejuif, France) in association with scientists at the Pasteur Institute (Paris), has demonstrated that the intestinal flora boosts the antitumor immune response during a treatment with cyclophosphamide, one of the widely used anti-cancer therapies. There is a synergy because the intestinal bacteria and the anti-cancer agent that starts when the drug facilitates the entry of some friendly bacteria (from Gram+), that enters both into the blood circulation and lymphatic ganglions, by stimulating the production of PTH17 anti-tumor cells. This type of cell works as the new immune defense system that helps the body to fight against cancer cells.

Simultaneously, other researchers from the National Cancer Institute (USA) have demonstrated that intestinal micro-flora reinforce the chemotherapeutic treatment with oxaliplatin by stimulation of the immune system. It has also shown that supplementation and stimulation of the intestinal flora while including a specific diet can reinforce the action of the anti-cancer treatment.

Overall in our daily life, good results could not be obtained with good diet and detoxification, while doctor's drugs and antibiotics cannot help, on the contrary, damage the intestinal micro-flora and favor infection and other diseases.

Elimination Organs

The colon is without a doubt the most important elimination organ of the human body although it is not the only one. Not many people are aware of the extraordinary elimination system our body possesses. Nature seems to have acted intelligently and preventatively to protect us against the accumulation of residue derived from the digestion of food.

We will see how these organs, called "emunctories," can help or compensate for one another when either one breaks down. This allows the organism to maintain a certain balance, although complications or crisis in elimination can arise and can be mistaken by patients as disease symptoms, which they are not.

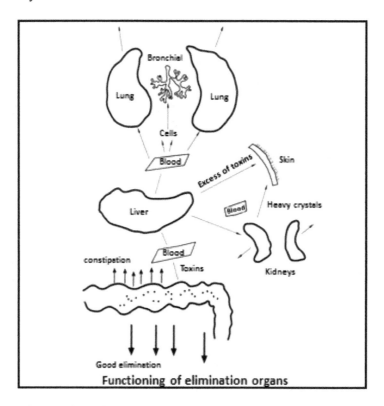

Functioning of elimination organs

Apart from the colon, other elimination organs are the kidneys, the lungs, the skin, and the liver. The liver is not really an elimination organ but simply a laboratory known as P450 using enzymes for transformation of chemicals and detoxification, acting as a filter that protects the organism against toxins capable of entering the blood stream. At this point, the liver detoxifies and reintroduces about six hundred liters of blood into circulation every twenty-four hours at an average of twenty-five liters an hour. This is an enormous task with the only aim of preserving the blood from accumulation of toxins and bacteria, by filtering the blood stream.

As we age, less blood enters the liver to be detoxified and the blood accumulates more toxins and bacteria, which explains why older aged people become increasingly subject to infections.

On the other hand, the liver stores various vitamins, such as beta-Carotene, releasing them according to need. If the brain is working, the liver supplies it with nutrients. But if the muscles are working, the liver also supplies them with nutrients.

The job of elimination through the colon, kidneys, skin, and lungs is not limited to expulsion on behalf of each of these organs. It is a real group effort among one another.

When colon elimination malfunctions, for example, when a bowel movement occurs only every two days, the blood begins to carry toxins that are supposed to be filtered by the liver, but if not, they accumulate in blood. The organism is going to find another means to get rid of the toxins. The skin, which is not only a defense barrier but an exterior filter, has a derivative role. The organism cleanses itself by sweating. In certain cases, in highly intoxicated people the skin produces unpleasant smells to indicate that the organism is trying to rid itself of toxins and putrefied substances, which are normally expelled through urine or feces. When the skin is dull, darker, with blackheads, pimples, or eczemas it is a sign that the intoxicated organism is trying to eliminate those substances through the skin. Macromolecules deriving from non-digested foods are captured by the immune cells like the macrophages and polynuclears, which move them to the skin. Indeed, the organism does not have enzymes capable of degrading these extremely solid substances.

The excessive concentration of white blood cells and dilated blood vessels under the skin shows that the body tries to eliminate these molecules through the skin in a tentative manner to detoxify the blood from excessive toxic waste, which in turn creates an inflammation in the skin.

Iridology is very important when you need to check on patient skin condition associated with colon intoxication, but also in case of lung disease. By always checking on the colon, the skin, and even the kidney, you may find some answers especially wherein to start your treatment. By observing the irises of patients with intoxicated skin we notice a darker ring around the periphery of the iris. This is known as the "skin ring" and its diameter and color vary according to the degree of intoxication and accumulation of toxins under the skin, coming from the colon and a sluggish liver, and circulating in blood, which the body is unable to eliminate. I often notice an extremely condensed skin ring in people with chronic constipation, respiratory disorders, or psoriasis.

We must understand that the organism provides us with all the outlets necessary to detoxify itself. Therefore, when the colon does not work properly and the skin is overloaded, the organism tries other ways of elimination through the bronchials and the lungs, even the nasal canals that help drain the mucous which blocks the lymphatic system. For example, if blood is intoxicated with heavy mucus, which is insoluble in water (this originates from the colon) and the emunctory organs are congested, the body will try to eliminate this through an alternate elimination pathway. We may call it the secondary emunctory, but I prefer to call this mechanism "Derivative Transference," which I first coined when giving lessons at the French School of Naturopathy in Paris, back in 1970. I realized that nasal secretions, uterine secretions, and even sinusitis were only a Derivative Transference from the normal elimination organs having been blocked up.

These nasal secretions are often derivative discharges of an intoxicated organism, triggered by a severe cold. It tries to move them through the lymphatic system to the respiratory system (In fact, there are various lymphatic vessels ending in the nose), which has a surface of 80m^2 and is full of cavities. When these substances get into these cavities they cause a certain amount of irritation and coughing attacks.

When these situations worsen, they can cause bronchitis, asthma attacks, or even infections. Indeed, certain bacteria or fungi have the tendency to adhere to these mucosities that reside in the cavities of the lungs and the bronchials triggering inflammation. Catarrh, we all know, is no more than an accumulation of mucus.

I treated the case of a woman who constantly coughed up greenish viscose substances, which showed a high degree of intoxication. Good results could not be obtained without detoxification. After many years of observing the iris I know that there is a relationship between the colon and bronchial disorders.

In chronic inflammation of the bronchials, the corresponding area of the iris appears darker in color just like the area of the colon, which is found exactly opposite. This shows the indirect relationship between the colon and the accumulation of toxins and inflammation in the bronchials.

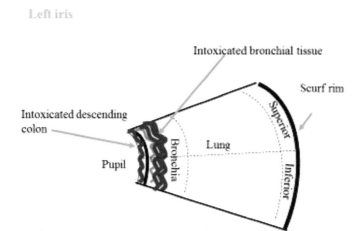

Elimination organs

In other words, if a person has an inflammatory condition of the bronchials, it is possible that the colon is involved in the pathology. Hippocrates stated correctly that the first thing we must know in order to treat an illness is understand the correct functioning of the organism.

Environmental Pollution

Currently, human beings are increasingly more preoccupied with the environmental pollution of cities. This pollution of the cities which has increased visibly is also directly responsible for the increase in respiratory illnesses and allergies. Pollution together with the internal mucous creates favorable conditions for the proliferation of bacteria and fungus in the respiratory system.

We must not be surprised to see what happens in hospitals, especially an alarming increase in highly resistant infections and number of deaths. Portugal makes no exception. In the last two years over 17,000 hospitalized patients died of infection. The unsanitary state of bed-ridden people causes infestation by colonies of resistant bacteria on patients with poor immune defense because of antibiotic overuse. Today hospitals are facing serious problems since many patients interned for disease or even only for checkup, die of infection and nothing is done about it.

Finally, there is the skin, which not many people really understand. The skin is an organ which produces immune cells, known as "lymphocytes," that protect us from external aggressions. Its essential mission is total immune defense and requires constant nutrition and hygiene. It has recently been discovered that there is a real language in the skin passing through the neurons with about two hundred receptors per square inch of skin. Damaged, dirty, and intoxicated skin can disrupt the work of communication from the skin which is linked to each one of our organs.

Modern thermography devices which capture the heat emanating from a particular area of the skin show where there are neurons leading to a specific organ, establishing a biological diagnosis. This proves that there is a complex system connecting the skin with the organs, or vice versa, through the nervous system. On various occasions I had the opportunity to observe skin problems linked to auto-intoxication in cases of severe bronchitis.

Let us consider the example of an eighteen-year-old girl who came to see me because of a severe skin problem on three fingers of her right hand, which were cracked and always suppurated with pus. She and her two sisters had a poor health status, and above all, a weak, nervous constitution, as observed in their irises. This is always considered an indication of further health problems.

The intestines were irregular and her deficient diet was not very good (she normally ate in university cafeterias). She had gone to France for a summer camp for fifteen days where their diet was based on meat and French fries, with no vegetables, which is a common way of feeding the youngest during the summer months. She returned to Portugal with severe constipation, having a real block-up of her intestine, with a bowel movement only every four or every five days. This meant a very serious accumulation of feces in the sigmoid colon and probably up to the descending colon, but at first I didn't realize how intoxicated she was and prescribed a homeopathic treatment focusing on the skin, but I was wrong obtaining only little result.

The toxic substances and amines produced by the daily ingestion of meat and the lack of fibers caused a decrease in intestinal elimination, retention of toxic feces, bacteria, and subsequently an auto-intoxication of the colon, with a derivative process of toxins passing through the skin.

It was then that I suggested an enema treatment from a mixture of various selected herbs and potassium salt that we have used exclusively for nearly forty years with patients of our clinic. The mixture is added to one liter of warm water and used as enema. It produces by reflex action, a strong discharge, and elimination of feces.

After three days of intestinal cleansing, we had instances where she eliminated incredible quantities of dark feces, residues, and mucous that intoxicated the colon, the blood, and the skin. This elimination occurred not just once but a second time. After one week's time, she started to improve. After two weeks the infection disappeared. Her skin cleared up and returned to a normal condition. This was for me a great lesson to learn even after practicing for so many years.

Many of the body's reactions are sometimes manifested in inflammation or pain but repressed forcefully with antibiotics or anti-inflammatory, drugs which is wrong.

The Function of the Kidneys in Detoxification

The kidneys are also essential organs for expulsion and elimination. They also act as cleansing filters with the help of more than a million filtering units called nephrons.

The kidneys carry out the enormous task of detoxifying seven liters of blood an hour or 53,280 liters a year. This is a gigantic task, if we consider all the dietary excesses, which constantly overload this magnificent organ, which, despite this, maintains the balance of the organism.

The kidneys filter heavy acids (uric acid, urea), which are defined as crystals as they are hard. The crystals are remains of the protein metabolism. They can also originate through an excess of acid food or refined white sugar. These are eliminated in great quantities through urine and in lesser quantities through the skin's sweat glands.

The kidneys also filter the organism's residue of toxic substances. These toxic substances, which are not properly metabolized, end up attacking the kidneys causing microscopic lacunas in the nephrons.

The accumulation of crystals, at first, compel the kidneys to accelerate their function and are then said to be hyperactive. In a second phase the kidneys get tired and become hypoactive. This is followed by the appearance of such classic disorders as kidney stones, sciatica, and nephritis. Alternatively, the kidneys provide another exit and divert the crystals to the skin, leading to more or less complex acne.

Situations like this seem inexplicable but are based on the theory of the emunctory organs. They are precise physiological functions, which are part of our organism's functionality.

It is always good to reflect on the natural functions of the organism equipped to defend itself. Many of the organism's reactions are sometimes manifested in pain and attacked with great force by antibiotics or anti-inflammatory drugs. Often healthy fevers, which are part of the immune and defense mechanisms built up 2 million years ago, are inevitably repressed. Fevers are a way for our body to defend itself against excess bacteria and toxins, having been scientifically proven. The fever allows the skin to eliminate up to several liters of sweat and to kill microbes. Sweat is overcharged with considerable toxins, uric acid, and urea.

If we constantly keep repressing temperature with antibiotics, resulting from a fever in children (and adolescents) this is not the best solution, except in the case of high fever. In this manner, we repress our natural detoxification process which further decreases in efficiency, each time the body's power is utilized to activate this defense mechanism. This situation may also indicate a deficiency in the intestinal immune system being unable to protect the body against microbial invasion. Overall the constant repression of fever may in turn weaken the entire defense system of our body, where we effectually eliminate the efficacy of the immune defense mechanism and detoxification process. Medicine does not make children and adults more healthy, but more vulnerable to disease.

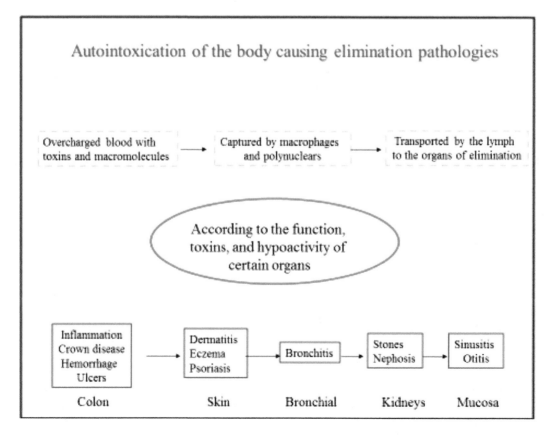

Part III

The Main Disorders of the Colon

Constipation
Flatulence and Spasmodic Colon
Diarrhea
Colon Irritation and Diverticulitis
Colitis
Prolapsed Colon
Colon Cancer

Currently, colon disorders are extremely common. Problems of this kind were already encountered at the beginning of my career, especially constipation, diverticulitis, or diarrhea, but never to the same extent as today.

It is very alarming since, instead of improving our health, we set the stage for increasingly more chronic disorders, and above all, degenerative diseases. Hospital emergencies and admissions for colon problems largely exceed those for any other illness. The patient is often hospitalized with severe pain, subsequently undergoing infinite tests, X-rays, and more without obtaining a concrete diagnosis. It is clearly a paradox that we consider ourselves a healthy society.

In 1992, America spent $950 billion on disease maintenance along with inefficient and unnecessary health care expenditures costing $100 billion annually. By 2014, total U.S. Healthcare spending soared to $3.8 trillion annually.

Is it really so difficult, or are we incapable of first understanding that colon disorder is not necessarily a pathology, and secondly that constipation, or a ballooned colon can be responsible for a variety of symptoms. What is the origin of these intestinal disorders and what solution should be taken?

I remember the case of a thirty-six-year-old man who suffered from frequent intestinal pains. He was admitted for five days and underwent all possible kinds of tests to no avail. He was sent home because everything appeared to be normal. However, this man's nervous system was really in a terrible condition, which affected his sleep, his gastrointestinal system, and also his waking behavior.

Iridology could be most useful when it comes to understanding these cases, and above all, in identifying their cause. In this particular case we prescribed for the patient a balanced diet, detoxification, and a treatment to strengthen his nervous system. He then went back to living a normal life, completely free from intestinal disorder and pain.

The colon is the most important part of our elimination system. It is subject to various complications that affect thousands of people. These problems are sometimes very painful and are reflected in our faces. In the same way, our emotions can also affect our colon.

Notwithstanding the criticism that unfortunately still exists, how important would understanding the connection or link between alternative medicine, nutritional therapy, and conventional medicine be for the patient!

Most causes of gastrointestinal problems point to wrong dietary styles, heavy meals, excess of animal proteins, mixtures at the same meal of meat and several carbohydrates, fried foods, and a diet poor in vegetables, fruits, whole cereals, and fibers. However bad a colon may be from a hereditary point of view, as we have observed in irises, it also serves as the basis for problems that start with bad dietary style. My personal practice with patients leaves no doubt about this understanding.

Most of the food bought at large supermarkets has dubious freshness without mentioning all the manipulations and chemical operations they underwent before reaching the shelves: the radiation, colorants, hydrogenation, pesticides, preservatives, and artificial flavors.

Modern society cares little about how an apple or a bunch of sprouts are farmed. Commercial farming is governed by the laws of profit using astronomical doses of insecticides and pesticides.

Our European laws are more preoccupied with the size of an apple for commercialization in supermarkets, where inspectors are measuring the size of the apple to check if it is according to ECC regulation, but nobody is interested in the excess insecticides found on the apple or how the apple gets to the consumer.

How many people have we seen with abdominal pains after having consumed these big and rosy apples? While in Canada back in 1968, I visited an organic apple grower whose farm was in Manitoba. The owner told me the story. In prior years, he was growing apples using a large quantity of insecticides, and he ate many apples himself, but developed intestinal pains. One day while spraying insecticides, he lost his senses and got sick. He woke up and said, "This cannot be the will of God using chemicals on food." He moved to start a new apple orchard growing on virgin land, importing an herb from Egypt to kill insects. This happened forty-four years ago, yet where are we today with insecticides?

If food has a determining role on colon disorders, we must not neglect to mention that chronic stress, nervous disorders, and emotional behavior which commonly affects our society is also responsible for a number of intestinal and digestive disorders.

In this context, women are as prone as men to gastrointestinal problems, which was not the case thirty or forty years ago. I also believe that today, the scales tip more towards women. They live under increasingly permanent stress, housework, and children without having time for themselves to cook healthy meals. Of course the modern woman doesn't worry too much about what they eat, where frozen and microwavable food is integral part of the busy-modern woman's lifestyle. In the end, these conditions cause very serious problems. As Dr. Bernard Jensen used to say so long ago, "A lot of killing is done in the kitchen." What about today after forty-five years? Dr. Jensen would certainly be horrified!

The most common problems affecting women are constipation, hemorrhoids, and fistulas, with or without hemorrhages or diarrhea. Colitis, ballooned colon, diarrhea, ulcers, not mention increasing percentage of colon cancer in middle age women can often be observed in our clinic. If we accept living with a lazy colon, and not worrying about poor elimination, such as a colon movement every two or three days, the consequences can become a problem ranging from colon disorders, inflammation, Crohn's disease, to the beginning of intoxicated blood, that with time may be driven to chronic and degenerative disease. In fact, I have often witnessed this in my clinic.

Recently, a new colon disorder has been appearing more often, known as "irritated bowel syndrome" (IBS) or colon irritation. This problem results directly from imbalancedfood on the table, industrial food, oxidative stress and low antioxidant enzyme status that protects the wall of the colon. Irritated bowel syndrome has spread itself very quickly through industrialized countries, without sparing women.

In this book we will often talk about these disorders in their respective chapters, especially when we speak about auto-intoxication, which is a determining factor. Auto-intoxication not only affects the colon or the intestinal system, it can give rise to an array of organic disorders and illnesses which compromise the entire organism.

Constipation

The human body is built in a way that it absorbs food, digests, assimilates, and expulses in a manner that nourishes our 60 trillion cells. Therefore, colon expulsions should occur each time we eat to expel undigested waste and bacteria. Each American eats approximately 19,996 pounds of food per year, 5 1/2 pounds per day, of which 2/3 is converted liquid, water, where two pounds of solid waste should pass out through the colon. If not, it accumulates, creating a situation known as constipation.

Since the 1920s and 1930s, there have been works with important references to this subject, referring and relating to constipation with health problems. Prof. Arnold Ehret's work is one good example. In 1922 he published a book called, *Chronic Constipation – Overcoming Constipation Naturally* that I was lucky to have bought in Los Angeles in 1963, a new edition reprinted several times over the years. I thought that this doctor was really explaining the cause of disease. Born in Germany, Arnold Ehret, at thirty-one years of age, was physically very weak and suffered from kidney trouble. He became so distraught and frustrated after consulting twenty-three doctors, with the result of "incurable," he literally felt like killing himself. Accidentally he heard of Naturopathy and was treated at the Kneipp Sanatorium, where he wanted to make himself well. Thereafter he moved to the USA.

Constipation is one of the greatest present-day internal dangers to health, to which we play little attention. Today 100 million North Americans suffer from some kind of intestinal disease and 70 million from chronic constipation. Indeed, constipation is the direct cause of toxemia and auto-intoxication which in turn are associated with many diseases. Some of the results of chronic constipation are to lower the body's resistance, increase fatigue, infection, and the initiation of many diseases. Constipation may also have a negative effect on excretory organs or emunctories by increasing their activity. These are the skin, kidneys, lungs, lymphatic system, and the liver. These organs and systems become hyperactive and overworked, but after some time from the overload of toxins, they decrease their activity, become less efficient, and more toxins start to accumulate resulting in a sluggish cellular metabolism. Iridology can show perfectly the condition of emunctory organs, and if they are slowing down their activity.

Unfortunately today, even after fifty years, only a few doctors associate constipation with health problems, and even common people do not associate certain diseases as a consequence of their constipation. Truly speaking, conventional medicine has never associated, and ignores, this as an important biological function of the human body for preserving our health. Many diseases are surely associated with chronic constipation and feces stagnation that poisons our body.

Usually these people of middle-age have either experienced the accumulation of physical symptoms associated with their constipation or have read some books about it that makes sense. Naturopathic doctors use to play a central role since they were the first to alert and teach patient about this problem. While today it seems to me that Naturopathy is no longer what it used to be, as far as "teaching the patient" is concerned. However, this is also very important, which is why I decided to write this book so all my patients, readers, and fellow health professionals can learn about this important topic.

During the past fifty years, society has confined itself to using laxatives so much that in the United States the sale of laxatives comes second to that of aspirin. If we imagine that 33 billion aspirin tablets are consumed in one year, that equates to a lot of headaches and a large quantity of laxatives.

According to my experience, modern day men and women have serious colon problems. An evacuation every two days is the norm, but every three to five days or more is still common, and nobody pays great attention about this fact.

A fifty-year-old woman says she only has a bowel movement every second day or at two- or three-day intervals. The illnesses she suffers from—hypertension, cholesterol, migraines, rheumatism—are not merely a question of bad luck! There are also more serious cases with one evacuation every three to five days. I had a serious case of a twenty-three-year-old girl who only had a bowel movement once every fifteen days. She was on the way to a nervous breakdown and was forced to abandon her studies.

We still live under misconceptions, because modern medicine never considered natural intestinal elimination as a biological factor of the human body and health. In an American book, which is actually a medical manual for patients (*The Physician Manual for His Patients*), the chapter on constipation literally says, "Remember, that a bowel movement a day is not essential for good health." How about that? Meaning you can have a bowel movement every three days, take laxatives if necessary, and you'll be OK, you are healthy. What about feces accumulation! Surely there are consequences to our health status.

The consequences of living with a lazy colon and with poor elimination can lead to serious intestinal disorders, colon dilation, and excess gases, fistulas, intestinal ulcers, diverticulosis, hemorrhoids, tumors, and various types of pains, not to mention in the middle or long term from multiple symptoms to serious chronic disorders, which we will discuss later on in the book.

I really believe that we should give more attention to this problem, which will keep escalating if we do nothing to correct it, especially where women are concerned. I have spent fifty years educating patients on this matter, yet this is only one important facet.

If this occurs, there are dietary styles involved together with sedentary life, which affects more women than men. It is easier for men to play a bit of sport or physical activity than for a woman. Even a hunter or a golfer exercises the intestinal muscles when walking. Women also have to contend with the hormonal factor, which cyclically causes congestion of the genital organs and of the lower abdomen, responsible for edemas, liquid retention, and worsening constipation, which may already exist.

Pregnancy slows down the process of feces elimination and many women suffer a lot during this period, apart from the problems it can cause to the unborn child. The pregnant woman's need to program a correct diet and adopt certain rules of hygiene in life in order to stimulate intestinal transit stands to reason.

It is a problem that must be understood and addressed, both for the specialist and for the patient that today has absolutely no knowledge or intuition about what to do, discharging all responsibility over the gynecologist.

I often have the opportunity to observe, with the live blood analysis system, the blood of pregnant women and this is tragic. We may observe some abnormal conditions that include bacterial growth (intestinal bacteria) fungal invasion, lipid plaques, excess of toxins, damaged red cells, all demonstrating bad dietary style, constipation, and oxidative stress status, all of this being unknown to the physician, which of course affects the unborn child.

Since ancient times, elimination of feces took place in a squatting position creating pressure on the abdomen, facilitating the expulsion of matter. Today, elimination takes place in a seated position on a comfortable seat no less, but without pressure which results in only partial elimination.

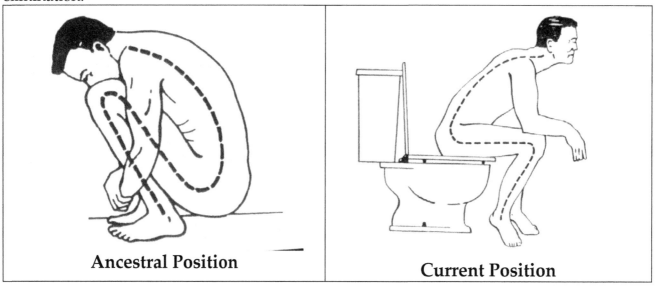

Ancestral Position   **Current Position**

However, the organism's physiology requires a complete elimination. There is a great difference between the squatting and the seated positions, which has a bearing on the weight of the eliminated matter. According to Dr. Ivan Popov, a Soviet specialist in gerontology, there is a 60g to 70g decrease in eliminated feces in the seating position. These feces can become impacted in the colon in large quantities.

When we eat it is necessary that waste and residues from absorbed food be eliminated when entering the large colon along with a large quantity of dead microbes. Then a peristaltic contraction of the colon takes place pushing the feces towards the rectum.

But everything is not that simple, an entire mechanism is necessary to concentrate the matter in an appropriate solid form. In order to do this, the intestinal mechanism uses liquids with incredible precision. It is necessary for 86% of water to be reabsorbed by the intestines so that the feces have a normal consistency.

If 88% of water is reabsorbed, the feces become too hard, causing difficulties in elimination with a tendency to stick to the terminal part of the colon.

With accumulation, the feces harden and adhere to the walls of the colon. Many women have almost liquid and yellowish feces but pay no attention to it. Yet, this is already problematic, as it must have a regular consistency; otherwise, only a small quantity is eliminated and it slowly accumulates in the colon or in the final tract. During or after every meal, we should feel the need to go to the bathroom to evacuate fecal matter left from previous meals.

If we eat three meals a day it would be logical to go to the bathroom three times a day. But this only happens for some people and two bowel movements a day is acceptable, indicating good intestinal function. If we usually eat three meals a day and we only go to the bathroom every three days or every four days, imagine what remains. Obviously we will accumulate nine or more meals in the colon. (See illustration next page).

Various Aspects of Intestinal Health and a Badly Intoxicated Colon

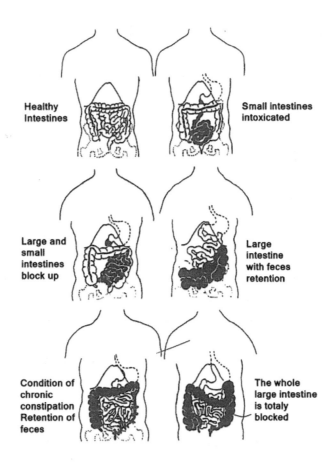

Healthy Intestines

Small intestines intoxicated

Large and small intestines block up

Large intestine with feces retention

Condition of chronic constipation Retention of feces

The whole large intestine is totaly blocked

Healthy and diseased states of the intestines

Therefore, it is understandable that after a few years, chronic constipation can cause an accumulation of dried feces layering the intestinal walls. Encrustations form which can reach several inches, progressively reducing the space in the intestine. This is the empty or hollow part.

According to Dr. Iron, a well-known American Naturopath famous for his works on the colon, we can accumulate up to seventeen pounds of feces in our intestines. We might think that this is an exaggeration or that it is only in extreme cases, yet in highly obese women who suffer from a multitude of organic disorders, it was possible to provoke expulsions of more than two pounds of feces and a large quantity of worms, utilizing a detox treatment taking my low-molecular antioxidant compound mixed with enzyme yeast cells and liquid chlorophyll three times a day. In other cases with the application of detox diet and colon irrigation, patients eliminated more than six pounds of feces.

The consequences of these accumulations not only affect the colon mucosa by creating micro lacunas, but in time they affect the entire organism. Fatigue, wrinkled face, deformed features, heavy legs, physical deformation, vertigo, migraines, and bad circulation are common factors. Diseases appear and we often ask ourselves why we are ill or why we feel sick and tired.

Most people, and I frequently see it in patients, do not pay attention to their intestinal condition. It is no surprise that they develop different symptoms, various pathologies leading to chronic or degenerative illnesses. Cholesterol can also be linked to constipation. When the intestinal transit becomes slower, it allows fat to stick to the intestinal walls and be absorbed into the blood stream.

More than fifteen years ago I had a patient who already at that time suffered from severe constipation. Today she has multiple physical symptoms and suffers from cognitive disorders. Recently she was diagnosed with the onset of Parkinson's. Aware of the problem, she admits that modern day living makes one forgetful of the hygiene rules for good living, disrupting a good diet, and not going often to the bathroom. Unfortunately, this is common, and apparently we are slaves of an unstable social life, wrong dietary style, and unhealthy industrial foods, which lead us to forget the most basic rules of health. We just build diseases with our teeth, since 40% of cancer cause is attributed to wrong dietary style, not to mention chronic and auto-immune disease including multiple sclerosis, with death as a consequence.

I am not exaggerating in saying that constipation may be a danger to our health and at the origin of organic disease, premature aging process and overall a variety of symptoms.

Currently two major afflictions may have an indirect link with constipation is colon cancer without doubt and breast cancer, although a personal theory for breast cancer not always accepted but lately formulated by Prof. Wolfgang Kosler, oncologist. I developed this theory after many years of clinical observation of irises, which I explain later in this book. Today, new lines of research are now focusing intestinal bacteria and pathogenic bacteria growing in the large colon as the cause of many diseases, but why not breast cancer!

In more primitive societies unspoiled by modern civilization and industrial foods, like the Hunzas for example, eating only natural, unprocessed foods, not only did intestinal problems and constipation not exist, but diseases as well, mainly cancer. Modern society, which is so proud of its technology, is mainly responsible for these problems and diseases we started to call "Diseases of Civilization," being itself the cause of these problems, creating even more gastrointestinal illnesses, including constipation. Sadly, we don't do much about them.

More recently I saw a program on TV about a region in China, a village where people live over 120 years without any disease. The government sent medical doctors to open an office for consultations, but they soon closed the office, because it had been without patients. As always, a medical science that denied the effect of natural food on health status sent a scientific team to analyze the "air" as the probable cause of longevity, but of course, not natural food.

Today, interest is slowly emerging in this problem relating to certain diseases of civilization. Some South African and English experts, for example, admit that constipation can cause certain disorders of the gallbladder, varicose veins, cardiovascular diseases, appendicitis, and hernia. These illnesses often require hospitalization, inflicting burdensome and unnecessary expenses on the governments. Yet another example typical of the appalling consequences of constipation, thyroid disorders, are increasingly more frequent, where we know that this gland regulates numerous functions of the organism. For example, it activates the production of hormones (T3) intended to regulate the cell's consumption of oxygen. An excess of toxins resulting from constipation diminishes the thyroid's functions. The cysts that often appear in the thyroid are the direct result of chronic and prolonged constipation.

In 1989 I carried out a specific study in my clinic in regard to the relationship between the different organic disorders common to women and stages of constipation with a group of 260 women, whose cases with elimination problems were analyzed:

50% suffered from nervous problems
52% suffered from insomnia
70% suffered from anxiety
36% had undergone surgery for gynecological problems: cysts, fibromas, etc.
50 cases of intestinal elimination 2 to 3 times a day were analyzed:
20% suffered from nervous problems
15% suffered from insomnia
10% suffered from anxiety

No Gynecological Problems Existed

A colon cleansing and detox diet expel a large quantity of fecal matter and toxins circulating in the blood, which accumulate in tissues that in turn decrease the production of free radicals triggered by these toxins, and therefore from oxidative stress. We also reduce the level of auto-intoxication, which simultaneously reduces the risk of other problems, symptoms such as pains, headache, nervousness, poor memory, and fatigue common in women today including the youngest ones suffering from chronic constipation.

A clean and healthy body depends mainly on our life style. Our health status is dependent on both healthy cells and mitochondria, which need the best nutritional food received from the quality of our blood. We cannot have healthy and clean blood with bad food, excess toxins from a bad colon, and poor liver and kidney function. Live Blood Analysis observation can prove this easily. This is a biological fact, a direct observation, and not some interpretation. This is what I have done for the past thirty-five years. A clean body depends mainly on how our body can detoxify the toxins from metabolic process. This is not only theory but rather the way our body is functioning. Our diet should provide all nutrients and be rich in vegetables and fruits, large quantities of fresh vegetable juice, and whole cereal fibers. A clean body depends mainly on the quality of blood, with the help of a diet rich in vegetables, fruits, whole cereals, and fibers revitalizing the intestinal flora, and wherever possible, some additional exercise. It cannot be any other way.

Laxative abuse is not a solution. On the contrary, this is why we are witnessing a constant increase in colon irritations and inflammations requiring treatments, which in extreme cases may lead to hospitalization. Indeed, laxatives are aggressive and irritate the intestinal mucosa in order to force elimination. However, feces are generally not totally eliminated and their consistency is also altered.

The abuse of laxatives ends up causing various problems such as irritation of the mucous membrane, a decrease in potassium, and an accumulation of feces in the sigmoid colon, since feces are only partially eliminated, and the colon gets used to laxatives. It can take an adult several months to regain a normal elimination rhythm with the help of correct dietary planning and the revitalization of the intestinal mucosa.

Consequences of constipation and Laxatives

```
Constipation
     │
  Laxative ──────── Suppressed natural ──────── Irritation of the
     │                 elimination                Intestinal Mucosa
     │                      │
 Dependency          Partial elimination      Acumulation of feces
     │                  of feces                 in the sigmoid
     │                                                │
Loss of liquids                               Autointoxication
 and sodium                                     Of the colon
     │                                                │
Reduction of potassium ── Muscular deficiency   Chronic and
                           And arrhythmia       Degenerative illness
```

It is almost impossible for elderly people to reverse poor colon functionality and regain a normal one, since over the years, colon tissue and muscle have become weaker and old, which is easily observed through iris diagnosis. However, I have obtained very good results with patients in their sixties through a diet of vegetables juice cocktails, probiotics, molasses, fibers, and supplementation from enzyme yeast cells rich in potassium, magnesium, and manganese, with the addition of nucleic acids to repair and strengthen the intestinal muscle. Some of my patients that I treated for over twenty and thirty years, at eighty to eighty-five years of age look healthier because they have a better diet and are concerned with their intestines.

Inconsistency in our modern society, lack of time, poor hygiene in certain bathrooms, being away all day from home, either in work offices or schools are certainly factors that prevent adults and adolescents from going to the bathroom when needed or more regularly.

I knew a case of a six-year-old girl who suffered from celiac illness. She had irregular intestines, as many children do. She only went to school in the morning, but to my surprise, she told me that the bathroom was dirty and that she held it in until she got home. By suppressing the natural function of elimination, the entire defecation mechanism is contracted and the colon begins to delay feces elimination, and as a result, the intestines will never be normal.

We worry about many diseases of which some are very serious and come with consequences. For instance, we are concerned with diabetes, especially juvenile diabetes, which is very prevalent, but what about chronic constipation that seems to have become a major problem that should be solved?

While we are asking this, we are going to see, from an embryonic standpoint, that the pancreas is part of the colon. There is a direct relationship between them, same as to the liver. In fact, since the pancreas is part of the colon, in many cases a bad pancreas is linked to bad colon tissue, so there is a direct relationship between the two, in fact the same as with the liver.

50

Combating Constipation

- Drink a lot of water and liquids (2 liters a day) including vegetable juices.
- Eliminate the toxins in the colon.
- Acidify the intestinal flora.

- Promote a good intestinal flora.
- Consume fibers.
- Practice some physical exercise: walking, swimming or cycling.
- Prevent and combat stress.

Breast Cancer and Colon Health

Over the past years breast cancer has become the #1 killer in women involving surgery, chemotherapy, very aggressive radiation, and depression, yet cancer often relapses with subsequent bone, lung, and liver metastases, which is still too high with about 70% disease recurrence within the first three years. This is why prevention is important by any means. Based upon my experience, Iridology is one of the best diagnostic tools that can determine breast cancer risk.

My interest in breast cancer began more than thirty-five years ago when I was diagnosing the irises of breast cancer patients and observed some links with the colon. Today, more than ever I believe there is an association between breast cancer and constipation as well as with the nervous system. We still do not know everything there is to know about cancer.

While we will not go into an in-depth discussion to scientifically describe cancer growth, but instead we can underscore that dietary lifestyle seems to have an implication in breast cancer development, especially when diet involves an intake of red meat in excess, hormones, sugar, pesticides from industrial farming (and nutritional deficiencies). It may modify genetic expression but also result in bad bowel function and constipation. The U.S. is a big consumer of animal hormones used to induce a baby cow to grow faster, but places the health of the consumer at a disadvantage.

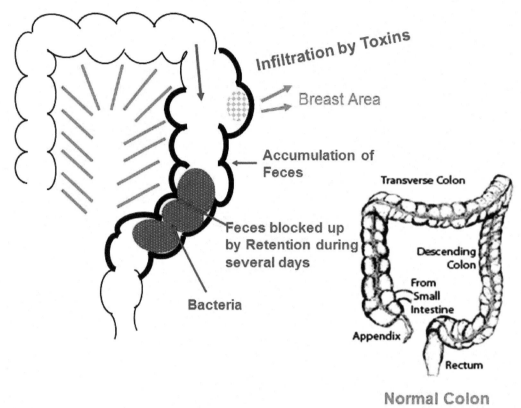

Bad and Toxic Colon in Breast Cancer (According to Iridology)

Serge Jurasunas 2012

Bad and Toxic Colon in Breast Cancer

Most breast cancer patients suffer from constipation. When we observe the left iris, the descending colon always looks darker than other parts of the colon, which indicates the retention of toxins and feces. The collarette appears to be also involved, look irregular, irritated, often pushing into the mammary area.

An irritated collarette coming from the colon and pointing to the mammary area indicate that the irritated nerve vessels send some abnormal vibration to the breast tissue. This is a reflex condition from the nerves to any of the body's organs, especially the ramification with the intestinal nerves that spread all over the body.

At the same time we can observe some iris signs such as inflammation, dark crypts, and genetic signs as transversals from 3:00 to 4:00 in the left iris and from 8:00 to 9:00 in the right iris, which may indicate some tumor risk. However, I would be cautious, before making any statement, to corroborate this with further testing.

An excess of red meat intake that we discuss further on in the book is a source of hormones, bad fat, and promote activation of cyclooxygenase 2. Cox2 is an enzyme that promotes inflammation, activated by excess free radicals such as peroxinitrite and hydroxyl radicals and also catalase. The conversion of arachidonic acid to prostaglandin 2, a molecule of fat which, when activated, works as a potent immune suppressor and induces the activation of the enzymes metalloproteinase MMP2 and MMP9 that tumors need for the degradation of the ECM and to further extend. Modern studies show that Cox2 expression is subsequently increased by 40% to 60% in breast

52

cancer leading to a down-regulation of apoptosis, inducing pro-angiogenic factors, and further impairing cellular immune defense. In turn, prostaglandin 2 (PGE2) stimulates aromatase transcription leading to increasing levels of estrogens.

We can thus imagine how an excess of red meat consumption contributes to increased breast cancer from several directions. This can lead to a series of cascading events. A plate of steak contains about ten carcinogenic pollutants and contains saturated fat and toxins where pollutants are already absorbed. I also have observed in many cases of breast cancer, oxidized lipids circulating in blood through the special Bradford microscope designed for Live Blood Analysis observation which supports the theory of high fat intake in the diet decreasing antioxidant levels in blood plasma, resulting from low vegetable and fruit intake and chronic constipation.

Auto-intoxication of the colon gives rise to the formation of intestinal carcinogenic bacteria that penetrates into the blood circulation, which may further disturb cell division, cell differentiation, along with decreasing apoptosis, leading to cause cancer. As previously mentioned in this book, Dr. J. Seignalet's theory also points out the role of both intracellular and extracellular intoxication from food macromolecules or bacteria coming from the colon. According to Dr. Seignalet, these macromolecules can penetrate the cells and block up certain mechanisms such as tyrosine kinase, associated with the membrane receptor, as well as some signal transduction pathways such RAS and other enzymatic cascades.

By using Live blood analysis with careful observation, I was able to observe intestinal bacteria circulating in the blood of cancer patients including cases of disease recurrence. According to Eric Enby, a Swedish doctor who wrote a book called *The Hidden Killers*, even some bacteria circulating in the blood can infect healthy body cells and contribute to uncontrolled division and malignant growth.

Recently I had participated at The 2012 Congress of Complementary Oncology in Munich, Germany. To my surprise, I heard Professor Wolfgang Kostler (President of the Austrian Society of Oncology), mention during his lecture that most breast cancer patients suffer from constipation. Incredible! My own theory, built thirty-five years ago, was no longer a nonsense factor but accredited by a progressive oncologist. What steps had taken place in the interim? One interesting factor to remember, that in fact motivated me to link a toxic colon with breast cancer, was because up to 90% of breast cancers occurred in the left breast. Tell me why?

Anatomically the descending colon is situated near the left breast. We can understand how vascularization permits a quick intoxication of the breast milieu by toxic waste and pathogenic bacteria. Compared to normal daily bowel movements, some breast cancer patients only have a bowel movement every three to six days, which strongly indicates auto-intoxication of the colon, which in turn irritates the nervous system (including the emotional brain). Furthermore, this nervous system ramification extends to our immune organs responsible for body defense against toxins and intruders, such as our thymus, Peyer's plates, amygdales, spleen, and lymphatic ganglions. This observation from an iris check-up permits us first to observe what I call a "breast cancer profile" and to underline the association of the nervous system with the various immune organs such as the spleen, thymus, Peyer's plates, and lymphatic ganglions, linked with breast cancer disease. This is why we cannot neglect the emotional factor that involves breast cancer and offer some psychological support.

I am working constantly with breast cancer patients, often after disease recurrence, which has really shown a peculiarity of being a very emotional disease which involves brain neurotransmitter imbalance, but often involving also the colon itself, our second brain. Emotional behavior and anxiety are associated with decreasing immune activity which may favor metastases invasion, since cancer cells can escape from inactivated immune cells. In fact, I have developed a breast cancer profile chart base on many years of iris observation and breast cancer detection, and I believe it is most helpful since we may underline the whole story of the disease and not only diagnose a local tumor. We may be surprised about how many factors may be involved with the disease.

Of course there is an apparent relationship with colon intoxication, excess dietary fat intake, and lymphopathy. The term "lymphopathy" means that oxidized lipids are blocking the lymphatic circulation. Having been blocked by oxidized lipids and even large macromolecules, as well explained by Dr. Majid Ali and the late famous French researcher Dr. Salmanoff, this also impairs detoxification of excess of hormones accumulated in mammary tissue and also impairs the circulation of immune cells to the breast tissue. As a result, lymph vessels are unable to detoxify breast tissue as a result of excess hormones contained in industrial foods, chemical additives, xenoestrogens from plastics, and pollution.

The study in the States of 1,481 non-nursing women revealed that chronic constipation was linked to abnormal cells found in breast fluids. My own research contribution includes irises diagnoses coupled with the Live Blood Analysis from breast cancer patients. Careful observation made at different time intervals such as 20, 30, 40 and 60 minutes revealed the presence of numerous pathogenic microorganisms, which grew and invaded the blood smear. The LBA observations may also show in patients with breast cancer oxidized lipid plates, conglomerates, damaged red cell membranes, platelet aggregation, and toxic blood plasma. This further shows an oxygen deficiency in the blood circulation leading to a condition of hypoxia in the connective tissue, which contributes to an accelerated process of tumor growth from active angiogenesis and down-regulation of apoptosis. Nobody knows about these early events, about which there are several hypotheses.

I personally have spent several decades studying and observing the correlation between dietary style, constipation, and breast cancer, concluding there is a strong link between the three. I also observed that 80% of cancer occurs in the left breast and why! If we observe the large sigmoid colon, we see that it appears very dark with retention of fecal matter opposite to the area of the breast in the iris. This is really the link between breast cancer and constipation from toxins, pathogenic bacteria, and even oxidized fat penetrating into the blood and lymphatic circulation to the mammary tissue.

We have also to consider emotional behavior associated with intestinal disorders. For about seven years I have been involved with the molecular markers related to cancer, such as the P53 tumor suppressor, known as our guardian against cancer. P53 mutation is the most commonly mutated gene and associated in more than 50% of all cancers, including breast cancer (See:www.sergejurasunas.com - Breast cancer diagnostic and prevention through the P53 tumor suppressor gene). P53 mutation is often caused by insecticides, pollution, viruses, and bacteria. This mutation also involves auto-intoxication of the colon, overstimulation of the immune system, and sometimes a severe nervous depression, which in turn depresses the neurotransmitters as well as the immune system, thus increasing the risk of infection. Again we need to further implicate lifestyle eating habits, nutritional deficiencies, and an excess of red meat in the diet.

Let us look at the difference of breast cancer risk and cancer incidence in countries like the USA, where each American eats about 125Kg of meat per year. This is incredible when compared to the French who eat only 37Kg per year and to countries like Sri Lanka or Japan which eat much less meat, especially with Sri Lanka having a much lower risk and incidence of cancer.

Breast cancer by itself probably needs a whole book, but I felt that I should explain some facts which relate to the subject matter of this book. However you can get more information on the Internet looking for my article, "An Integrative and Naturopathic Approach to Breast Cancer" including several other articles, or in the *International Journal of Iridology*, issue 8, volume 3, #2 or on my website, www.sergejurasunas.com.

An important recommendation for women with breast cancer risk who already know they have irregularity and a sluggish colon should be to improve their colon function, first with detox, and then with better dietary food intake and nutrition, which I suggest in this book. This helps fight constipation. Performing regular hospital check-ups does not protect anyone from cancer, because when it starts to develop and grow, nobody knows about detecting this early on. Therefore, the best way is to be proactive and take preventative measures so as not to give your body any opportunity to develop cancer by improving your bowel function, changing your diet by reducing fat intake, reducing white sugar, and fighting inner pollution.

Among the many examples I could present is a woman who recently came to my clinic after seven years of absence. In fact, she came only once before and was not convinced when I told her, after looking at her irises, that she had a high risk of breast cancer, particularly on her left breast because of specific iris marks associated with her chronic constipation and other visible factors. Now she came back with a developed breast cancer, which already had spread into the lymph nodes along with a swollen arm, which is not a good prognosis.

We can only regret her first response and failure to take proactive steps. Unfortunately, many people are not prepared to hear this prognosis and prevention is not important to them. In fact, on my Internet site, I have some interesting articles about breast cancer prevention that link with Iridology and the molecular markers test. Curiously my documents on how to treat cancer are downloaded and read by thousands of people. When it came to prevention there were only few hundred readers, but with time I believe that prevention of breast cancer will increase in interest, especially among women. Breast cancer recurrence is still too high, as much as 70% within the first three years, no matter the surgery and treatment. This requires the patient to better understand about a food-diet prevention, to detox, to activate the colon function, and to utilize the molecular markers test. According to my experience, this is the only way to anticipate disease recurrence.

Preventive Testing

One of the barriers to real prevention is the common mistake that people make who still believe that hospital check-ups are sufficient by themselves to prevent a disease recurrence, which is wrong, since there is no medical diagnosis available to prevent primary cancer development or its recurrence but only to diagnose an already-active tumor. At best we ought not to depend on early cancer diagnosis but to prevent it before it is declared. This is what we actually do with the help of Iridology. I have spent considerable time over the last twenty-five years to profile breast cancer risk during iris observation, having been lucky to observe thousands of breast cancer cases. However, Iridology could not predict and prevent from disease recurrence, which to me was an obstacle. About ten years ago, I decided to start the study and investigation of molecular markers and started to include in my diagnostic and preventive level of the P53 tumor suppressor test alone with other innovative diagnostics.

Today I am now using the P53 tumor suppressor gene test along with other molecular markers to show the correlation between the two, either a risk of cancer or an already-existing tumor activity.

This is already a very important victory, being able to anticipate a cancer mechanism, detect tumors earlier, and prevent disease recurrence.

For more information read,
1. **"Breast Cancer, Prevention, Detection, Targeting Molecular Markers"** at www.sergejurasunas.com
2. **"A Naturopathic Approach to Breast Cancer," by Prof Serge Jurasunas. Townsend letter June 2003 (available online)**

Flatulence and Spasmodic Colon

One of the most common problems of intestinal disorders is flatulence accompanied by a dilated abdomen. Colon dilatation affects one area, generally the descending colon, which may literally swell up like a balloon.

The causes of flatulence are many, arising from an excessive accumulation of intestinal gas, and lack of intestinal tonus, which favors colon dilation. It has been often stated that an accumulation of intestinal gas is insignificant or that it has no consequences for the colon.

But I have to emphatically differ. In the first place, an excess of intestinal gas is already a sign of digestive disorder, which can trigger a variety of symptoms. Accumulation of gas over a period of years may have consequences not only on the colon but our welfare. For example, people who complain of bad breath could have intestinal problems. I remember a case of a woman, more or less forty years old, who constantly suffered from very bad breath. She went to see the dentist who, after careful analysis of the mouth, could not find anything that could cause this. Obviously he could not solve this case as the woman suffered from severe constipation, accompanied by hemorrhoids and intestinal gas.

The gasses infiltrate through the blood stream, circulate up to the lungs where they are expelled through the respiratory tract. This is the explanation for the bad breath.

The bloating and size of the colon, often seen in middle aged men and women, are the result of retention of gasses, which cause strong pressure and could also cause severe intestinal pain.

Putrefactions are generally the cause of these symptoms and of accumulated gasses. These are reabsorbed as toxins by the blood stream and are often responsible for migraines, headaches, vertigo, and even nervous disorders.

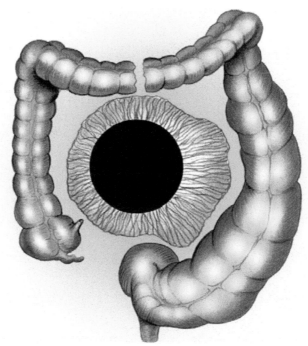

Swollen and Hypotonic Descending Colon with Respective Iridology Observation

The main problem is to correct for the wrong diet and heavy food for the digestion, which is responsible for gas formation in one person, while the same wrong diet doesn't cause those problems for another person. Sometimes a pancreatic deficiency decreases the production of digestive enzymes followed by poor degradation, digestion, and in turn, you have gas formation in the colon.

In our modern society, and here in Portugal, most people at lunch time eat in restaurants, including shopping centers not really serving fresh food, have a plate of meat with French fries, white rice, gravy, bread, other greasy food, spaghetti, pizza etc..., which are really heavy foods and especially with no vegetables in the plate. Of course, some people are trying better food like Japanese style, but only a small percentage. Not everyone has the same digestive capacity, or the same hereditary profile, which is another interesting topic for further research. Sooner or later one suffers from the consequences of eating such foods for several years. These heavy foods, over the years, dilate the colon causing a ballooned colon, a prolapse, diverticulosis, or other problems. Unfortunately medicine neglects totally or ignores this problem that is at the root of many symptoms and diseases in our society.

Eating food is one thing while digestion is another thing, because badly digested food and proteins, for instance, become food for intestinal bacteria such as Escherichia Coli, being responsible for putrefaction and are breeding grounds for a greater number of bacteria. Now, since a great number of these toxic bacteria are undesirable in the colon, it is necessary to destroy them or keep them at bay by increasing the level of friendly bacteria in the intestine with a good source of probiotic supplementation.

We also have to keep an acid/alkaline balance in the colon and have a clean colon in order to keep down toxic bacteria as much as possible. We are still tied up with the theory of calories, which was for decades the only preoccupation of medical doctors. In measuring calories, any food can serve, not just the quality of the food; whether sausage, spaghetti, or pizza, but quality and nutritional value also make an important nutritional difference.

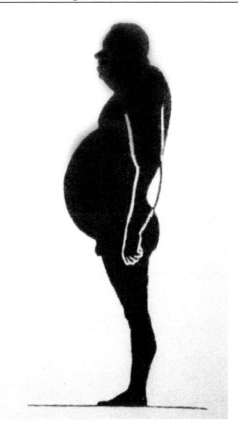

Spinal Deformation caused by an Intoxicated Colon and Abdominal Swelling

In an intoxicated environment with intestinal putrefaction, the friendly bacteria of the microbiome are not active and are often destroyed.

The distention of gases produced essentially by middle-aged people is mostly associated with poorly digested food and a lack of digestive enzymes. Probably this is linked with bad dietary lifestyle over the years that overtax digestive enzymes. It is true that with age, the production of digestive enzymes in saliva, stomach, and pancreas decrease. The young can eat any heavy food and not feel inconvenienced because they have a good digestive enzymatic system. However, up to a certain age, if we continue to abuse foods such as pork, meat, pasta, white bread, gravy, and fried foods, these dietary excesses can eventually catch up with us.

We overtax the enzymatic system because we force the organism to constantly produce digestive enzymes. We just abuse our genetic mechanism that slows down the production of enzymes. Under these conditions, ingested food passes rapidly through the small intestine towards the large intestine, but the food is only partially digested which causes intestinal putrefaction and flatulence. I remember a middle age couple coming from Africa for consultation. Both had large, dilated abdomens, especially the husband, but the wife weighed 98 Kg (216 lbs.), a lot weight for a person 1.58m (5 ft. 2″) high. Both were big eaters without restriction but seemed not to understand the relationship between their physical symptoms and what they ate being related to the condition of their colon. Their eating habits included of a lot of meat, white rice, yellow potatoes, very little vegetables, and some fruits. The woman drank about 1 liter of Coca-Cola per day, and they also frequently traveled by plane eating even more junk food.

When food is cooked with water at a high temperature, this destroys not only a quantity of certain vitamins but also the enzymes. Some people are more susceptible to bad digestion and gas formation than others. Certain vegetables such as onion, cauliflower, cabbage, and sometimes broccoli when cooked, produce gas because they contain sulfur. In this case, when consumed raw or even steamed, this does not occur or only produces only small quantity of intestinal gas.

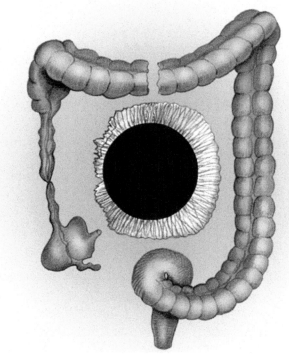

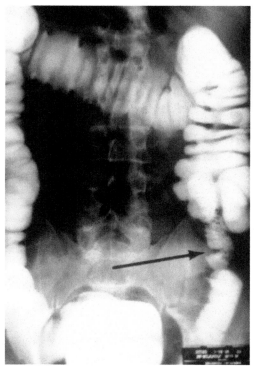

Spasms of the Ascending Colon with Respective Iridology Observation

Intestinal Spasms in the Descending Colon

Intestinal Spasms in the Ascending and Descending Colon with the Related Observation in Iridology

Spasms are the opposite of abdominal bloating. They are caused by hyperactivity of the tiny nerve that controls the muscle of the colon walls. It is evident that hereditary build as well as a bad diet are also determining factors. Being related to the condition of the colon, intestinal spasms often occur in the descending colon, in the ascending colon, and sometimes in the transverse colon. As constipation is always the root cause, and feces are blocked in the descending colon, we can understand why spasms manifest above all within this space.

Often the colon feels ballooned from excessive feces retention and accumulation of gases. The muscles of the descending colon are extremely stressed; they become irritated, tense, and end up causing spasms. The accumulation of feces in these weakened walls combined with a state of permanent stress causes strong pressure on the colon walls. In observing the iris of patients I always find an association between nervous conditions, stress, and colon spasms. And these abnormal conditions of the colon negatively influence the nervous impulses that go from the colon to the brain. Therefore, periods of anxiety are repeated and complicated. The hectic rhythm of modern life including that of young students increases the percentage of intestinal problems such as colitis spasms and flatulence.

I remember the case of a forty-six-year-old woman who suffered from anxiety, nerve depression, insomnia, and muscular pains. She had a bowel movement every five to six days and felt ballooned from accumulating gases. She even said to me, "Sometimes I look like a pregnant woman." A change in the dietary program adapted to each case, just as a certain disciplined practice of Yoga and relaxation may be able to decrease nervous tension and stress and could even combat disorders of this kind.

Early on, as I began my career in Canada, I was presented with a complicated case of ulcerous colitis with diarrhea in a fifty-year-old man. He had consulted over twenty-four physicians with the result of "incurable" and wanted to kill himself. He already tried all the medical drugs, which seemed ineffective in resolving his problem or stopping the frequent diarrhea. Even after forty years, similar situations still arise and baffling cases of diarrhea are frequent.

At that time a natural food, therapeutic diet with functional food was practically unknown. Canadians were used to eating heavy foods and they were not educated at all on good diet and colon function. No one had suggested to this man to change his diet consisting mostly of pork meat, beans, white rice, white bread, etc. This was the popular food habit in Quebec (French Canada), at that time.

Still quite inexperienced at the time, yet with some experience from Dr. Bernard Jensen at Hidden Valley Health Center, I also put my trust in the wise words of Hippocrates, "Let food be your medicine," which I had also observed with patients at Hidden Valley Health Center. After consulting a few books, including Dr. Bernard Jensen's, I created a personalized special food diet for this patient. The poor man was willing to do anything to not end up with this chronic daily diarrhea that was certain to kill him.

The basis of this diet was made from a mixture of several vegetables, first steamed then mashed in puree, to which we added one egg yolk, 100g of white fish, one tablespoon of pollen, and mixed together.
This "vegetarian puree," as I call it, is still included with much success today in my practice.

The man was directed to eat this vegetable puree twice a day and nothing else. After eight days on this special diet, his diarrhea became intermittent, and later, his intestines slowly returned to their normal function. It was, in brief, my first victory in a case of intestinal illness using food as a means of healing.

Generally, there are two categories of diarrhea, although there is a need to emphasize that currently constipation is predominant both in adults and adolescents.

1st - Acute diarrhea with an unpleasant appearance, often linked to a viral or bacterial infection. Note that acute diarrhea is common in babies. In France, more than 50,000 hospitalizations are reported a year, in some cases fatal.

2nd - Chronic diarrhea like colitis or caused by parasites. Chronic diarrhea also has its origin in the inflammation of the digestive canal caused by allergies originated by certain foods.

Acute diarrhea can be caused by bad quality food, or by deteriorated food served in restaurants, or by food from take-out fast-food establishments, or from supermarkets selling low-priced foods. More recently we have had instances in France of children becoming ill and having diarrhea from eating hamburgers bought in supermarkets at very cheap prices, which is not always the best for our health. A few years ago, McDonalds Europe destroyed 1 million hamburgers containing harmful bacteria after children had been intoxicated from eating these poisoned hamburgers.

Diarrhea can become very serious as long as there is proliferation of Candida during an infection or colon irritation, or in the case of severe pathologies such as Crohn's disease and ulcerous colitis. The absorption of toxic metals which accumulate can, in time, cause a significant intestinal discharge. It is a means the organism needs to detoxify itself from undesirable substances.

I had the case of a forty-year-old lady who, for fifteen days prior to her visit, went to the bathroom at least six times a day. This woman was debilitated, nervous, and irritable. She was completely infected by candidiasis with vaginal and mouth infections.

The role of Candida is underestimated in many cases, above all in digestive disorders. Candida, after taking the form of mycelium, grips onto cells of the mucosa of the small intestine. The consequences can result in primary inflammation and an increase of permeability of the intestinal barrier.

Going back to the aforementioned case, the woman lived under permanent stress, constantly taking antibiotics, antidepressants, and a contraceptive pill, which stimulates the growth of Candida. In brief, a classic case in our era that fills up today's hospitals. Nothing seemed to alleviate this patient, but rather every change of medication seemed to worsen her situation. Often drugs from medical prescriptions can have toxic effects on already-inflamed intestinal mucosa. Chronic diarrhea is dangerous, among severe consequences, causing a loss of electrolytes and weakening the patient even more. Approximately after twenty-five days of treatment, with a specific diet and restoration of the nervous system, the diarrhea began to diminish and space itself out. After two months she no longer had diarrhea.

Diarrhea in babies and children can often be the result of consuming of cow's milk, which is responsible for allergies and inflammation of the gastrointestinal mucosa. According to studies published by English scientists, cow's milk is largely responsible for Crohn's disease, which is often accompanied by violent diarrhea, but not always. The molecules of cow's milk are transformed and digested with difficulty by the human organism, and even more so for babies. This can be even more serious if they are born with intestinal deficiencies, since the human digestive tract is not programmed to metabolize the larger protein molecules from cow's milk.

In cases of severe and prolonged diarrhea, it is absolutely necessary to determine its causes and test for parasites, Candida, salmonella, or other bacteria. If blood is observed in liquid feces, a specialist must be consulted immediately. Sometimes, this is a warning sign of a tumor that may have been forming for years without any manifestation. It is known and I repeat often, in cases of a tumor in the colon, pain is often nonexistent and can lead to serious errors. In conclusion, diarrhea, no matter from what source, is a defense and detoxification factor or a process of inflammation requiring precise identification and adequate therapeutic intervention.

At the same time, diarrhea underlines an incompatibility between ingested food and the quality and state of the digestive tract, including the nervous system, which often influences the intestinal discharge.

Colon Irritation and Diverticulitis

Irritated Bowel Syndrome is one of the new manifestations of the abnormal and degenerative conditions of the intestine. It has various causes and can provoke various symptoms. The main symptoms are as listed:

- Gas and flatulence
- Bloated abdomen
- Diarrhea
- Pain

A diet badly adapted to the intestinal mucosa, combined with hereditary factors and nervous disorder, are probably the main factors linked with the irritated colon syndrome.

The next figures on page 64 and 65 illustrate the mechanism of free radicals combined with the intestinal inflammation and the decreasing induction of the antioxidant enzyme superoxide dismutase (Cu-Zn S.O.D.) in the intestinal tissue.

> *A study of Crohn's disease showed that a dietary detoxification gives the patient an 80% improvement.*
>
> *—Dr. J. Hunter, Addenbrooke Hospital, USA*

Besides allergic substances, cow's milk contains a substance called nitric oxide, which human and animal organisms use for certain functions (relaxing muscles of the blood vessels and reducing blood pressure). However, in the presence of iron or free radicals, nitric oxide may form extremely toxic free radicals known as peroxinitrite, which may cause severe damage, inflammation of the intestinal mucosa, and irritated colon syndrome, just to mention some examples, about which most people know very little.

Modern society, influenced by TV advertising and medical advice, consumes too much dairy food, especially milk, forgetting that pasteurized milk is no longer natural milk and not well tolerated and absorbed by the body. Cow's milk causes alkaline feces, while mother's milk causes acidic feces. Raw milk after a few days at room temperature turns into cheese, while pasteurized milk turns rancid. Therefore, it is not a healthy food and causes allergies, inflammation of the intestine, catarrh, respiratory disorders, and even auto-immune diseases. Recently, several books published on milk authored by medical doctors made strong accusations against the value of milk.

This is when such problems such as intestinal disorders, constipation, diarrhea, or infections arise. Modern women also bear quite a few babies that are not given breast milk but start immediately with formula, canned, or powdered milk. Their babies are not given any chance to build up their intestinal flora from the mother's milk, and therefore become subject to symptoms or diseases.

I remember the case of a six-year-old girl suffering from diarrhea since eighteen months of age, which started to worsen, becoming acute diarrhea with up to ten to fifteen bowel evacuations per day. Not even large doses of antibiotics could relieve the diarrhea. The child was getting worse every day. I then prescribed a special food diet, one from my own formula in vial made from trace elements, silver, copper, magnesium and potassium, extract of red beets, herbs, organic germanium, and ginseng. After one week, the diarrhea began to decrease, and after one month, she was completely relieved from this diarrhea. I saw the child during the coming months over the next year. Twenty years later, she came to visit me as young woman for some minor health problems, but she never suffered any further from diarrhea as a result of following my dietary food advice over the ensuing years (see her case page 311).

Stress and its Devastating Effects

A diet which is badly adapted to the intestinal mucosa, hereditary factors, and variations and alterations of the nervous system, are other factors linked to the irritated colon syndrome.

Stress and Antioxidant Experiments

"Various groups of researchers have recently associated the causes of intestinal inflammation to oxidative stress and the decreasing activity of antioxidant defenses in the intestinal mucosa."

Antioxidants Prevent an Excess of Free Radicals

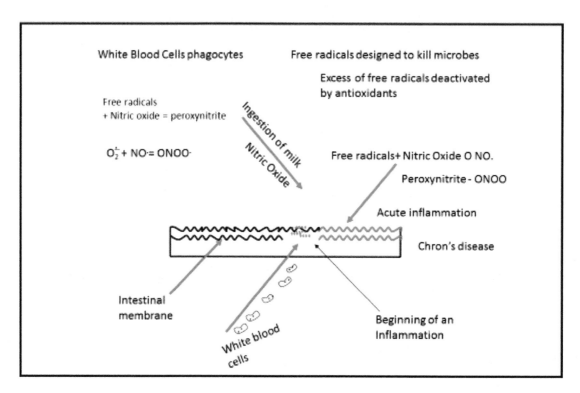

Biopsies of the intestinal mucosa of patients suffering from chronic intestinal inflammation were studied at the free radical and antioxidant level, both being indicators of oxidative stress.

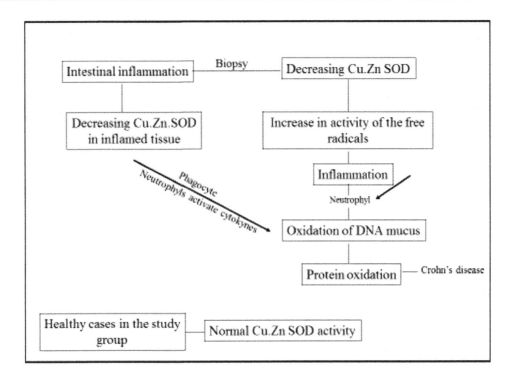

When comparing test results of the study group with those of healthy individuals, a slight increase in the level of free radicals and protein oxidation was noticed in the samples of the patient's mucosa.

These same characteristics can be observed in all inflammatory pathologies of the colon and especially in ulcerous colitis. In these cases, besides the increase of free radicals, iron was found in the inflamed tissues, which consequently increases their production further.

The Metabolic Blood Test (MBT)

For many years I have been involved with the science of oxidative stress and antioxidants. I spent over ten years researching the antioxidant enzyme, Superoxide Dismutase Enzyme (SOD), our most important antioxidant defense, which I discuss in this book. I also wrote a separate book on this subject.

(Visit www.sergejurasunas.com or search Google: Serge Jurasunas (S.O.D.)

In order to monitor the imbalance that exists between antioxidants and stressful substances, meaning a situation we call oxidative stress, we use in our clinic two main blood tests, which are the Metabolic Blood Test (MBT, also known in the USA as the Oxidative Stress Test or Oxidative Dried Blood Test), and the Live Blood Microscopy Analysis (LBA) to monitor oxidative stress and nutritional deficiency.

We developed the MBT technique that examines the blood coagulation taken from a small amount of blood expressed from a fingertip, transferred to a clean microscope slide, and allowed to air-dry for few minutes. The resulting fibrin web structure is then examined microscopically using a multiphase contrast microscope with high-definition amplification to monitor morphological changes or any alteration of the fibrin nets in the blood smear.

The MBT basically monitors oxidative stress status, both physical and emotional, plus offers valuable information on a number of topics such as allergies, vitamin C deficiency, bowel intoxication, stages of inflammation and disease progression, overall organic dysfunction, metal toxicity, and hormonal imbalances. These results need careful interpretation.

The Live Blood Analysis is quite different from hospital blood observation, since it uses fresh blood, without stains or colorants. This is our main methodology for demonstrating, as well as documenting, the condition of oxidative stress in the blood. We may also at this point explain that the LBA test is also an important tool to monitor the effect of wrong dietary style, excess bad fats, as well as an intoxicated colon in regard to blood health status.

Actually, it offers a direct view of whole blood, including the red blood cell status, where you can view their shape according to oxidative stress conditions and pollution, and also observe blood viscosity, micro clots, and micro-plaques. LBA may warn you about potential risks of brain stroke, phlebitis, and thrombosis. It also shows how the blood is intoxicated as a result of poor liver and kidney detox which includes chronic constipation.

Valuable information gained from monitoring a fresh drop of blood:

Abnormal shaped red blood cells (from oxidation)
Lipid plaques
Lipid ribbons
Platelet aggregation
Red blood cells in rouleaux or aggregation

LBA observation provides information on nutrient deficiencies plus many more types of information. Both of these tests offer over valuable information on over thirty-six conditions in a matter of 30-40 minutes, which would take several days or more in a hospital. Once again, LBA and MBT observation need careful interpretation and a good level of clinical experience; however, they should not be considered a substitute for medical check-ups.

How Morphological Changes Appear in the Peripheral Clotted Blood Sample

One of the causes of these morphological changes is attributed to an excessive free radical activity damaging cell membranes, oxidized fat forming peroxidation, or pathologies affecting the individual. During the process of degenerative disease and high oxidation, the blood carries fragments from the degradation of the extracellular matrix (ECM), releasing fragments into the blood. Heavy metals, polymerized proteins, and bacterial or fungal invasion may deteriorate blood components, modify the fibrin nets which in turn make a deviation from a natural blood pattern, observed after the blood coagulates to an abnormal one visible in the blood layers drops.

How to Evaluate the MBT

Breaks in the fibrin web, or the absence of a web are important factors to note when evaluating the results of this test. Under free radical activity and toxic families such as hydrogen peroxidase or hydroxyl radicals, white clots are mostly observed and referred to as Polymerized Protein Puddles (PPPs), being the result of cellular disorganization from metabolic disturbance factors and stressors. These are not clear holes but rather contain a white material that is the result of an excess of free radical activity. Each white footprint represents an inflammatory process ranging from an acute to a degenerative condition. It is now well established that PPPs seen in the layers of hard-clotted blood indicate oxidative stress conditions ranging from acute to chronic stages.

These results, within the presence of the dried blood drops, show the number and position of white blood clots. These appear in different sizes, shapes, and color, indicating the stage of inflammation and/or the disease. Sizes may vary from the smallest round PPPs of 2 microns, an indication of allergy sensitivity, to a larger size of 30 microns, an indication of physical stress, psychological and associated stress, or other trauma. However, depending how these appear, the large 30-micron PPPs could be seen as a cancer condition. The next layer size of 40 to 50 microns, being more visible in the case of advanced cancer or other degenerative process, indicates an advanced stage as well. For instance, breast cancer at first diagnostic has shown four times more free radical activity than an earlier detected stage II cancer. This can be observed with the MBT showing large PPPs of 30 to 40 microns. Each of the PPPs requires a careful interpretation. After many years of practice, seminars, exchanges of information, and collaboration with other colleagues, we have divided the pathological conditions as shown in the dried blood layers into a series of general categories.

The Metabolic Blood Test can monitor:

- Chronic vs. acute conditions
- Inflammation
- Physical stress or localized trauma
- Psychological stress
- Hormonal disturbance
- Degenerative disease indications
- Toxicity from polluted environment
- Allergy

While the MBT is not a substitution for regular hospital check-ups to diagnose pathologies, the fact is that in a few minutes you will know so much more about your patient's condition. More important, reversing the process from broken fibrin nets and the presence of PPPs of several shapes, sizes, and their dissemination to a normal blood pattern, is a real challenge but advantageous since it shows, step by step, the result of the applied treatment and a return to a better health status. MBT provides an excellent tool to monitor patient improvement and progress.

Description and Origin of the Test

The idea of examining a drop of dried blood to diagnose a disease is not new. It was backed in Europe as early as 1920 by several medical practitioners from Germany and France, who were able to implement a similar method of blood observation. After WWII, a German doctor established in Paris made hospital observations from the blood of cancer patients and wounded persons, and then discovered that their blood was morphologically different from a healthy person. Unfortunately, Dr. Heitan died without writing any explanation except for only few notes.

While in Paris, just after my return from the USA and Canada, I collaborated with the French School of Naturopathy. We then organized a congress where I met Dr. Lagarde, who knew Heitan, and became acquainted with the test he called the H.L. Test. However, he limited himself to observing cancer patients, but did not offer any precise explanation about his findings. He used a regular biologist's microscope, quite limited compared to what we use today. One year later I moved to Portugal, had been busy settling myself, and for the moment forgot about this blood test. Two years later I travelled to Germany and someone told me about a curious blood test called the "Aura-Blood Test" or "Aurascopy" discovered by Dr. Karlheinz Blank and his wife, Mrs. Hannelore Aurus-Blank. This particular test was from a drop of dried blood as well, but technically much different, not easily accessible, and to register for the course, the fee was quite expensive. One would have to sign a document with the statement that you will not personally teach the test anyone. The real problem was the German language usage for this course. However, I managed to collect some illustrated documents along with some limited explanation.

One of the main approaches of the Aura-Test was to diagnose between cancer and non-cancer, while in addition, some organs of the body could be observed in this blood test. Later on I bought a small microscope to start observing dried drops of blood according to Heitan's discovery and tried different approaches and manipulation to see if I could observe something unique. At that moment, I could not explain the results very well, but only from the standpoint of metabolic disturbance, toxins, and necrotic tissue circulating in the blood from the tumor itself. In the meantime, Dr. Robert Bradford from American Biologics (California) was interested in this test and travelled to Paris and met Dr. Lagarde during a congress and subsequently imported the test into the USA. Later on (1979) I flew to San Francisco and stayed few days with Bob, who was really working to find some further explanation for this blood test. With the help of some biologists, he was in position to offer a hypothesis concerning the blood pattern modification associated with oxidative stress, which is the reason it is known today as the Oxidative Dried Blood Test.

However being engaged in my own research and clinical practice I decided to call it the Metabolic Blood Test (MBT), since it not only monitored oxidative stress but metabolic dysfunction as well, which made more sense. A couple of years later I was thinking again about the theory of the "Aura-Test" and became further intrigued by some observations made from the layers of the dried blood in the drop. One day the insight came to my mind, that just like in the irises, certain organs of the body could be also observed and positioned in the dried blood drop layer, the same as in an iris chart.

According to Dr. Blank, the blood circulating through all the organs therefore carried their biophysical vibrations according to their specific functions. I decided to investigate further, where my first interest was to see if I could put in a sector for the colon, the same as in the iris, the skin, and the breast since I was very much interested at that time with the disease of breast cancer. I immediately had the presentiment that the topographical arrangement could be similar to the iris chart.

Simultaneously I used one iris microscope along with one microscope for the blood test, both with a video camera, and additionally the Vega DFM-722 electromagnetic field testing device. Hospital X-rays were utilized to double check on colon and breast findings. Two other medical doctors further assisted me. One day I had a group of eighteen Dutch doctors, who came to my clinic to learn about my work on cancer, organized by Dr. H. Oswald, who personally was intrigued by MBT. I tried to further explain about my new theories and the new discovery, concerning localization of the organs. One of the Dutch doctors offered to come back later on and help me. He did, and subsequently we spent a couple of weeks working together with patients trying to define the position of the dried blood layers relating to several additional organs.

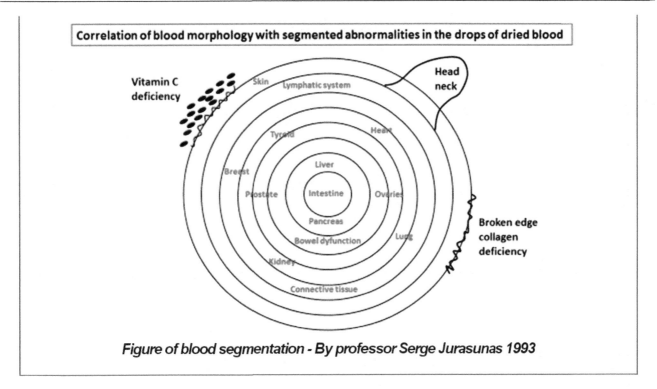

Correlation of blood morphology with segmented abnormalities in the drops of dried blood

Figure of blood segmentation - By professor Serge Jurasunas 1993

In 1987, after three years of work and experimentation documenting correlations with the body organs from the Iridology studies from that period, along with blood tests taken from a population of several hundred patients, I began to formulate my conclusions and theory. This process evoked strong feelings and insights from my discoveries. I then produced the first blood layer segmentation by organ position, just like in an iris chart. Although it was probably not 100% certain, it became the basis of a new discovery in the field of alternative diagnosis. This test is relatively easy to administer, but requires proper training and knowledge. The results however are immediately available and interpretable in the clinic setting.

One year later I made my first presentation of my discovery showing the correlation between Iridology and the oxidative dried blood test, also called H.L.B. by Robert Bradford, during a seminar sponsored by American Biologics in San Diego. In this kind of seminar, Iridology was at that time not well understood or accepted. While the seminar was also focusing on the oxidative dried blood test, it was apparently too soon for doctors to understand my discovery. Very few doctors if any had shown interest. But what do you know! As usual, later on other doctors, and particularly Bob Bradford, who with the help of some biologists and biochemists, started to seriously investigate my work. In 1993, I made a new and more complete chart on dried blood layer rings, with most body organs positioned the same as in the iris chart.

Today the oxidative dried blood test and the examination of the dried layer rings is widely spread in countries like the USA, Australia, Brazil, and to an extent in Europe, through promulgating further seminars and teaching. However probable, nobody knew about the origin or the discovery of the ability to monitor organ dysfunctions through the dried blood test, and indeed, I was the one who made the discovery. I had been waiting many years for the opportunity to explain the story.

I really believe that the MBT, as I call it, is very important since it not only monitors oxidative stress conditions, but also may show situations linked with a toxic colon, inflammation of the intestine, liver dysfunction, lymphatic congestion, or kidney trouble. More importantly MBT can monitor the stage of inflammation and/or disease. This test can be done in a matter of 15-20 minutes, which is a substantial convenience for a patient that has no need to run to various medical specialists, who more often than not, are unable to make a diagnosis.

Permit me to present the following case that offers an example illustrating the importance and consequences from a disturbed colon, wrong dietary style, and high oxidation. Recently, I found an example, one among many where a patient came to me with an advanced stage of stomach cancer. In summer of 2012, the patient felt considerable stomach discomfort, where the doctor told him it was only acidity and not to worry. He only gave him a prescription, but then only a few months later, the news about the patient came back to me. He felt so bad that he was hospitalized. I believe that the MBT, which is interesting to monitor the inflammatory process including the grade of inflammation, could have informed us about some abnormal condition especially along with an iris examination and therefore inclined the patient for an additional medical examination. The MBT is neither a medical test nor a substitute for a hospital check-up, but it is very useful to monitor oxidative stress and increasing inflammation from pathological conditions, abuse of pharmaceutical drugs, or even excessive oxidation after chemotherapy. The test can offer more valuable information as well as compliment regular conventional diagnostic procedures.

In order to illustrate the importance of food and the imbalance between antioxidants and stressors, let me present the following case of a sixty-year old patient suffering from severe diarrhea and frequent bleeding. An ultrasound followed by a biopsy of the colon diagnosed an ulcerous colitis located in the sigmoid colon.

Live Blood Analysis Observation (LBA)

At the same time, the level of oxidative stress and abnormal blood condition was observed through Live Blood Analysis observation. We obtained reliable confirmation about the existence of stressful factors and the lack or decreasing activity of antioxidants.

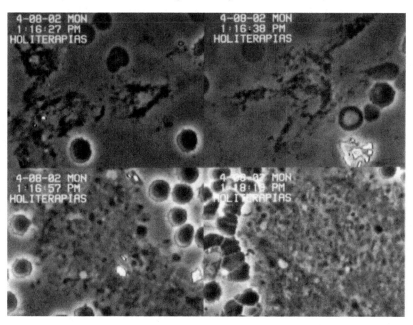

1st LBA Test

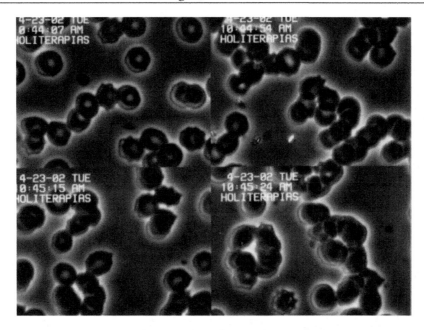

2ⁿᵈ LBA Test after treatment

We performed a live blood analysis monitoring a fresh drop of blood under an American Biologics microscope, developed by Robert Bradford, with a high definition magnification of 40 x 15000, which permits the observation of tiny particles up to 5 microns in length, red cell membrane morphology, white cells, platelets, immune cells, and any other abnormal condition. Increasing free radical and decreasing antioxidant levels in the blood circulation are quite visible through abnormal/damaged red cellular membranes. Other interesting observations are lipid peroxidation, excess toxins, heavy crystals, bacterial or fungal invasion, which underlines a bad colon condition, and bad eating style.

The LBA observation, as shown in the 1st figure, indicates a condition of oxidative stress, lipid strands, fungal growth, and a major decreasing activity of antioxidants levels in the blood circulation.

We decided to treat the patient on a twelve-day basis, but with no specific diet, only my special low-molecular antioxidant compound (Anoxe) made from modified vegetables and seed, having a SOD-like activity (that contains vitamins A, C, E, beta-Carotene, catalase, glutathione, polyphenols, flavonoids, and riboflavin from modified vegetables and seeds), with pharmacological properties as well as an anti-inflammatory effect. The aim of this treatment was to test the efficacy of this antioxidant compound on oxidative stress levels both in blood circulation and inflamed mucosa.

At the end of the twelve-day treatment, the patient came back very happy because he no longer had diarrhea. The new LBA test which we can observe on the 2nd figure showed a modification of the blood status, better shaped red cells, and elimination of the large clusters of oxidized lipids and yeast forms like Candida. This demonstrated that, first and foremost, our special antioxidant compound is very powerful with a strong anti-inflammatory action. This definitively demonstrates the need for antioxidants to help correct any abnormal situation that may occur in any part of our body, including the colon.

In a similar way we have reason to believe, in case of irritated bowel syndrome or ulcerous colitis, an effective treatment first requires a special diet, food and/or supplementation rich in antioxidants increase the immune defense and detoxify the body.

Live Blood Analysis from the Author's Clinical Research

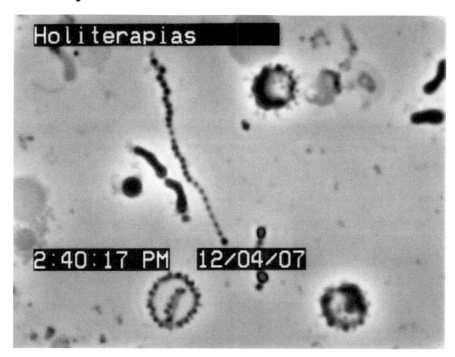

Figure 1

Figure of normal spiral of spirochete (*Borrelia burgdorferi*) length of approximately 30u with elongated bleeds along its membrane.

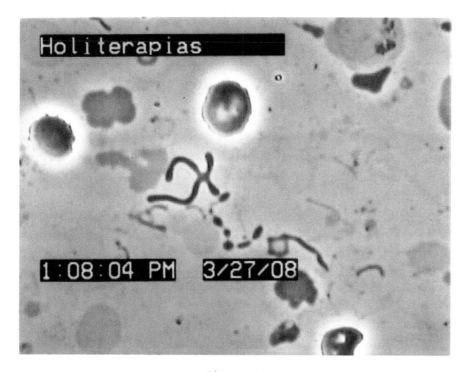

Figure 2

Figure of a normal spiral of spirochete, and below, the elongated form double back on itself, forming close-packed multiple dusters. On the left of the spirochete we observe a giant fungal form.

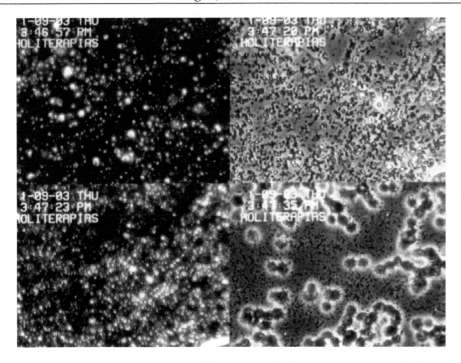

Figure 3

HIV – We observe a major bacterial invasion on the whole drop of blood, which suggests that HIV is not only just associated with a virus.

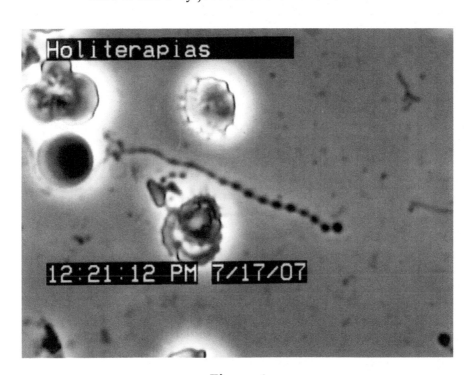

Figure 4

Bright field 8.000 X
Elongated bleed form of the spirochete (*Borrelia burgdorferi*) Lyme disease

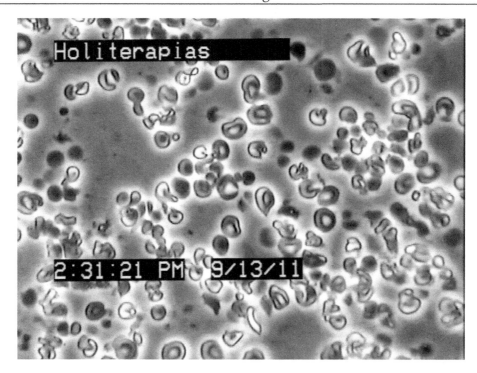

Figure 5

1 Fragmented and distorted red cell membranes from high free-radical activity and low antioxidants status – S.O.D. Glutathione, vitamin E, beta-Carotene.

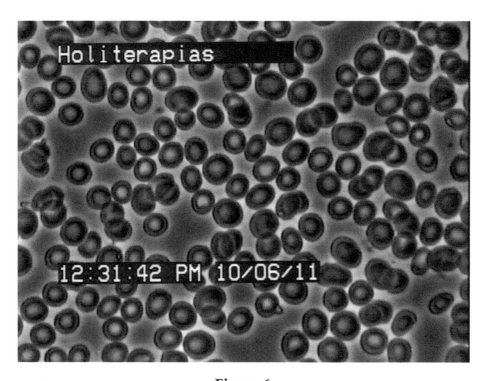

Figure 6

2 The same case after about one month taking Enzyme Yeast Cells supplementation, Sun-Chlorella, revitalizing drink with apple, kiwi, pineapple, etc. and a nutritional food diet. This is a 100% improvement of the blood status.

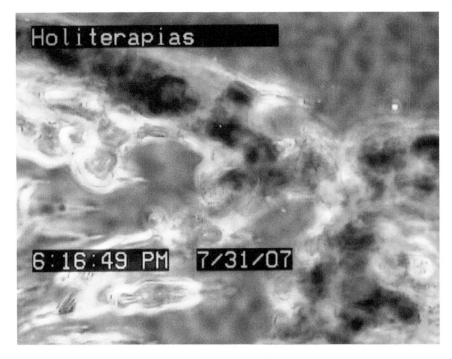

Figure 7

Figure 7 shows intoxicated blood with large clusters of mucous, toxins and accumulation of pharmaceutical drugs (in red) where none had been detoxified by the body.

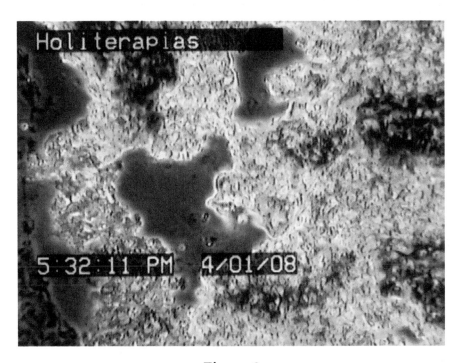

Figure 8

Figure 8 shows a major accumulation of heavy crystals in blood circulation from an aged person. It indicates bad kidney function but also bad dietary style. Heavy crystals are responsible for pains in the bones, inflammation in the tissue, and may, in return, block kidney functions.

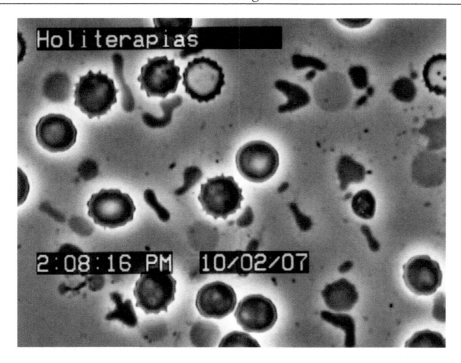

Figure 9

Bacterial overgrowth. We observe many fungal forms spread all over the photo: poor liver defense, poor immune system, oxygen deficiency.

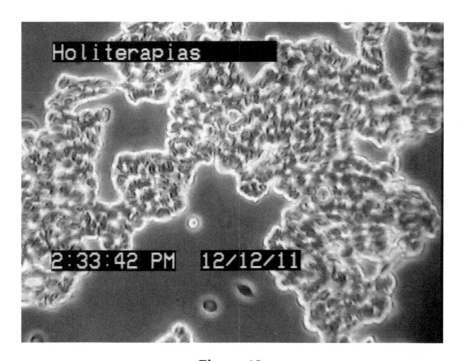

Figure 10

Red blood cells concentrate in strong rouleaux. Blood viscosity. Poor circulation and a lower oxygen supply for cellular requirements and brain neurons. May develop cognitive disorders. Strong rouleaux are visible in the case of chronic fatigue, poor health status, and chronic/degenerative disease.

Before

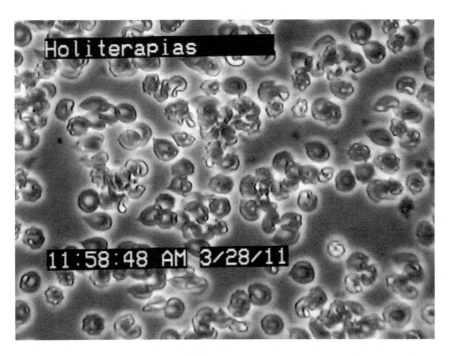

Figure 11

Before: High oxidative stress. Bad dietary style.

After

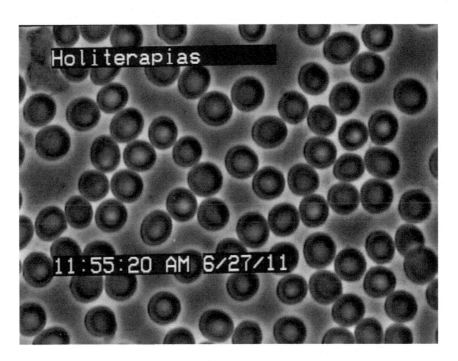

Figure 12

After: Detoxification and treatment.

We observe a 100% modification with the condition of the red blood cells, which now show a very normal shape. The patient followed a two-month treatment that includes enzyme yeast cells, Sun-Chlorella, probiotics, and organic fresh vegetable juices.

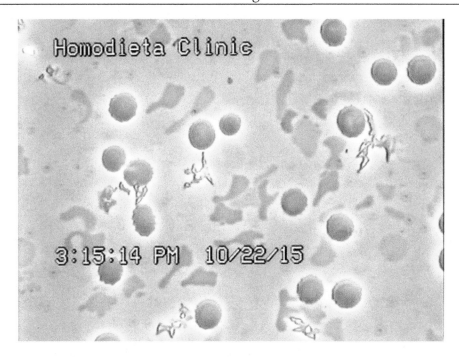

Figure 13

This slide indicates a major fungal invasion, bowel dysfunction, constipation, immune deficiency, and low O₂ status.

More cases may be viewed at www.sergejurasunas.com   (Click on "Blood Tests")

Oxidative Dried Blood Layer Test

This is only a short introduction about this technique. Here it shows the intake of a drop of blood taken from the small finger and transferred onto seven layers of blood smears on glass slides and allowed to dry and coagulate at air temperature. After the various dried blood layer are carefully examined under a microscope, each layer represents specific characteristics with different sizes and shapes of PPPs (Polymerized protein puddles). Here is the research I developed after hundreds of examinations, clinical work-ups, and correlations with other diagnostics including Iridology that has permitted the localized organ body dysfunction in the various dried drops of blood and segmentations (For instruction contact: sergejurasunas@ hotmail.com).

A classification of the study of the Metabolic Blood Test includes:

    A – Increased number of white clot areas and the leaking of fibrin nets.
    B – Density and size of white clot area.
    C – Localization of white clot area within the drops of blood.
    D – The presence of metabolic by-products such as necrotic tissue, degenerating red cells, within the white blood clot.
    E – The density or destruction of the fibrin network.
    F – Any additional colors inside the white blood clot.

The 7 dried blood layer

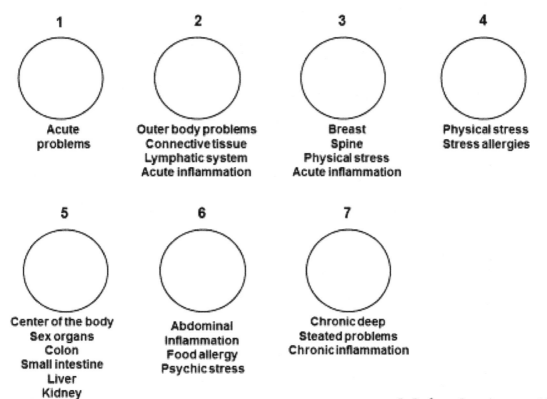

1

Acute
problems

2

Outer body problems
Connective tissue
Lymphatic system
Acute inflammation

3

Breast
Spine
Physical stress
Acute inflammation

4

Physical stress
Stress allergies

5

Center of the body
Sex organs
Colon
Small intestine
Liver
Kidney
Panceras

6

Abdominal
Inflammation
Food allergy
Psychic stress

7

Chronic deep
Steated problems
Chronic inflammation

By Professor Serge Jurasunas 1998

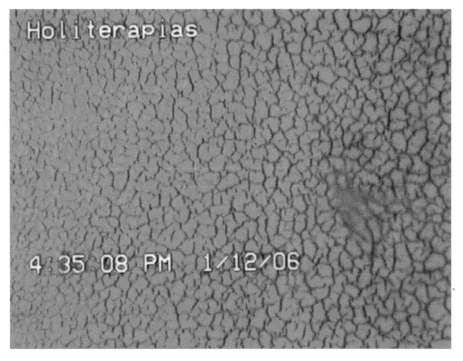

Figure 1

Normal blood pattern

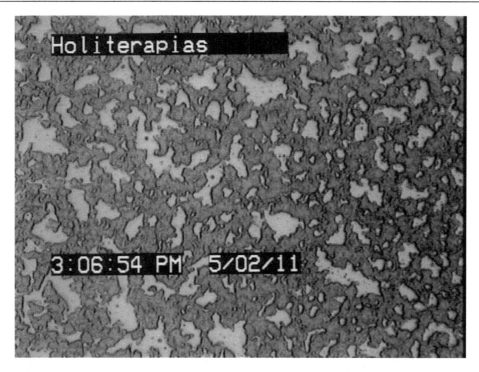

Figure 2

We observe a total dissemination of PPPs from 20 to 30 microns size showing a major inflammatory process in a prostate cancer. Very small PPPs of 2 microns are associated with allergy.

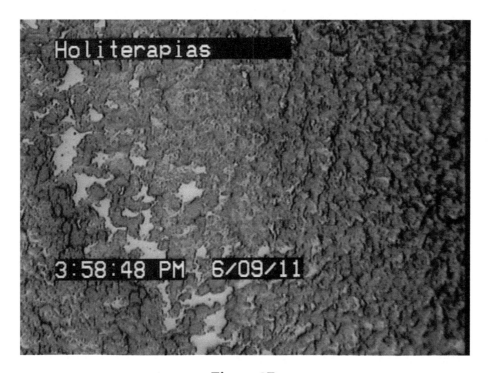

Figure 2B

After about one month of treatment we observe an improvement with a significant decrease of the PPPs and inflammatory process.

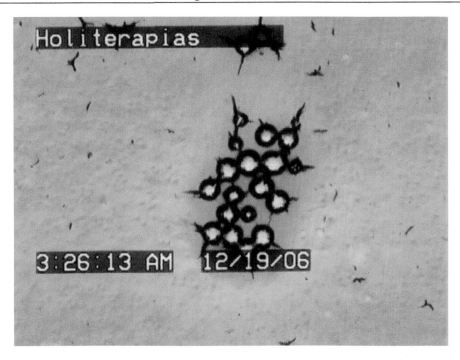

Figure 3

6th drop layer of dried blood – intestinal polyps – fibrin nets are totally non-existent showing deficiency of proteins and hormones.

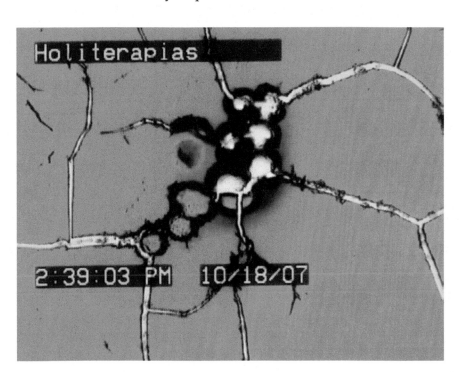

Figure 4

Liver congestion with congested lymph circulation.

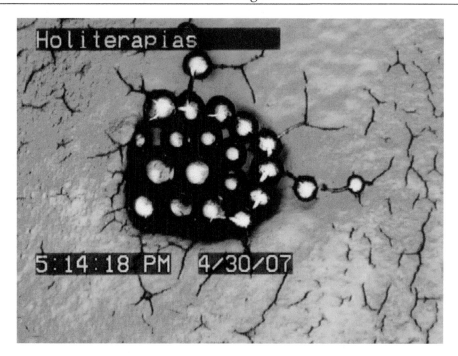

Figure 5

Chronic constipation and a toxic colon.

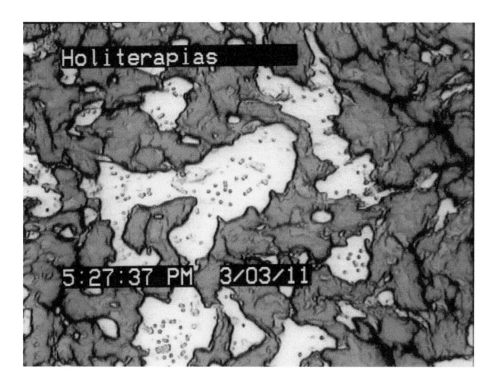

Figure 6

Well defined appearance of large 40 microns PPPs with a defined edge, typical of cancer disease.

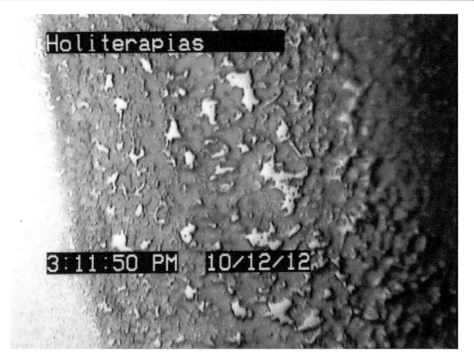

Figure 7

Middle-aged physical stress – PPPs of 20 microns.

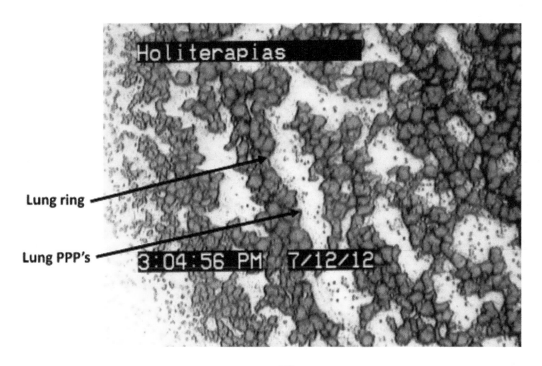

Figure 8

Lung cancer stage III with metastases to liver.
Large 40 micron PPPs. Elongated PPPs forming connections between each other underline lung cancer. This is a very high inflammatory process; denatured RBCs and free radical footprint is visible inside of the PPPs.

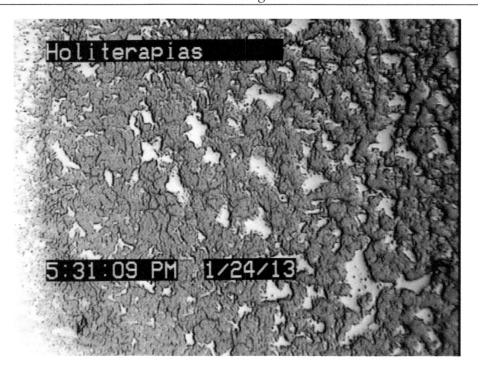

Figure 9

F. Twenty-nine years – PPPs from 20 to 30 microns, physical and psychological stress-decreasing antioxidant status.

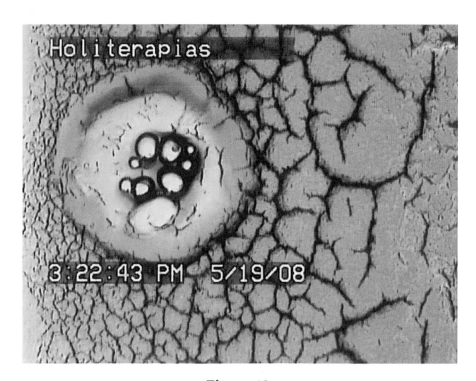

Figure 10

5th drop layer, 6th - 7th ring representing the colon and liver. Indeed, it shows a very toxic colon and liver toxicity.

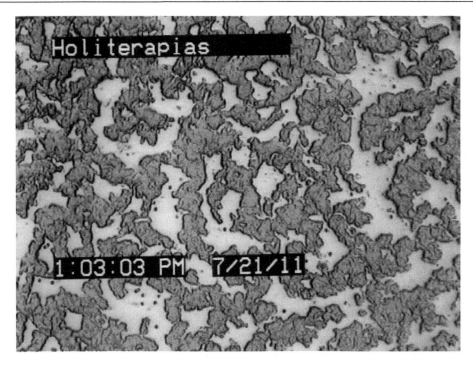

Figure 11

Colon cancer stage 3. PPPs from 30 to 40 microns. High oxidative stress – after chemotherapy.

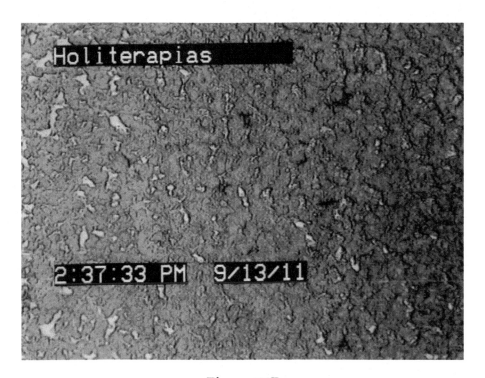

Figure 11B

After two months of treatment and diet, we observe a reversal process, and almost a total disappearance of the PPPs.

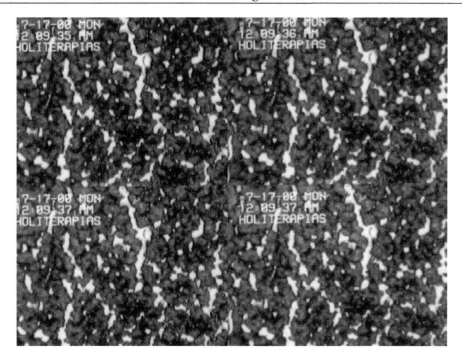

Figure 12

Major acute intestinal inflammation, 5th-6th layer, 6th segmentation, very small, elongated PPPs from allergy condition and free activity.

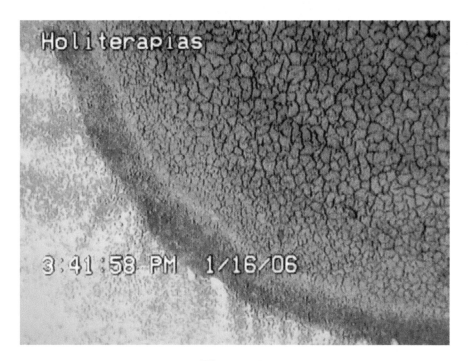

Figure 13

The dark ring around the periphery of the dried drop layer blood shows an intoxication of heavy metals. The blood is also dark from excess of toxins.

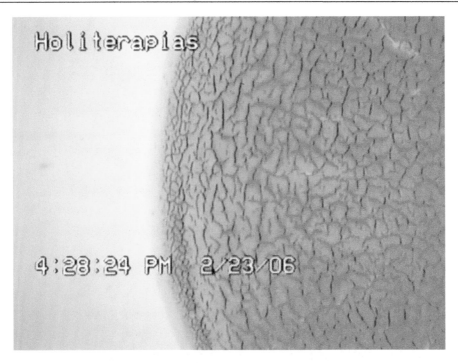

Figure 13b (Oxidative dried blood test)

After about forty days of treatment with chlorella extract, the new observation shows a normal periphery and elimination of the toxic metals. The blood is also cleaner and much brighter.

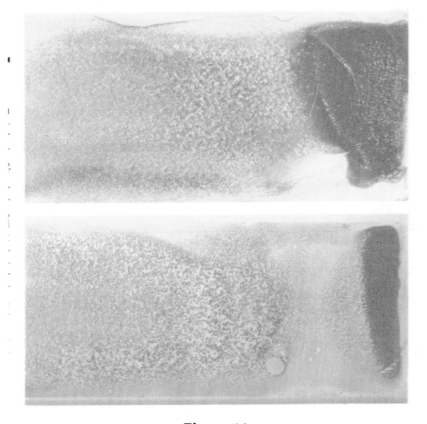

Figure 14

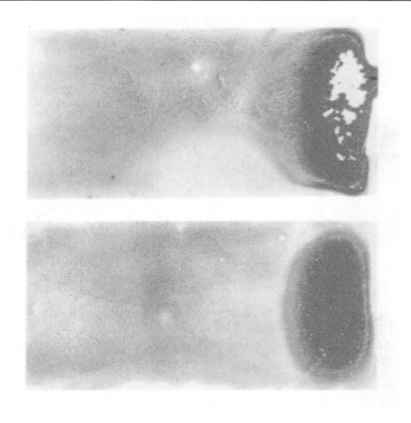

Figure 15

Above: Glass slides with dried blood from Aura-Test (Aurascopy) – Germany
A typical example of cancer disease.

Below: Professor Jurasunas in his clinic.

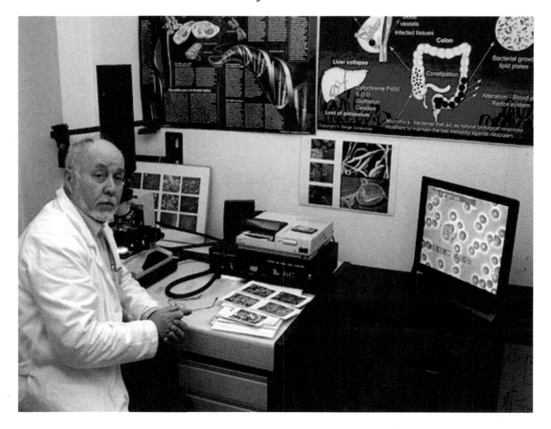

Diverticula

The diverticula are anomalies, only recently taken into consideration by medicine as they are essentially linked to modern eating habits and food style preferences.

Diverticula look like small sacs found in the interior wall of the colon. They can be compared to small mushrooms, hollows that burst in the tree bark. The word "diverticulum" comes from the Latin root *divertu* which means "turn aside." They result from of the deviation of normal structure in the colon wall tissue.

The sigmoid colon retains more fecal matter than the descending colon, hence, in cases of diverticula, the feces enter there. Many people have diverticula but are not aware of it. The complications appear when an inflammatory condition arises.

If the diverticula are inflamed, the condition is called diverticulitis. Under pressure, they swell and transform into actual hotbeds of infections. For example, if muscle fibers are weaker in a particular area of the colon, a small hernia may be formed, which subsequently can be transformed into diverticula. In the most serious conditions of the colon with putrefactions and chronic diverticula, worms can proliferate, penetrate into the diverticula sacs, and secrete virulent toxins.

I remember the case of a fifty-year-old man with severe colon problems. The X-ray of the descending colon up to the end of the sigmoid colon showed more than one hundred diverticula.

I constantly warn patients about the dangers of constipation and of its consequences, one of which is precisely diverticula. Once constipation is linked to eating habits, it becomes one of the main factors for the onset of bad health and disease. As long as our diet is deficient in vegetables, fruit, and whole cereals, we need good muscle function in the colon. This is especially true for the sigmoid colon, being very necessary in order to make the hardened feces advance toward expulsion. A colon being already weakened from pressure exhorted on various parts of the colon walls, as well as from a hereditary standpoint, along with a poor mineral supply, makes for a combination that can definitely cause the formation of diverticula spreading throughout the sigmoid colon (90%), asymptomatic until they become inflamed which can be a probable risk factor for acute peritonitis. Diverticula situated in the sigmoid colon represent a greater risk than for those which are formed in the descending colon. The possible formation of toxins, often virulent, increases the auto-intoxication of the colon causing further undetermined disorders. Unfortunately, should a diverticula burst, the bacteria and other toxic matter spreads throughout the abdominal chamber possibly causing acute peritonitis. This would be an extreme case; however, many problems can occur before one reaches such a serious situation. Hitherto, diverticula were considered a consequence of age, that is, they only existed in older people. Why only in older people? It is simply the result of many years of work, fatigue, and often dietary abuse. Meanwhile, we must appreciate that our ancestors were stronger and hardier than our generation. Hereditarily speaking, they certainly had a stronger body and access to a more natural, healthy food supply, rich in vitamins, minerals, enzymes, and fibers. They were not bombarded with an excess of pharmaceutical drugs, whereas today we simply abuse our bodies with so many "miraculous" drugs such as antibiotics, even at an early age, not to mention the youngest, including babies.

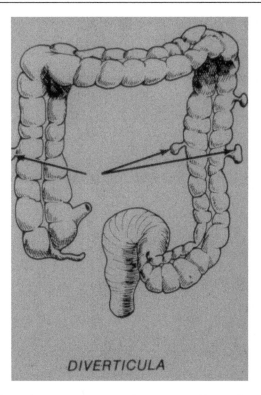

DIVERTICULA

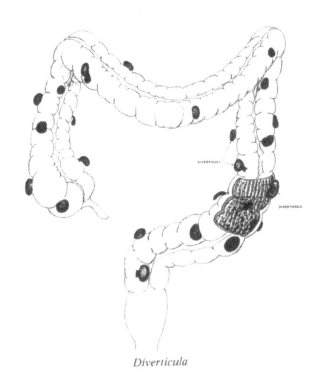

Diverticula

Therefore most people especially sick people seem to follow a bad dietary style, eating heavy meals without knowing if their intestinal system accepts such food. Recently it has been shown by experts that the wrong foods can alter the gut microbiota very rapidly and increase the risk to develop colon cancer and probably some other diseases. Eating habits do not get better as we grow older, they become increasingly worse, which makes today's adolescent a good Candidate for intestinal disease, diverticula, IBS, infection, and possibly even cancer. Unfortunately, there are no vaccines against diverticula, prolapsed colon, abdominal bloating, or diarrhea, just as there are none against fatigue and stress.

When diverticula are present a correct diet, detoxification and physical exercise seem to be the best and most appropriate solution. While one waits for an X-ray, why not opt for an Iridology test? Iridology is extremely precise in detecting and localizing diverticula in the colon. In the iris, the diverticula appear as small dark lacunas arranged along the rays of the sun. It is not rare for me to see the presence of diverticula in patients without them having ever suspected the problem.

This is simply because they feel no pain, do not expect any problems, and have no outward signs. However with aging and bad dietary lifestyle the colon may soon deteriorate, depending also on hereditary status. In these cases, Iridology can be a great help and becomes an essential test, as it can easily trace the exact profile of the intestines, detect the weak points and prompt corrective action before it is too late. Consequently, we can resort to X-rays to confirm what has been detected by Iridology and then create a correct dietary regimen.

Superoxide Dismutase (SOD)

For many years I have been involved with the science of oxidative stress and antioxidants. I spent over ten years researching Superoxide Dismutase Enzyme (SOD), our most important antioxidant defense, and wrote a book on this subject. When I traveled in 1978 back to the USA, I met with some knowledgeable men in this new science, such as Dr. Bruce Alstead M.D., PhD, Larry W. Oberley, Ph.D., an authority in SOD enzyme research and later on, Dr. Y. Niwa MD, immunologist, laboratory researcher, a world authority in SOD, and author of many scientific publications, from Japan.

SOD is probably our most important antioxidant enzyme defense, being genetically produced in every cell and tissue of aerobic life including animals and humans. SOD is specially produced in our mitochondria, the main source of free radicals in our body. SOD is a metallic enzyme which includes cu-zinc SOD or SOD 1 and manganese SOD, MnSOD or SOD 2. The origin of SOD goes back about 2.5 billion of years ago when oxygen invaded the planet and became a poison for primitive anaerobic bacteria and prokaryotic cells.

Oxygen was the first step to stress and imperil anaerobic bacteria. Neither died, some bacteria escaped by going deep into the earth, while other bacteria penetrated the host cells and adapted themselves by developing a system that could use oxygen to produce energy, and at the same time, synthesize a defense system against the corrosive action of oxygen, for which we know SOD and glutathione are the two main antioxidant defenses. Mitochondria are born at the same time as the Eucaryotic or aerobic cells. SOD is the only enzyme synthesized by mitochondria, as I said before, which may explain as a missing link in cancer, since we know today that MT DNA mutation is involved in cancer. You can read more about this topic by consulting my article published in *Townsend Letter* August/Sept 2006, "Oxygen, Mitochondria and Cancer."

SOD is the first antioxidant defense line that converts superoxide in hydrogen peroxide that, in turn, is converted into water by glutathione or catalase. In other words, SOD prevents them from an accumulation of superoxide, which in turn may mix with other toxic compounds and become a cellular poison . However, it is not so simple since if a high level of free radicals can damage tissue or a cell membrane, since at low concentrations free radicals are necessary to modulate cellular signaling pathways. In other words, SOD activity keeps superoxide at low concentrations and converts the excess of hydrogen peroxide into water.

This is why SOD has even more biological effects and may even have a link with cancer. Many lines of research have shown that SOD expression can suppress tumor cell growth in-vitro by using large doses that convert superoxide into hydrogen peroxidase that conjointly with chemotherapy increases the toxicity. We know that in cancer the cellular SOD activity is greatly decreased; however and therefore, the conversion of superoxide into hydrogen peroxidase is compromised. Other lines of investigation have shown that SOD may modulate the activation of redox-sensitive transcription factors such as Nuclear Factor-Kappa B (NF-KB and API). MnSOD maintains intracellular redox and redox balance in our body and thus there remains more that we need to understand about what is an antioxidant.

The induction of SOD protects our cells against the bad effects of pollutants, which when penetrating our lipid cell membranes, generate free radicals with genotoxic consequences. It is the same for smokers, however with age SOD production is decreases, a reduction affecting each individual that becomes much lower in older people, where they are more subject to inflammatory diseases, chronic diseases, the harmful consequences of pollution, and to cancer risk.

Now the problem is that SOD is a big molecule, and exogenous SOD, orally ingested, is not well absorbed by our body and is quickly eliminated by the kidney. Many plants contain SOD, but trapped in large polymer chains, which our digestive system cannot break down. However, after studying the work of the Japanese, I subsequently became involved in manufacturing my own antioxidant compound from vegetable sources, using a system that breaks down the large molecules. In other words, I managed to produce a low molecular antioxidant compound having a SOD-like activity.

Several follow-up investigations, in-vivo, and in-vitro tests showed the pharmaceutical properties of my antioxidant compound that decreased COX 2 activity along with strong anti-inflammatory and even anti-cancer properties. I am using my antioxidant compound Anoxe widely, which in fact, I presented in St. Petersburg, Russia during an International Congress on free radical pathology (see: Therapeutic Application of a New Low Molecular Antioxidant and Cyclooxygenase Enzyme Inhibitory Property of Anoxe online at, www.sergejurasunas.com).

This low molecular antioxidant, SOD-like acting compound, offers therapeutic application with quick results. Anoxe when taken orally is very quickly absorbed by the body where it starts to be active about one hour after ingestion. Free radical activity decreased 50% after one hour and remained active after twenty-four hours, as demonstrated through in-vitro and in-vivo chemiluminescence testing in a German hospital.

Anoxe Shows Strong Therapeutic Application
Two Studies Available on the Internet at:
www.sergejurasunas.com

-Therapeutic Application of a New Molecular Antioxidant and Cyclooxygenase Enzyme Inhibitory Property.

- Effects of the Natural SOD-like Compounds on Redox Potential and Free Radical Generation in Venous Blood and Plasma.

However, Anoxe has also demonstrated, besides strong antioxidant properties and targeting inflammatory mediators and restoration of P53 function, efficiency in detoxification treatment. Anoxe is useful in any situation that involves pain, inflammation, asthma and of course as a support in cancer treatment.

More information is available, along with at least two studies that we have conducted, on the Internet, but what you need to remember is that exogenous SOD in tablets orally taken is rapidly expelled by the kidneys about one hour after ingestion. The same occurs for the enzyme catalase. The difference is that my antioxidant can be used in Therapeutic Application with some beneficial biological effect and offer a therapeutic response.

Colitis

Colitis is essentially characterized by an inflammatory factor which manifests itself in various forms. It can be dry with constipation or humid with diarrhea. In its acute form it can cause an acute diarrhea crisis with frequent eliminations per day.

Colitis can be associated with pain, loss of appetite, high fever, anemia, and loss of weight, sometimes necessitating hospitalization. On occasion, colitis can progress to a form of ulcerous colitis, developing in various areas of the colon.

I remember the case of a twenty-five year-old man with a severe case of ulcerous colitis whose life was constantly affected by this illness. He had lost thirty-seven pounds and, medically speaking, there was not much hope for a cure. This can be very traumatic for a patient not knowing where to turn to for help. At the time of his first visit, he had just spent thirty-six days in the hospital, then forty days recuperating at home, followed by relapse with an additional thirty days in hospital, then another three months at home, and finally, another fifteen days in hospital.

He constantly suffered from diarrhea with five to nine bowel movements per day, which completely debilitated him. During hospitalization the patient underwent all the regular tests that one can imagine, which always came out negative. Tentative treatment consisted of transfusions of serum and cortisone injections to stop the diarrhea. What is amazing is that nothing in particular was done in respect to improve a deficient diet, which was seriously needed. The patient was subjected to about the same institutional food that all patients are served, which is usually bad food.

Causes of Colitis

There are various known or still-unknown causes capable of triggering colitis or ulcerative colitis. The most well-known causes are diet and sensitivity of the mucosa. The most common causes of colitis are wrong food and sensitivity of the mucosa to food. Psychological stress is another known cause, which has a great influence over the tissue structure of the colon. This stress can strangle and even inflame certain areas of the colon, inducing the production of free radicals, which in turn increase inflammation of the intestinal mucosa.

Problems, worries, and emotions associated with the errors of the modern diet favor an inflamed colon, which today manifests itself in people of all ages. Younger generations are also victims of this problem.

Heavy and irritating foods, chemical substances, a lack of vegetables and fruits rich in antioxidants, and a lack of mucilage destined to protect the mucosa are some additional factors that contribute to colitis.

In cases of ulcerous colitis, there seems to be a true intoxication of the colon which results in the abnormal elimination process of mucous, toxins, and often some bleeding and diarrhea.

Conventional medicine has difficulty in resolving these kinds of acute and chronic disorders of the colon. If we limit ourselves to hospitalization without correcting the life style of the patient, they will hardly be spared from further relapse. A good dietary program or detoxification, as well as a new attitude or flexibility towards stress and social problems, yields good and effective results in correcting colitis and also ulcerous colitis.

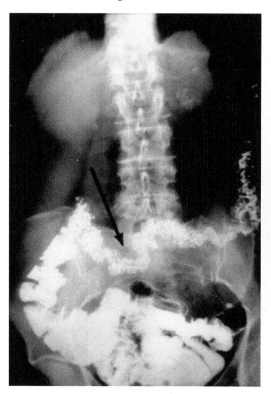 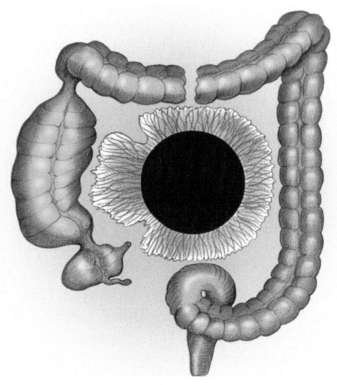

X-ray of a case of colitis with severe nervous colitis in the ascending colon with detection through Iridology, showing Tension throughout the entire intestine.

Prolapsed Colon

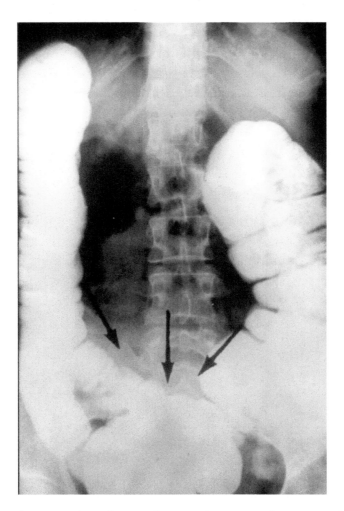

This X-ray clearly shows a prolapsed transverse colon exerting pressure on the organs in the lower abdomen.

A prolapsed colon is one of the most interesting things to observe in a person's iris. Its meaning can shed new light on disorders of unknown cause.

I have been particularly interested in this factor to which I have given much thought since my early career in Canada. First of all, this prolapse is located in the transverse colon which extends across the upper abdomen, in most cases. We can imagine the pressure such a prolapse would put on the abdomen which at the same time exerts considerable pressure on the lower organs, while preventing the transverse colon from descending into the lower part of the abdomen. This pressure is harmful to the colon and likely may also contribute to causing the prolapse to form.

First, let us briefly examine the cause of this prolapse. There are at least three main factors. The first one is essentially linked to an imbalance of minerals, and the second is an excess of food, and the third is constipation. These two factors are equally linked to the permanent force of gravity, which acts on the organism and causes a tendency for this part of the colon to collapse and drop.

Let us not forget that we spend most of our time standing up on our feet and we are subject to the pressure that the earth's atmosphere exerts on our entire body.

Moreover, the transverse colon is made up of soft tissue that crosses the upper abdomen horizontally from one side to the other. It is therefore understandable that the colon has a tendency to drop.

The intestines are supported by fine ligaments and a covering of highly resistant fatty tissue called "omentum." This cover, or rather this type of tissue, protects the intestines against vibrations and other traumas. But in truth, these ligaments keep the upper part of the colon in a horizontal position preventing it from descending onto the lower part of the abdomen. The ligaments, just as any other tissues, have nutritional needs, which primarily are minerals such as potassium, magnesium, manganese, and other substances designed to repair and regenerate the tissues. If the organism receives the substances necessary for it to repair itself, for example DNA or other enzymes, then, initially the colon remains in its position without dropping.

We often talk about the need for vitamins and antioxidants, forgetting about minerals except for calcium for the bones. In the same way, we still do not have the knowledge needed to fully understand calcium and its metabolism. Minerals are the main components of the tissue's structure. We can, for example, cite those often forgotten: magnesium, potassium, silica, copper, and sodium.

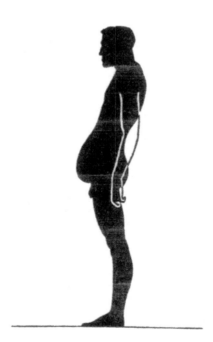

Deformed Backbone causing Abdominal Relaxation

Magnesium is very important for maintaining the vertebral ligaments, but above all for maintaining the colon and preventing its prolapse. When the vertebral spine curves, the position causes pressure on the abdominal organs. This pressure is harmful to the colon leading it to drop. When we are at the beach, we can observe curved vertebral spines of people who walk around and which almost always correspond to dilated and dropped colons.

Constipation can also contribute to the prolapse of the transverse colon. Indeed, when fecal matter accumulates, it dries, mixes with mucous deposits and creates pressure causing a lapse of the abdomen. At the same time, this deficiency of nutritious substances weakens the muscles and ligaments. Our modern life style, constant fatigue, and a bad diet are the main causes of deficiencies in the colon. Stress and fatigue that the modern woman is constantly under, even when young, significantly affects the muscular tone influencing the position of the skeleton. A prolapsed colon also contributes to further slowing the transit of feces, leading to a greater accumulation of toxic substances in this area of the colon.

This situation, along with the intoxication of the transverse colon, can have from an Iridology standpoint, repercussions on the brain, causing neurological disorders, headaches, and poor memory.

In women, the prolapse of the transverse colon exhorts pressure on the ovaries and the uterus simultaneously causing circulatory disorders in the lower limbs. Some young women considered sterile for no apparent reason, find an explanation and origin associated with the prolapse of the transverse colon.

In men and women, hemorrhoids, rectal lacunas and similar situations are often related to the prolapse of the transverse colon. Urinary disorders, ovarian pains, are often further associated with this prolapse. The observation of the iris leaves no doubt in this respect, showing the transverse colon with the radiating fibers of the organs it influences.

Obviously the correction of this anomaly provides great relief to the functions of these organs.

You will find suggestions about and solutions to this problem throughout this book. I, once again, repeat that this is a problem to be taken very seriously, and not one to be underestimated. It must be identified through specific tests. Iridology gives a clue that can easily be confirmed by an X-ray. An Iridology exam also shows the other organs influenced by the prolapsed colon, giving a more concrete idea of the state of stress, fatigue, and nutritional deficiencies.

Right   **Left**

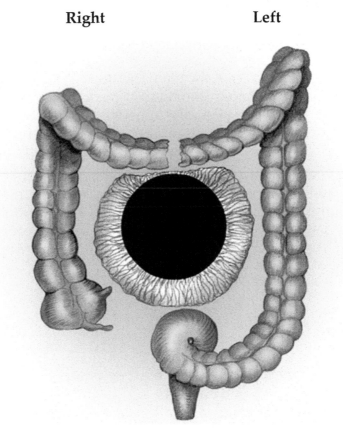

Prolapse of the Transverse Colon and its Detection through Iridology.

Colon Cancer

In the United States, the second highest cause of mortality after heart disease is cancer. 100,000 Americans die of colon cancer each year, but 200,000 more die from various other intestinal diseases. In 2014 in the US alone, an estimated 1,665 new cancer cases were diagnosed, and over 585,722 cancer deaths.

In Portugal, only 3,000 people died from oncologic problems of the colon up until 1999, a much more modest number compared to American statistics, although it tends to increase over time. The latest results pointed to 5,000 annual deaths, but probably much more today, since the first Portuguese printing of this book was released in 2009. In 2012 Portugal had 24,100 cancer deaths.

How did we get to this point? The simple answer is over the years food has become more industrialized, junk food has spread all over the country, not only in the U.S. but also throughout Europe as well. Meat consumption has particularly increased, and over the past several decades, we have alerted our patients and the public about the necessity to eat less meat. More lately in October, 2015 the World Health Organization made an announcement, reporting a large survey about the direct link between red meat and cancer. Large articles in major European newspapers about the association between meat and cancer have created a wave of shock in the population. According to the report, grilled meat develops some chemical carcinogens, as well as aromatic polycyclic hydrocarbons having high risk of cancer. Of course, some meat can be eaten, but with a larger variety of vegetables like broccoli.

One other problem is the transformed cured meats such as sausage, salami, smoked ham etc., that also contain colorants, preservatives, nitrates etc., all of which are carcinogens. Chemical fertilizers along with nitrates may also be associated with colon cancer.

Secondly, diet was not considered to be of the main factors involved. People have only recently, and sadly, belatedly (with reserve), started admitting (in theory) that diet plays an important role in colon cancer. In its past few publications the American Cancer Society has underlined the benefit of fresh fruit, green vegetables, vegetables such as broccoli and Brussel sprouts eaten raw or slightly cooked. These are the so-called "functional foods," foods that contain substances capable of activating the vital functions of the organism or blocking aggressive mechanisms. Page 492 of the latest work entitled *Nutritional Oncology* written by a group of researchers from the prestigious Harvard Medical School, contains a list of food that is hazardous for colon cancer and must be consumed in moderation. Here is the list:

Red meat (including overcooked or old meat)
White sugar
Animal fat
Fried Foods (Especially cooked in bad oils?)
Charcuteries

In this work we can also find the importance and great emphasis given to the insufficient quantity of the following supplements in our diets:

Vitamin C, D, E
Folate
Methionine

Emphasis is also put on the daily intake of fresh fruit and vegetables, as suggested by new medical research, which is increasingly more orientated towards prevention.

Besides the importance given to these foods, I am convinced that it is also extremely important to know where to buy these fruits and vegetables and where they are grown. In Portugal, the quality of agriculture has considerably diminished during the past few years, the result highly industrialized agriculture. Some examples of this are shown throughout this book, especially in the chapter dedicated to the use of chemical substances in food products. With the increase of commercialized foods, the increase of chemical substances added (to conserve, preserve, flavor, etc...) is not helping to stop the incidence of cancer. Just imagine what happens when these toxic substances become stagnated in a lazy intestine!

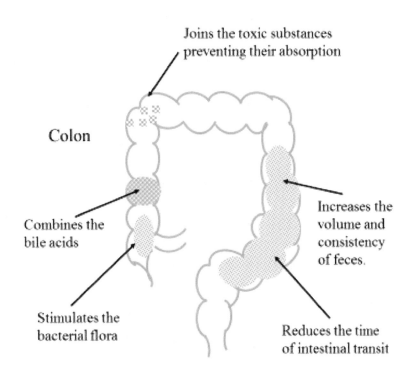

Effect of fibers in the colon's flora

According to some research and observation, colon cancer may also be associated with a lack of fiber, along with nitrates found in food and water. An excess of bad fats is also associated with colon cancer. By performing LBA (Live Blood Analysis) I often easily observe an excess of oxidized lipid accumulation in the blood of colon cancer patients, but also visible in other diseases and non-sick patients including juveniles with bad dietary style, which can be a problem and increase the risk of disease.

This underlines a diet low in vegetable intake, high fat intake, red meat, pizzas, fast foods, etc. Indeed, colon and breast cancer patients are the ones showing more oxidized fat in their blood. Also involved in this process are low amounts of antioxidants and vitamin intake such as vitamins A, E, C, folic acid, and beta-Carotene, important to protect from carcinogenesis.

Excess of heavy food, red meat, and low fiber intake can modify the metabolic activity of the intestinal micro-flora, which in turn play an important role in the conversion of bile acids and neutral sterols into reactive metabolites that may act as carcinogens.

We must emphasize the meaning of prevention before this disease blows up. More recently I had a fifty-eight-year-old male patient in my clinic come in for minor complaints. His irises really showed a very bad colon, and in my judgment, an increased risk of cancer. The patient was really worried and ready to take a P53 test. What do you think came up? A P53 mutation, along with a high level of mutated protein. It was a smart move for the patient since there was a 90% probability that he would have developed a cancer were nothing done.

When fecal matter accumulates, this favors putrefaction and stimulates pathogenic and carcinogenic bacteria producing some very toxic substances that may attack membrane cell tissue and turn a normal cell into a cancer cell.

An increase in genotoxic free radical activity may induce not only damage to the DNA cells of the mucosa but can increase the risk of P53 mutation which is one of the main "Hallmarks of Cancer."

Indeed, the fecal analysis of patients with colon cancer shows a high level of destructive free radicals in the hydroxyl radical family, which are extremely toxic. While medical checkups only concentrate on the local pathology, fecal analysis, and blood analysis of free radicals, this could probably serve to alert on any abnormal condition, which in conjunction with a good iris analysis, could indicate in certain persons, a risk of colon cancer. Additionally, a molecular markers test, which includes the P53 tumor suppressor gene, may eventually indicate a pro-tumor condition or a cancer process, which has already been activated.

Often I have observed this condition in patient iris profiles and warned them accordingly. The last case came back to me after seven years along with a cancer of the colon, while undergoing chemotherapy. Unfortunately the patient didn't believe sufficiently about my warning and here was a result, which could have been prevented. People still do not understand fully about the meaning of prevention before this disease blows up. For them, blood parameters and scans are more reliable while these cannot prevent but only help diagnose a tumor. Indeed, these women run to a medical doctor who prescribes some hospital checkups, which found nothing wrong with them. How can we explain this? They then feel relieved and never come back and keep following the same wrong diet.

Science increasingly associates colon cancer with a lack of fibers. The effect of fibers is easily explained as the by-products of fiber digestion through the colon's bacteria, which transform the acid environment and strengthening the mucosa making it more resistant to carcinogenic substances. This defense barrier from a balanced intestinal flora and fiber intake increase the elimination of fecal matter, prevent the colon from constipation and auto-intoxication resulting from a diet poor in vegetables.

In 80% of cases, colon cancers are located in the sigmoid colon and rectum and 20% in the ascending colon or transverse colon. We know that a great amount of feces and toxins are concentrated in the sigmoid colon, especially in the upper part of the rectum. Most colon cancer is formed in these two main areas.

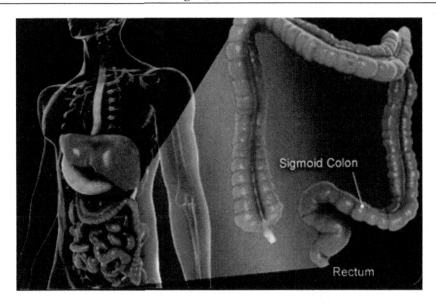

When people poorly eliminate stagnated feces, this tells me one of the main reasons for cancer risk.

Wherever feces stagnate, it develops into pathological hotbeds of bacteria and carcinogenic toxins and it surely increases the risk of colon cancer in some populations with fewer defenses. The other cause of colon cancer risk is associated with nitrates from modern agriculture found in food, water, and bad fat.

However, it is important to mention that an excessive consumption of red meat and pork associate with a poor intake of fruits and vegetables, which surely accounts for the increase of colon cancer, especially in women. In a region of Portugal called Alentejo, it is still very wild with rural farmers who eat more red meat and smoked sausages, where colon cancer runs very high in men but also with women eating the same wrong food.

A diet poor in vegetables and fruit intake, whole cereals, and fibers creates a problem, which is worsened when several types of food are combined, especially carbohydrates and fried foods. Some years ago I visited Costa Rica and saw the fantastic wild life and asked our driver, "What was the typical dish people eat?" It is called "Casado" (married). This plate is composed of meat, rice, beans, potatoes, eggs, and eaten along with more bread, but without vegetables. Indeed this is what he eats when we stop for lunch, on the road. What a bad and heavy combination. No wonder Costa Rica has high rates of colon cancer but also in Argentina, because of a high consumption of red meat. The same goes for Hungary, where people practically do not eat fish.

Red meat is also a leading cause of colon cancer since it may induce several biological responses that are responsible for the increased risk of the disease. First, red meat consumption increases the level of free radical activity resulting in DNA damage, P53, and Kras gene mutations further leading to the proliferation of abnormal cells and the initiation and progression of carcinogenesis.

Alternatively, heme (an iron porphyrin pigment of red meat) catalysis can also lead to generation of lipid peroxidation end products, such as malondialdehyde (MDA) along with other aldehydes. The urine of cancer patients contains a six times greater presence of MDA compared to healthy persons. MDA exposure can result in DNA-addictive formations leading to DNA mutation and aberrant proliferation. Heme is present tenfold higher in red meat compared to white meat such as turkey or chicken, not speaking of the excess of arachidonic acid that increases inflammation. However, eating white meat is healthier and limits the risk of colon or breast cancer, especially if you have a high intake of vegetables. Meat intake is also linked with excess hormones, especially in U.S., now forbidden in Europe. Meats cannot be exported unless a certificate can show it is hormone free. Cooked meat leads to the degradation of animal amino acids which is converted in the formation of many toxic substances such as ammonia. Ammonia decreases the growth of normal cells, but not of cancerous cells. Therefore, when the concentration of ammonia increases in the colon, it also increases the risk of cancer.

Of course colon cancer develops more easily where the tissues are weaker and toxic, and often iris observation shows some specific hereditary marks that increase the risk during lifetime. I have been observing cancer patients all year round. I am very well experienced about irises of cancer patients but particularly colon cancer. Probably I have taken iris photos of several thousand cases and keep in my papers a large number as examples. Many non-cancer patients also may show a risk of colon cancer indicated in their iris.

I remember a case of a man with an iris observation indicating to me a risk of colon cancer, localized in the area of the sigmoid together with other chronic dysfunction such as the liver and various dark toxemic spots. Under my advice the patient agreed to do a complete molecular markers test, where the result revealed a P53 mutation with high level of mutated protein and over-expressed BCL2. Definitely it was a case of a pro-tumor activity mechanism, leading to cancer. This is why Iridology is so important in the prevention of a disease like cancer.

Another important problem is that of nitrates which are commonly used in agriculture. The nitrates are metabolized by the body and transformed into nitrosamines, which are highly carcinogenic substances.

Nitrates are also used as one of the preservatives in canned food, especially with frozen fish, but above all in charcuterie or cured meats. Previously I explained that the people from Portugal's Alentejo region were eating too much charcuterie, fish in brine and preserved frozen fish.

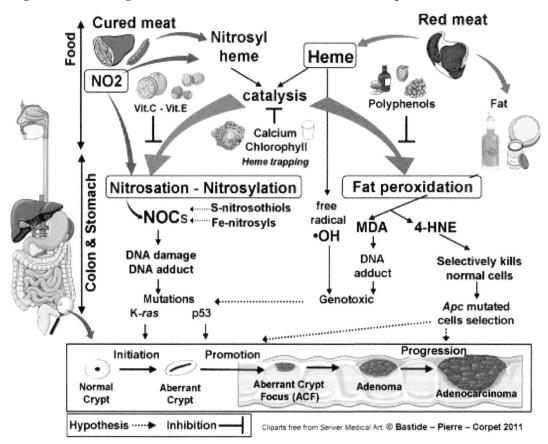

Hypothesis of Cancer Caused by Red Meat, Excess Free Radicals, and P53 Mutation.

How to Prevent Colon Cancer

This disease manifests itself in a perplexing way. There are hardly no signs, or pains, or lack of appetite, only often intestinal gases or flatulence which are not problematic, being paid little attention by individuals or doctors. I have presented many colon cancer cases reports including of a thirty-eight-year-old woman who was diagnosed with an advanced colon cancer and multiple large nodules to her liver, while yearly medical checkups found nothing wrong with her.

I recently had the case of a sixty-three-year-old man, suddenly diagnosed while on holiday in Spain with a colon cancer 15cm (5.9") in size localized in the ascending colon, with a 7cm (2.76") secondary lesion on the liver. How can this happen without symptoms?

Let me give you one example about the case of the husband of a patient that I knew for over twenty-five years who visited me regularly. The husband was never ill and felt following his wife's healthy regime was useless. However, four years earlier he came for a consultation under pressure from his wife but refused to follow a special diet and advice. His iris diagnosis revealed signs of gastrointestinal problems and especially indicated two small dark lacunas observed at the upper part of the rectum.

I saw these two small lacunas were an indication of degeneration in tissue, probably corresponding to polyps, which later on were confirmed by medical checkup. The man paid no attention but I warned the wife of the possible risk of cancer. One year later these two polyps degenerated into a cancer, which manifested through hemorrhage. Once again this man did not take this symptom seriously, which was a great mistake. The surgeon removed the tumor but the metastasis had already reached the liver and the man went for chemotherapy. Fortunately, the man decided to follow my treatment and diet. Even after eight years he is still in remission, because his wife carefully looked after their diet and proper food supplementation.

First, the presence of blood in the feces is suspicious and can indicate the presence of a tumor. Medically speaking it is then difficult to prevent the disease. Excess of gases may be also one indication of intestinal disorders. Thus it is important to take any abnormal intestinal symptoms very seriously. In this case it was important to change the bad dietary style, reduce the consumption of red meats, fats, cured meats, and increase the intake of protective vegetables such as broccoli, Brussel sprouts, cauliflower, spinach, watercress, and yellow peppers. This meant more fibers, more vitamins such A, C, E, and beta-Carotene.

The colon should eliminate twice a day, otherwise a diet rich in fibers, probiotics, and whole cereals is indicated, and otherwise a colon cleansing program to eliminate fecal accumulation is highly suggested. Iridology checkups are, from my perspective, a good way to profile a patient especially in regard to the colon. I have observed thousands and thousands of patients and there is no doubt about what the iris may reveal. The disease may develop more rapidly where the tissues in some area of the colon are weaker, become more vulnerable, and pick up more toxins. Iridology is perfectly suited to profile weak, degenerate tissue in the colon, along with eventual cancer risk. You may observe this in the upcoming chapter on iris clinical cases. We could then prevent many people from developing cancer by putting these principles into practice.

Most everyone walks along the street thinking that they are healthy, often because of the wrong medical conception. Prevention to me is more important in decreasing the incidence of colon cancer, than spending time and money to treat the disease, which often kills the patient. The time has come for authorities to take their heads out of the sand, who believe that by building more hospitals (and socialized medicine) they will solve the problem. This is not the case, and these (very expensive) measures will not change the way of life of people, who in reality need to be educated. We have the chance to take this responsibility and change our conception of living by changing our dietary habits, even if it is sometimes not easy to give up eating hamburgers and French fries. We have to be aware of our errors, the potential risks, and what can be done about correcting them.

Speaking truly, we must believe that governments are poorly informed and do not understand the true issues involved in the current cancer epidemic. On one hand, our governments are alarmed by the increasing number of colon cancer cases, but on the other hand they make vicious laws to restrict the use of vitamins and antioxidants essential for cancer prevention. There is a certain degree of irresponsibility and hypocrisy in this, since European lawmakers are also working to limit acceptable dosages of vitamins, most probably to an unacceptable level so people get no benefit from them.

On the contrary, we do need higher vitamin dosages in supplementation, since people are, on the contrary, are deficient. For instance, a large dose of vitamin C, and not the minimal 50mg daily as suggested by medical doctors, is not only important to boost white cell activity but to counteract the excess of nitrates in the intestine. This is only one example of the incoherence of government but usually politicians who themselves are ignorant and are pleased to follow blindly what they have been told by the medical cartel. But politicians themselves are also subject to disease and death.

I remember one Portuguese senator, a brilliant politician with a responsibility in the ECC in Brussels, who I believed to be an honest man. He was a good eater, habitual smoker, and overweight. He declared himself against vitamin supplementation and antioxidants, which he knew nothing about. One day on an official trip traveling through Portugal by car with his driver, he suddenly died of a heart attack. Surely a better diet, less animal fats, and some antioxidant supplementation would have avoided this tragedy at forty-six years of age.

On one hand, for most people we are face to face with a major deficiency of vitamins, minerals, and amino acids, especially with the elderly. On the other hand, we have to face the increased quantity of chemical substances present in the food chain, which includes an excess of nitrates and pesticides from modern corporate agriculture.

Our blood carries an amount of these chemical substances, which requires more vitamin protection especially to increase detoxification and reduce oxidative stress. Inequitable laws were adopted to keep the consumer ignorant, from being able to understand the meaning of a supplement label, or tell us what the true purpose of most vitamins is. But at the same time some politicians and health authorities seem to worry because cancer is increasing. What then is the purpose of this game?

Since I started writing a similar book I Portugal back in 2009, I have had in my clinic an increasing number of consultations, both male and female patients with colon cancer and metastatic colon cancer, although more in females. This has shown that our conception of eating or what we need to eat to be healthy has been getting much worse having been increasingly influenced by TV advertisements for industrially processed foods. We are told we no longer need to buy fresh vegetables to make homemade soup, just to buy it in a can or package at your supermarket. Our new generation of married women is cooking less and less, but prefer, for the sake of ease, time saving, and convenience to buy packaged food already prepared, such as pizzas and frozen dishes ready to put in the microwave. We are just preparing ourselves for more future diseases, more cancer, and more suffering. Remember that it takes ten to fifteen years to develop a cancer, while this just refers to what we are doing now.

We have to build rules and understand that our body requires some natural food instead of making life too easy with industrialized foods that you conveniently microwave. We are not going to see colon cancer decrease but instead increase as we pursue this misleading belief in ease and convenience. Each time, the increased incidence of colon cancer becomes more costly to the government and creates tragedy and sadness especially in elderly people who now are increasingly diagnosed with colon cancer, which I can really speak about with experience.

In conclusion, we can probably do much better in preventing colon cancer by changing our dietary style and pay more attention to our colon health. Auto-intoxication of the colon results from chronic constipation, accumulation of feces, toxins, pathogenic bacteria, and free radical activity. This situation originates from harmful substances with carcinogenic effects. While some people may have degenerative tissue from inherited colon weakness, this condition first requires a detoxification program followed by a healthy food diet, along with the support of nutritional supplementation that I present in this book.

Factors that Influence Colon Cancer

- Increase in the period of contact from toxins in the colon.

- Increase in the concentration of toxins.
- Saturated fats stagnating in the colon.
- Excess of red meat is associated with higher risk of colon cancer.
- Dietary regime poor in fibers.
- Dietary regime lacking in antioxidants.

Part IV

Colon Auto-Intoxication
Consequences of Auto-Intoxication of the Organism
Diagnosis of the Colon through the Tongue

Colon Auto-Intoxication

In the middle of the nineteenth century, a new medical system was born in the USA under a campaign of war and domination against Homeopathic medicine, later on becoming totally dominated by Pasteur's theory. It started first to treat disease by cutting up the body in slices, utilizing the privileged theory of localized diseases, along with the misconceived view of the role that microbes and viruses play in disease pathology.

The medical doctor became an engineer that sought to strangle the symptom (or disease) rather than working to resolve it by treating the cause. With the discovery of penicillin, antibiotics, and cortisone, modern medicine thought it had discovered the panacea for all disease, while at the beginning these saved millions of lives. While we still need them in an emergency, at the time, there was no further reason to go into a deeper understanding of how to protect or increase the body's defense against infection.

From this moment other medical systems like Homeopathy and Naturopathy became undesirable. The conception of the whole body, its self-defense systems, vitalism, auto-regulation, the role of food as medicine, along with detoxification and fasting, became heresy and were cast into total nonexistence. This is why today we still have real barriers in recognizing nutrition, for instance, as an important factor with therapeutic value. Similarly, our immune system is ignored by most medical doctors and oncologists as well.

The treatment of diseases was limited solely to the study of the possible mechanisms and symptoms rather than the study of the possible causes, both endogenously and exogenously, being based above all on the erroneous principle that diseases arise in healthy individuals. This is why today even cancer patients, who are at the beginning of their disease, are considered healthy, which is absolute nonsense.

Autointoxicated and aged colon

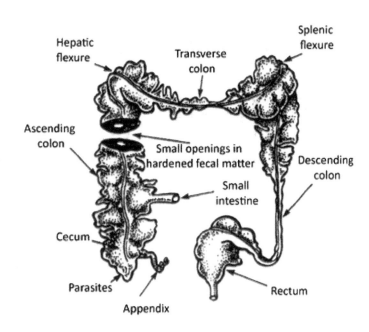

However, at the beginning of the twenty-first century, we have become more concerned with health and more preoccupied with the disaster we face from a medical community unable to fight diseases, as well as the alarming increase in chronic and degenerative diseases such as cancer, Alzheimer's, multiple sclerosis, Parkinson's, and autism.

We may also point out what affects our society even more is depression, anxiety, panic attacks, insomnia, and increasing suicides. These are also alarming. This does not even consider the impact of viral diseases, increasing and alarming infection from antibiotic resistant bacteria, and the return of tuberculosis, despite our vaccination programs.

In 1900, on a scale from one to ten, cancer was number eight. In 1997, it went up to number two. The death rate for kidney diseases in 1900 was sixth in this list of ten, but in 1997, it was in ninth position. In 1900, liver diseases were not on the list of the ten most deadly diseases, neither was suicide, which rose to number eight in 1997. Today Suicide is much higher, several husbands have killed their wife and children, later themselves, something about which society doesn't see or care to ask. Chronic and degenerative diseases are clearly increasing and coming from Western medicine. Why are they incurable? Where is the mistake? We must be facing a real failure in the medical system!

Principal Causes of Death in the United States of America	
1900	1997
1. Pneumonia and colds	1. Cardiac diseases
2. Tuberculosis	2. Cancer
3.Diarrhea and intestinal illnesses	3. Brain stroke
4. Cardiac diseases	4. Lung diseases
5. Brain stroke	5. Accidents
6. Lung Disease	6. Pneumonia and colds
7. Accidents	7. Diabetes
8. Cancer	8. Suicide
9. Senility	9. Kidney inflammations
10. Diphtheria	10. Liver diseases
New threats: purified water and immunizations reduce the basic illnesses, making way for	

In spite of our indisputable progress of medicine in certain types of diseases (or rather in better controlled organic dysfunctions), severe diseases are clearly increasing. Moreover, we do not even know why we are ill.

Some 2,500 years ago, Hippocrates understood why it was that we became ill. He condensed his incredible knowledge in some works which are still current. Today, when we speak of diets and new discoveries capable of treating diseases without resorting to medicines, we are actually limiting ourselves to rediscovering the dietary principles of Hippocrates.

Between these problems and the diseases that preoccupied the patients, we find it was rather from toxemia and auto-intoxication of the colon that illnesses were created. When the colon functions badly or in an irregular fashion, an abnormal condition arises which is called constipation, which is responsible for the accumulation of feces, food residues, and toxins in the colon that may, in turn, intoxicate the blood and create an unfavorable condition for the beneficial functioning of the entire organism.

There are at least three common factors capable of being an obstacle to a good healthy colon. They are hereditary profile, bad diet and chronic constipation. There are also social factors, and heavy stress, often responsible for intestinal disorder, colitis or even a block up of bowel movements, when the colon gives the signal for an expulsion.

It is rare to establish a relationship between chronic constipation, colon auto-intoxication, and diseases such as cardiovascular disorders, cardiac palpitations, arterial hypertension, high cholesterol, fatigue, and other disorders that arise as a consequence. Normally cardiologists, dermatologists, or oncologists never bother to pay attention to these situations, nor do they take their conclusions from these multiple symptoms. They rarely ask, "Do you suffer from constipation?" "How many days do you go without having a bowel movement?" It's a pity, because they could reach conclusions and offer treatment that could certainly benefit the patients. Of course you could tell me this is not scientific, especially in pathology, along with modern medical analysis and checkups. Just read how the media proclaims the miracle of medicine. We are looking for a localized, precise pathology and not for the cause of disease, which has been of non-interest. Is there any current medical teaching on this subject?

What is certain is that the theory of colon auto-intoxication actually provides an interesting answer to a number of explicable or inexplicable illnesses. Around 1972, I began researching the history of medicine and auto-intoxication of the colon with special focus on better understanding its implication in modern illnesses. When I started my practice in Canada, I found some books on constipation and auto-intoxication, such as those of Dr. N. W. Walker, Arnold Ehret, Dr. Tilden, and those by Dr. Max Gerson, an Austrian medical doctor, who immigrated to the United States famous for his book, entitled, *A Cancer Therapy – The Result of Fifty Cases*.

Max Gerson did not want to use analgesics for his patients in his New York hospital. If one of them complained of pain, although generally, the cancer patients are highly intoxicated and are in a lot of pain, he would prescribe one or two enemas a day, which calmed their pain. Currently, people depend on analgesics which destroy them just like antidepressants do, without realizing that this dependency reduces their quality of life.

Hippocrates' slogan was not to harm or damage patients, and all doctors should, supposedly, know this and practice it once they take the Hippocratic Oath at the beginning of their career, but of course today it means nothing since the new medical Oath is probably, "First, I will harm my patient," tragic, but only too true.

Every year in my clinic I had the opportunity to see a great number of people with the most varied health issues, from acute to degenerative disease, including all kinds and grades of cancer. Yet, there is a common element that frequently appears, and this is chronic constipation, auto-intoxication, and quite a number of other intestinal disorders. But curiously, this is not or is rarely the reason for the visit. Using Iridology as a means of observation or diagnosis of the gastrointestinal system, I quickly noticed the relationship between this problem and the disease that preoccupied the patient. At the same time, a questionnaire was used in order to verify the common elements existing between the written answers and the result of various diagnoses, including those of the iris. This is how I managed to establish statistics of the chronic and degenerative diseases, which are caused by bad dietary style and auto-intoxication of the colon. At the question, "Answer about your usual diet," this was no surprise for most patients that their diet was based on meat, bread, white rice, or spaghetti. Over time, I was able to develop and adopt modern, new testing techniques, where I could double check results and correlate outcomes between one test and another, which we will have the opportunity to talk about further on in this book.

Years ago I tried to gain better knowledge on the subject and undertook some historical medical research, since Europe is rich in medical development. I also tried to find arguments in favor of auto-intoxication and constipation as causes of disease. This path led me to researching chronic disease. I managed to discover some very important works, such as a treaty from the eighteenth century entitled, "Research on Chronic Illnesses" by Theophile Bordeu, published at the end of that century. An interesting phrase caught my attention and I quote, "One of the main causes close to diseases and which we can notice are the imperfections of the abdominal organs which communicate with all the other parts of the body through reciprocal correspondence." Throughout this book we will notice that there is a communication/relationship between the colon and all the other organs of the body. It is no less remarkable that this theory was already mentioned two hundred years ago, notwithstanding the limited means whereby it could be verified and proven. Many theories have been built under clinical work based upon the old books of medicine coming from the antiquities such the works of Galen, Avicenna, and Peracelcius.

Auto-intoxication, an Ancient Theory - The Pioneers

Before talking about more ancient medical works, I think the pioneers who enriched the end of the twentieth and the beginning of the twenty-first century should not be forgotten. Among them: Louis Khune, Benedict Lust, Paul Carton, Charles H. Kellog, and later Max Gerson and Bernard Jensen. We may also mention Dr. J. H. Tilden (1851-1940), who wrote several books on toxemia and disease. *Toxemia* was published in 1926, a few years before Dr. Jensen opened his first consulting office, and indeed, he learned much from Dr. Tilden, who opened a school in Denver, Colorado in 1935. He had been known as the Father of Natural Hygiene, on prevention of diseases, and for his writing on toxemia, although, as we explain further, toxemia was mentioned in Europe as early as the middle of the nineteenth century.

A special mention should be made of Dr. Catherine Kousmine, a great doctor and researcher, well known for her work on diet, the organism's defenses, and detoxification. Dr. Kousmine died in Switzerland in 1992 at the age of 96, not long before Dr. Bernard Jensen.

I had the privilege of meeting this wonderful lady, who invited me to see her at her home in Switzerland, for discussion about our research. We previously had met during a seminar, but she also heard about my work in the field of cancer and read my book on germanium and cancer when I first introduced organic germanium to Europe in 1974. At the time, my book created major interest, attracting large audiences to attend my lectures. The purpose for this meeting was to exchange our experience and ideas. I told her about my recommendations about toxemia and treating cancer with germanium and diet. Dr. Kousmine also pointed out the need to detoxify the body, a healthy diet, and intestinal hygiene, but especially the necessity of EFAs to protect cellular membranes in the body. She especially underscored the difference between dead and living oils. She authored several important books such as, *Save Your Body, Prevention and Cure of Modern Diseases, Be Healthy at 80 Years of Age,* and *Multiple Sclerosis is Curable,* which influenced many health professionals and doctors at the time in Switzerland and France. Thank God her work was not lost since the Kousmine Foundation continues to educate Naturopaths and medical doctors throughout Europe. Personally, she gave me precious information for my practice, proving that there are great similarities in the conception of theories and treatment of patients.

Dr. Kousmine was a Russian doctor, who immigrated to Switzerland, and she was perhaps the first in Europe to focus on the permeability of the colon and how non-digested food could cross a damaged intestinal barrier. Her principles were to choose natural quality foods that needed to be digested and assimilated, which indeed was a theory of Bernard Jensen's as well.

Dr. Kousmine stated that our first line of defense against cancer is our intestinal mucus; the second line, the liver; while our third line of defense is our cellular membranes that protect our cells against the penetration of toxic and carcinogenic agents. According to her, PGE 1 is the one strong anti-cancer agent that protects the intestinal mucus. Also, science discovered that some prostaglandins derived from gamma lineolic acid (GLA) boosts lymphocytes, T function, and in-vitro can transform cancer cells into normal cells. She calls the polyunsaturated fats such as vitamin F important for the good functioning of our body and even prescribed retention enemas with sunflower oil to strengthen the intestinal mucus membrane.

Dr. Kousmine spent many years on cancer research linked to nutrition and has done many experiments on groups of rats, feeding one group with natural food and the other with denatured food, to see which group developed cancer—of course it was the ones fed on industrial food. She particularly spent time to teaching us about how pollution can harm our body and entered into a war against several chemical companies for which she was strongly criticized.

Dr. Kousmine developed many types of food diets and made up a type of cream-cereal whose purpose was to protect the intestinal mucous, activate the intestinal function, and increase our immune defense. The composition is called "Budwig Cream," named in honor of Dr. Johanna Budwig from Germany (1908-2003), who was considered one of the world's leading authorities on fats and oils. She was nominated seven times for Nobel Prize, but unfortunately only medical discoveries (and markets) can win the Nobel Prize. The Budwig recipe is easy to find on Internet.

A fundamental principle of Dr. Kousmine is the importance of the four emunctory organs that I referenced myself over the past decades: intestine, kidney, lung, skin, and of course the liver as the main detoxifying organ. According to Dr. Kousmine, these represent our defense system against the invasion of bacteria and accumulation of toxins to preserve the integrity of our cells.

We realize that no matter the country or the researcher, the same identical principle of health is always taught, because health is only possible if we eat the proper food and properly detox. A site in French devoted to Dr. Kousmine, may be found at: www.solvida.org . Her book in English is available for download at the following link:
http://www.solvida.org/assets/plugindata/poola/the-kousmine-method.pdf.

And later, Max Gerson, Bernard Jensen, and Catherine Kousmine gained even greater acceptance. Perhaps few words about Dr. Bernard Jensen are not superfluous as he was truly a genius in the field of natural medicine and has influenced most Naturopaths, not only in USA, but all over the world. Hidden Valley Health Ranch was for decades the mecca of natural treatments. Vegetables and fruits were grown organically to be immediately served to patients, cooked, raw, and in juices during detoxification.

Back in the years 1964-1967, while learning at Hidden Valley Health Ranch with Dr. Bernard Jensen, I met Dr. John Arnold, D.C., an Iridologist who founded the World Iridology Fellowship Association and started a journal, *Iridology International*. Dr. Jensen had also learned from him. Dr. Arnold was eighty-five-years old at the time, but very active. He kept me at his side during consultations.

I first became acquainted about nutrition and diet, colonic therapy, Kneipp water-baths, chlorophyll, whey, goat milk, beetroot and juice, as well as how to detoxify, strengthen the liver, and to build up a clean and rich blood supply. I learned how to do exercises, about the colema slant-board, used to strengthen the abdominal muscles, combat colon prolapse, and to help to clean out diverticula.

I learned about Iridology by standing next to Dr. Jensen during iris examinations, telling me what he saw and, most important, how to see. Then he suggested I start drawing irises in color on a blank iris chart, from some patients showing the lacunas and other iris signs. This is the way I started with Iridology and became acquainted with nature-cure. There were no schools back then. Where to learn Iridology was an important question. This is why later on I travelled back to Europe and Germany to learn with the great German Iridologists, such as Professor J. Deck. But at Hidden Valley Health Center, all of this I mentioned did not even include the weekly lecture on spirituality by Dr. Jensen for the guests of the Ranch. As a man of health, during his weekly conference, Dr. Jensen often referred to the Bible or even Buddha during his lectures.

Bernard Jensen was truly a Master and we owe him a lot. With my own eyes I saw patients coming in with poor health condition, even unable to walk, and saw how they improved day after day using Dr. Jensen's Nature-Cure methodology. In fact, when I met him, he called himself on his business card, "Doctor of Natural Medicine." He used to say, "Iridology belongs to nutrition," meaning if you practice Iridology, you observe the dietary style of people, with the understanding only nutrition can change something in their bodies, but only after you can observe change in the stroma of the iris. Dr. Jensen stressed that in order to recover from a disease, we need first to clean up our body, and to accomplish that, we start with colon cleansing, liver detox, and blood detox. A second important thing he believed was the importance of vitamins and minerals necessary to make good, healthy tissues and activate cellular function. Above all, Bernard Jensen was a great teacher not only in the field of natural health, nutrition, and Iridology, but philosophy and spirituality as well. Among the many books Dr. Jensen published, his two master books, *Food Healing for Man* and *The Chemistry of Man*, are still valuable references.

Another important work I would like to cite as an example comes from two doctors: *Therapeutic Compendium* (1902), by doctors Bouget and Rabow. Both were professors at the Lausane Medical Faculty in Switzerland. The way in which these two doctors warn people about the risk of toxic substances, which can infiltrate the organism and cause illnesses, is admirable.

Indeed, I always give such advice as, "Besides the conviction that the relationship between the colon and illnesses exists, I believe in the hypothesis of the correlation between colon intoxication and cancerous terrain." It was this hypothesis, which I have been expounding for years, that has recently led me to include a chapter in this book on the involvement of intestinal toxins in the development of breast cancer.

This theory has ancient roots, which lacked concrete proof. For example, in an older work extremely rich in teachings, "Lessons on Auto-Intoxication and Illnesses" (1885), issued by the Faculty of Medicine in Paris by Dr. Bouchard, professor of pathology and general medicine, we can read as follows:

> *"The body has an interesting tendency to accumulate toxins and develop toxemia if not detoxified by the liver which forms an active defense barrier against excess poisons from the digestive tract. Thus, man is constantly under the threat of poisoning. He contributes to his own destruction, and incessantly tries to commit suicide through auto-intoxication."*

In 1913 a French medical doctor, Guillaume Guelpa, wrote a book called *The Guelpa Method – Detoxification of the Body*. His view was that disease and its symptoms were simply the result of an excess of toxins in our body, from auto-intoxication of the colon, and excessive food. In his book he claimed that medicine lost the whole vision of the body and its interaction with the environment. He attacked the theory of Pasteur that prioritized microbes as the cause of disease over the body's defense mechanism and the use of vaccines instead of revitalizing the body. Dr. Guelpa advocated diet, fasting, and intestinal enemas to detoxify the body.

There are long held theories which we cannot ignore until they are disproved by science, for example, the function of the liver in the transformation of toxins and xenobiotics. As for self-destruction through auto-intoxication, Bouchard was always correct, as cancer, a deadly disease has deep-seated basis in auto-intoxication. It is with good reason Dr. Tilden, also refers to malignant toxemia in his book.

Speaking from my own experience, there are hardly any cancers with a good colon having proper elimination. According to Dr. Kousmine, to whom I referred above, as well as from my own observation, 85% of cancer patients are unhealthy and about 90% suffer from constipation. I developed this theory some thirty-five years ago after observing several hundreds of cases about which I had lectured and published some documents, especially in relation to breast cancer and constipation.

This theory was explained in detail in one of my important books entitled, *The Health Revolution*, printed about ten years ago, which subsequently led me to recently publish additional articles on its involvement.

In his book *Predicative Medicine: A Fantastic Expectation*, (Albin Michel, Paris, 1990 edition) Dr. Alain Carnic, a graduate in oncological studies, wrote as follows: "A bad diet, through putrefactions, will destabilize the intestinal barrier (defense mechanism) effect, attack the immune system, and lead to degenerative diseases and many cancers." This cannot be clearer coming from a graduate oncology medical doctor, most probably having an open mind with an interest in the cause of degenerative diseases.

In the past, auto-intoxication was intrinsic in the teaching of the faculties of medicine in various European countries, but today it has totally disappeared in medical research. A return to it would certainly be useful since conventional medical practice has not yet managed, through its system, to reduce illnesses in humans and make them healthier.

I cited some pioneering doctors who supported these theories, most of them were authors of works which are unknown or ignored today. By the same token, one can argue that in spite of everything, we have no concrete proof regarding auto-intoxication, yet through observation and experience we are in a favorable position to hypothesize on colon auto-intoxication and intoxication of the organism. Moreover today, there are laboratory tests which can monitor any bad functional condition, such as liver detox, intestinal membrane permeability, and kidney elimination, to quote some examples.

Looking back, we cannot ignore the works of Alexis Carrel, who indeed made the major contribution to the theory of organic intoxication that came precisely from his scientific research.

Who was Alexis Carrel?

A French surgical doctor and Nobel Prize winner for Medicine and Physiology in 1912, Alexis Carrel became famous through his book distributed world-wide, which harmoniously mixes medicine, sociology, and philosophy: *Man is Unknown*.

There are only a few people who still remember Alexis Carrel, yet for those of us younger than forty, his name is unknown. I had only vaguely heard about Alexis Carrel until I was lucky enough to meet at a seminar, a medical homeopathic doctor, Dr. Ribolet. Strangely enough, he was also the president of the association called "Friends of Dr. Alexis Carrel," destined to keep his image and works alive. Dr. Ribolet was a fervent practitioner of Kneipp's hydrotherapy treatments, running his practice within a French spa. Thanks to him, I managed at the same time, to study some of Alexis Carrel's works. I further improved my knowledge on hydrotherapy, which I first discovered at Dr. Bernard Jensen's Hidden Valley Health Ranch.

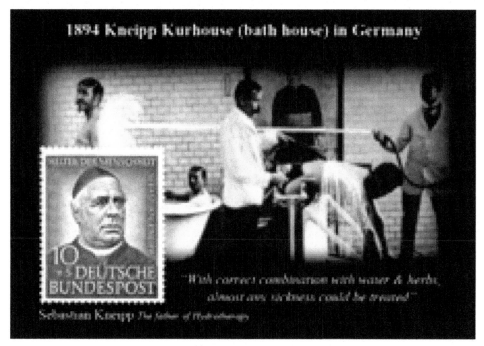

Abbot Sebastian Kneipp

Dr. Jensen had even traveled to Germany's Bad Warishofen's city spa to learn about the hydrotherapy methods of Abbot Sebastian Kneipp, known as the Father of Modern Hydrotherapy. Abbot Kneip himself had been very sick. He discovered in a book by Vincent Priessnitz (1799-1851), the benefit of water-cure. In 1822, he set up the first nature-cure and water treatment institute in Grafenburg. Even today, this old medicine technique is still used in many German and Swiss clinics, being very beneficial in treating many intestinal disorders.

Alexis Carrel, who worked at the Rockefeller Institute in New York, became known for his laboratory experiments with chicken embryos and tissues. Whereby he proved that when one harvests a live tissue grown in a test tube, it was necessary to provide it with a volume of liquid that is equal to two thousand times its own volume in order for it not to be poisoned by the food residues. Moreover, it required a gaseous atmosphere ten times higher than its liquid means. If we calculated the same proportions in relation to the human body, 200,000 liters of nutritive liquid would be required. We use seven to eight liters of blood a day and twenty liters of lymph, and even so, we are not poisoned. The truth is that water seems to be indispensable for life as the human body is made up of 60% to 70% water. Unfortunately, Dr. Alexis Carrel's discoveries were not consistent with the current level of medical conception based on local disease, or for that matter sterile blood. This doctrine unfortunately continues to dominate the international medical community's thinking and theory.

Today new discoveries through the observation of a drop of fresh blood through the Live Blood Analysis microscopy system, using amplification up to 18,000X, such as the one designed by my colleague and friend, the late Robert Bradford Ph.D. This special microscope was able to show many types of microorganisms, intestinal bacteria, fungus-like Candida, even Borrelia in the blood of patients with disease and even those considered healthy at the moment. This doesn't mean that you have or will have a cancer. While Candida overgrowth from a deficient immune system and poor oxygen status can cause some serious problems, they are of more consequence, but not the cause of cancer. Often I observe candidiasis, a bacterial invasion in pregnant women, where regular blood analysis certainly misses something since it may affect the future unborn child. However, current researchers are starting increasingly to reconsider the theory of intoxication based upon Alexis Carrel's works.

Alexis Carrel's Predictions

Alexis Carrel (1973-1944) predicted the crisis of modern civilization, future wars, criminality, social behavioral and psychological disorders, especially the current fall in birthrates in Western countries. He stressed that our civilization is in a danger that simultaneously menaces race, nations, and individuals. Each one suffers already from existing confusion in our life, our social institutions, and from a general weakening of our moral sense, as well as from economic insecurity, and from diseases that have become a major industry in our modern society, involved more in multi-billion dollar profits but not in improving the health status of mankind, especially our children.

Each one of us is a cause and consequence in our modern society. With science, we continue to ignore ourselves, having lost the development of our physiological, intellectual, and spiritual potentialities. Alexis Carrel predicted the decline of our civilization similar to that of the Roman Empire. With good reason Alexis Carrel stressed that our ignorance is profound. What about today's society, just seventy-five years later? In one way we have been the victims of a disastrous illusion that we can live and forget our natural laws, building our lives based upon materialism. We have totally ignored the laws that regulate our bodies, our minds, and our health. We just rely upon pharmaceutical drugs to bombard our sick bodies, but we are not really any healthier or happier.

The loss of morality is probably responsible for what is going on in the world of science and medicine, where without morals a doctor becomes dangerous for others, since health and well-being is not a priority to him but rather how he can make more money. It is scary to realize that the U.S. nation is now in decline, and that disease is now a multi-billion dollar industry. $3.8 trillion health spending by the U.S. government was projected in 2013, while in 2012 the spending was $2.8 trillion, yet to the contrary, the American people are far from being healthier. This is why we have to forget a little bit about science, about what we have learned in universities, learned from a cadaver cut in few pieces, and our indoctrination by medical academicians and the pharmaceutical industry. Perhaps we can put our mind on Alexis Carrel's book, heed his advice, so we may act with more sense, more morals, and really try to be good doctors.

Fortunately, these great advances in biology throw new light on the human body. They have already indicated that the human body contains the incredible number of 60 thousand billion cells which are literally floating in an internal sea made up of cellular serum in which there are currents capable of nourishing and detoxifying. These are the blood and lymphatic systems.

Obviously, extra cellular liquids, just as in the circulatory system, must always be free of toxins and rich in nutrients. How can we ever figure that intoxicated blood and poor nutrient levels can nourish cells and activate their function? Intoxicated blood also intoxicates tissues and cells. It also decreases the oxygen level in blood circulation, especially if viscosity coats red cells. One can be surprised by looking at the blood of intoxicated patients taking excessive medical prescriptions, through Live Blood Microscopy analysis. It can reveal heavy mucous, as well as red, green, blue, or black colored crystals, which can also cause more serious consequences by damaging the kidneys (You can see a few more examples on my website but modern medicine seems not to worry about these facts).

Our body is a masterpiece. If it were to be completely unfolded and laid out, the cellular tissues would occupy a surface area of 492 acres with 60,000 miles of blood capillaries serving as a channel to irrigate this enormous surface. What if a gardener were to water his vegetable garden with drain water? He would run the risk of poisoning himself, would he not? How could he not become self- intoxicated with industrial, polluted food from modern agriculture? Fortunately, the liquids circulate through the body at different speeds, according to our life style, in particular the lymphatic stream, which has the task of capturing the intracellular and extra cellular toxins and other metabolic waste in order to eliminate them. In order to prevent congestion, the lymphatic system provides for some waste disposal—the ganglia—which allows for the establishment of a barrier against an excess of microbes and other toxins.

But not everything is that simple since the lymphatic current can stagnate and clog. As a consequence, we have lymphatic disorders that are the cause of numerous problems such as severe fatigue, swollen legs, obesity, liquid retention, arthritis, and even more severe lymphatic illnesses.

Yet, our body is wonderfully conceived. It possesses an incredible group of organs called the emunctory organs: the kidneys, the skin, the lungs, and the colon, with special filters, which are the liver and the lymphatic system. This system has the task of eliminating the intracellular and extracellular waste, to eventually be eliminated by the kidney, and cleaning our organism in order to prevent overload and intoxication. If this were not the case, then why would the human body have been endowed with such organs capable of filtering and detoxifying? According to logical thought, this concept also suggests that in case of these organs malfunctioning, intoxication would then be possible.

We begin to realize this when we change the way we maintain and take care of the body, usually in the wrong way and sometimes with tragic consequences.

We have to agree that every one of us must look after our body with respect and intelligence. This is a conversation I always have with my patients. We must give some value to our body, which was what Dr. Jensen taught me. If you keep eating hot dogs, and this is the only value you give to your body, there will be a price to pay. Being healthy and disease prevention necessitates adopting a more balanced way of living and eating, as well as developing a different attitude about what should be done if we want to prevent disease. Our body is not a garbage bin, but overeating junk food soon turns it to garbage, meaning an intoxicated body.

Science places prime importance on chemistry and industrial food forgetting the basis of life that is sustained through a balanced, natural and appropriate dietary style based on nutritional value, since it has greatly affected our immune system and our other defense mechanisms leading to the chronic and degenerative diseases that we know today. Unfortunately, we have forgotten the basis of live, natural food and appropriate dietary style based on nutritional value. This can be disastrous since we forget about our body's own defenses and rely totally on medical care. "Let food be your medicine and medicine your food" was proclaimed both by Hippocrates and Avicenna.

Not long ago I received a visit from a cancer patient whose last tests were disturbing as the tumoral markers had increased disastrously. Her main worry was whether or not to get the flu shot, but she was in a critical situation and suffering from chemotherapy side effects. We continue to live with false hopes, following fixed ideas of not considering the human body or its nutritional needs, while continuing in the search for an easy remedy which can solve everything.

The thymus is the gland in charge of the maturation of lymphocytes produced in the bone marrow and the so-called T-lymphocytes, important for fighting infections. Our intestine also produces lymphocytes as part of the local immune defense. As a consequence of the constant attacks, pollution, stress and bad diets, we reduce our immune resistance and open the door to all viruses and bacteria. Every individual is genetically different in the face of pollution or faced with viral infection. Every individual creates their own auto-intoxication, which in turn reduces immune defenses and creates a fertile ground for bacteria and viruses.

Indeed, when blood is intoxicated, some big white cells, such as macrophages, are in charge of capturing food waste, bacteria, and dead cells in order to transport them to the elimination organs. The French doctor Jean Seignalet M.D., Immunologist and Biologist, carried out and published various works on this subject. Considering that blood is constantly being intoxicated by today's life style, the immune system is easily worn out leaving it open to possible cancerous cell development.

In truth, there is still no logical explanation why a tumor evolves in the organism when it is supposedly capable of inhibiting or destroying it through specific immune cells. This is why the hypothesis of colon auto-intoxication becomes logical in the pathogenesis of cancer, also involving the liver which filters toxins but fails to eliminate the excess of toxic substances because of a lack of detoxifying enzymes.

In conclusion, we can say that auto-intoxication is the direct result of a chronic intoxication of the colon, which is incapable of purifying itself. In truth, it starts with the accumulation of a quantity of harmful substances, which will overflow beyond the borders of the colon to be absorbed by the organism.

The Origin of Intestinal Putrefaction

We know that all foods have the tendency to deteriorate in the presence of light, oxygen, and heat. That is why we keep them in the refrigerator in the cold and far from light. Remember that it is the free radicals of oxygen present in the atmosphere that are responsible for food deterioration.

Industrially grown vegetables have a greater tendency towards putrefaction, even if kept in the refrigerator, because they lack antioxidants and quickly deteriorate from the action of oxy-radicals. Another example of food deterioration is as follows: if we leave a plate of fruit on the table it will begin to deteriorate after a few days, and rot in the end. The time the fruit remains fresh depends on their quality and richness in antioxidants.

Daylight along with oxygen causes an interaction, giving rise to free radicals when combined with the environmental temperature lead to food putrefaction.

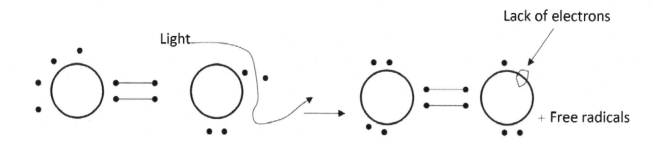

Light absorbing the electron of a molecule of oxygen = radical of oxygen

Another modern day phenomenon is farmers harvesting green unripe fruits, in order to prevent losses, which are also deficient in antioxidants. People buy these fruits and after a few days they rot without having ripened.

It is obvious that temperature also plays an important role in conservation or putrefaction of food. In the intestines where the temperature is elevated, when certain foods such as meat, charcuterie, fish, and eggs are kept for longer than necessary for absorption, they will quickly begin to alter. Moreover, foods such as dairy products and eggs also have the tendency to form mucous in the intestines making good absorption of nutrients difficult, where this mucous sticks to the intestinal walls preventing transformed foods from penetrating the blood stream. For the best results, food must quickly transit through the intestinal tract to be transformed, and immediately after, absorbed by the blood stream. A slow digestion or badly digested food, when combined with high temperature, will produce intestinal putrefactions.

Cooked foods are not so good since most enzymes are destroyed during cooking and take longer to be digested. If you eat raw foods, you'll get hungry much quicker since it's already been proven these foods are quickly digested and absorbed. And the problem is worsened when foods are combined, for example: meat + rice + French fries, or even additional fried eggs, which are popular in Portugal. These dietary errors may be responsible for causing intestinal putrefactions with toxic bacteria, which become concentrated, feasting on the food residues and their favorite source of food. Intestinal gasses are simply the consequence of bacterial action on hotbeds of putrefaction.

Badly digested food can remain in the intestine for several hours, even days, before the organism can absorb or eliminate them. But there are still some residues that are not completely eliminated which are a result of daily meals, heavy meals, and abuse of certain unhealthy foods.

If once in a while we overeat, but immediately after return to the correct diet, it is not serious. But if we habitually and daily abuse food, causing a permanent accumulation of putrefied food residues and unwanted bacteria, we can end up developing serious intestinal problems, and consequently diseases which follow. We seriously need to think about avoiding these bad eating habits.

The accumulation of toxins can easily enter the blood stream. Fortunately, we have a key organ capable of defending us against the invasion of toxins in the blood stream. This is the liver. Our liver defends us and plays an important detoxifying role, which can remove the flow of toxic residue, kill bacteria, prevent blood intoxication, and as a consequence, cellular intoxication.

The Attack of Pollutants on the Liver

There is little doubt that the alarming increase in chronic and degenerative illnesses, including cancer, are in part linked to the liver's incapacity to detoxify from exogenous chemical agents and the continual flow of toxins from the intestine. Moreover, the lack of certain vitamins such as vitamins A, C, E, methionine, sulfur, and other nutrients in today's diet, reduce the liver's ability to detoxify pollutants. Besides endogenous toxins, the liver still has to face an incredible number of chemical substances from the excess of pharmaceutical drugs, which is characteristic of our times.

We try to ignore this situation, without giving much thought to the consequences, but what is certain is that this situation is responsible for many diseases of which we do not know the origin and for the increase in hospitalizations and thousands of deaths per year in industrialized countries. In the USA, statistics show that pharmaceutical drugs are responsible for the death of over 200,000 persons per year. The late Senator Ted Kennedy stressed this was an insult to the American people. How many people are killed every year by weapons in the USA, compared with pharmaceutical drugs that kill over one hundred thousand people? Yet, the government still keeps very silent about these numbers.

Over the past decades, I have become increasingly aware of the fact that almost 80% of the patients who come and see me have liver problems. We observe first from a hereditary standpoint, as seen in their irises, coming from our life style which has led us to a great number of dietary errors.

Ever more popular airplane trips, where the quality of the food is increasingly poor, organized holidays in hotels with prices so low that they can only serve low quality food, road trips with stops at road side restaurants, meals in malls, even wedding dinners; these everyday situations result in colon intoxication and may lead to overtaxing and damaging the liver function, and a poor health condition. According to some German pioneers of biological medicine and cancer, such as Dr. Issel and even Dr. Vogel, all the cancer patients harbor a very bad liver.

Not only is the liver involved in most of the chronic and degenerative diseases of persons of middle age, but it is increasingly more apparent in younger people. This means that we are all under the threat of degenerative illnesses from one generation to another. We are not yet sufficiently aware, firstly, of the importance of food in our physical and psychological health, and secondly, of the protective role that the liver plays as a defensive barrier.

I remember the case of a young twenty-eight-year-old woman who suffered from a chronic infection of the bladder of which she could not seem to rid herself. When I began talking to her about her diet, she told me, without thinking, that she ate at restaurants every morning and evening, even on the weekends. Therefore, I gave her a complete dietary regime including advice on life hygiene. To my great surprise, although suffering from considerable inconvenience and a urinary problem, she thought the diet was very complicated. When I asked her what she thought of the importance of the liver in maintaining one's health, she confessed she was completely ignorant on the subject.

As I already mentioned, not many people are aware of the role played by the elimination organs and by the liver being a protective filter. Moreover, the liver also plays a fundamental role in digesting food, storing vitamin A, synthesizing proteins and hormones, and participates in the production of good red blood cells. If we keep eating unbalanced and very heavy meals, over time this may overtax the liver, reduce its function and capacity to detoxify, and become even more harmful to the liver over time. It may then lose its ability because of the increasing exogenous substances the subtly penetrate the organism through food, water, and air.

Let us examine this example, which illustrates the liver's ability to protect the organism against toxic substances. If we inject a toxic substance into the portal vein of a dog, it would not die. This would require three or four repeated injections. On the contrary, if we were to inject a poisonous substance into a normal vein of the dog, he would die within a few minutes of the injection. It is therefore understandable that our liver is a real barrier of defense against exogenous pollutants and endogenous toxins.

But, over the years, the liver starts to wear out and loose its ability because of the numerous external substances that subtly penetrate the organism. In the long run, these consequences are unforeseeable and in most cases are severe, since many of these substances are carcinogenic where it all depends on our genetic ability to metabolize and eliminate them.

The list is enormous among the 60,000 chemicals used on the market that include: artificial colors, artificial flavors, preserving agents, pesticides, and herbicides. All of these are dangerous and all have the approval of the Food and Drug Administration or the European Health Agency, both being under the control of Big Pharma. Toxic metals, such as mercury in particular, are dangerous for health and are found in water, in sea and fresh water fish, as well as in vaccines. Aluminum, containing excessive quantities of hydrocarbons, is being used ever more frequently for packing food, meats, smoked fish, and poses a further attack against correct liver function.

How the Intestine Reacts to Pollutants

There are certain exogenous chemical substances given the technical name of "xenobiotics," which include detergents that are liposoluble in the cellular membranes. This means that they can easily enter the membranes of cells that are rich in fatty acids. Their behavior is varied. They can, for example, produce free radicals when entering the membrane. These free radicals damage the structure of the cellular membrane, puncture its surface, and increase permeability disturbing its function. Not only does the membrane protect the interior of the cells, but through external receptor cells, form a communication network from one point to another or from one cell to many others.

The intestinal mucosa in our organism is constantly under attack, and is responsible for what we call a "leaky gut" or permeability of the membrane, allowing non-digested protein and bacteria to enter into blood circulation, as explained previously. However, the body is not equipped with enzymes to break up these large molecules which can migrate to tissue organs and trigger disease, as explained previously.

Allergy as well as a number of auto-immune diseases may originate from a hyper permeability of the mucous membrane, including rheumatoid arthritis. Non digested food entering into the blood induces an immune response, after which immune cells start to attack the body. This topic will be discussed further on in this chapter.

There are already private testing labs, like Great Smokies Diagnostic laboratory, that offer tests to check on intestinal permeability, liver detox, and heavy metal intoxication, which is useful when it comes to improving health status or treating disease. This may be important after an Iridology check-up that empirically can detect such situations, which, of course, require clinical experience and dialogue with patients. A check up with the Vega computerized system can also underline heavy metal intoxication, activate liver detoxification or poor liver or colon function. I always use first the Vega check up with patients before they enter for consultation. Usually, the Vega machine report matches up with the Iridology exam results.

We cannot separate out the colon from a variety of symptoms, because accumulated toxins in some specific area of the colon, created by a condition of irritation, which by reflex may affect other organs such as some local dysfunction or by causing pain, for which we don't know the cause. Iris observation has always shown in this case; darker tissue in the portion of the colon involving the collarette when pointing toward a specific organ, indicating the cause of the problem.

Intestinal Bacteria

Our body can be intoxicated by excess toxins and macromolecules from non-digested food, but also by intestinal bacteria that penetrate the barrier because of its hyperpermeability and invade the blood stream and cause, not only infection, but also, according to the Nobel Prize in Medicine, Professor Luc Montagnier, can be associated with diseases such as Parkinson's, Alzheimer's, diabetes, and cancer.

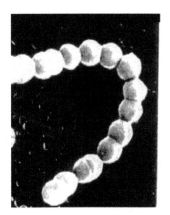 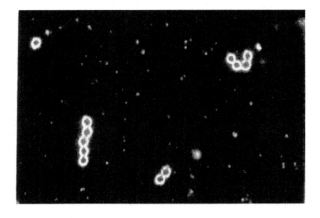

Intestinal bacteria in fresh blood specimens

This problem has never been well thought out, as it is difficult for currently accepted medical thinking to accept that the intestine could become permeable. We have, for many years, observed intestinal bacteria in fresh blood specimens. My book was published several years before Professor Montagnier delivered his lecture in Lisbon. At the time he gave an interview with local journalists who published an article in the most popular Portuguese daily newspaper called, "Alzheimer's Has an Origin In The Intestine," which indeed was a great support to my own work and theory. According to Professor Montagnier, micoplasma are the co-activator of the AIDS virus, but of course this theory was not accepted by official virologists, in charge of manipulating the media, their understanding of this disease in the public eye. This was also related to the billions of dollars generated by anti-viral drug sales.

Alzheimer's may well have an origin in the intestine, which justifies the following question in my book regarding whether the disease had its origin first in the brain, or in the colon.

Today, because of our increasingly artificial diet, we ourselves assist in the growth of bacteria and their migration into the blood stream, crossing the intestinal barrier. Once in the blood stream, they can multiply in excess, adhere to and damage epithelial cells, freeing toxins that are the source of many inflammatory processes. Amongst the most dangerous bacteria we can cite are staphylococcus, streptobacillus, clostridium, shigella, and salmonella. In an alkaline terrain these bacteria can take on an even more aggressive form.

It is true that this new theory debunks the classic medical dogma based on Pasteur's research that stipulates disease is caused by exogenous microbes, being opposite of the theory of Antoine Bechamps, the enemy of Pasteur. In fact, Pasteur took advantage of Bechamps who discovered a tiny microorganism in blood he called Microzima. More popular at the time, Pasteur made a presentation at the Academy of Medicine and said that he had discovered exogenous microorganisms that he called Microbes, derived from Microzima. Bechamps was attacked with such fanaticism that he could not publish his book in France. Before he died, he gave the document to an English doctor, Montague R. Leverson M.D. PhD, who, in 1912, published the book in England and was later republished in Australia in 1988, *The Blood and Its Third Anatomical Element*, is still forbidden in France even today. Amen!

Previously I had explained about what we call a leaky gut, which allows harmful bacteria to penetrate into the bloodstream. Today it is already possible to establish and point out the presence of Candida in blood. Thirty years ago, we faced strong criticism when my colleagues Bob Bradford, Majid Ali, M.D., and I demonstrated, through the observation of a drop of fresh blood, the presence of Candida. Today, however, the question of Candida hotbeds in the blood circulation is accepted and beyond the shadow of a doubt.

In order to balance the acid-base terrain, nature has provided us with fruits and vegetables with a pH. value that can vary between approximately pH. 6.80 to pH. 3.20 depending on the food we eat. This pH. range includes moderately to middle alkaline vegetables or moderately to middle acidic, while some foods like dairy, meat, and shellfish are highly acidic. We should keep a balance and never eat an excess of highly alkaline food or highly acidic food. Basically, by eating large portions of varied vegetables, we develop infections less frequently because this keeps the blood slightly alkaline. Moderately acidic food is also necessary to maintain this balance.

Candida

The role of Candida, a kind of fungus, the most common form of which is *Candida albicans*, and its involvement in physical and nervous disorders is still fairly recent. They are considered to be responsible, among other problems, for chronic fatigue, nervousness, headaches, aggressiveness, and digestive disorders.

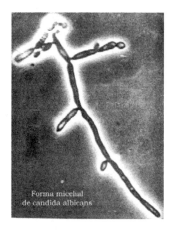

Forma micelial de candida albicans

Normally yeast forms like Candida, live in the intestine and in the body's mucus, *Candida albicans* being the most common. Inside the intestines, Candida adopts a mycelium form, sticking to the intestinal walls, and spreads its tentacles between the mucus cells, thereby increasing the permeability of the intestinal barrier.

The intestinal balance always forms a barrier against the dangerous proliferation of Candida, but under the effect of intoxication, the barrier is altered and becomes imbalanced. In this way, the Candida manages to enter the blood stream, dragging other bacteria along with it. In the blood Candida produces some toxins which associate with a number of symptoms and diseases including rheumatoid arthritis, nervousness, aggressivity, muscular pains, headache, fatigue, and menstrual pains. Something that we never think about, which needs some correction is food style, oxygen supply, and immune stimulation.

Intoxicated Blood

Resulting from an intoxicated colon, toxins further intoxicate the blood along with heavy crystals, oxidized fats, bacteria, yeast-form like Candida, and other microorganisms. Majid Ali M.D., refers to this in his book, *Oxygen and Aging*, as Primordial Life Forms (PLFs). An LBA observation may show major bacterial invasion, amongst which are micoplasma (very common today) that may penetrate tissues and cells of the body and be associated with additional symptoms and diseases. It is incredible that medical doctors are not only totally ignorant about what can be observed in a small drop of fresh blood, but they simply show no interest to learn something new and relevant.

If the body is unable to detoxify and expulse excess toxins produced by bacteria, they keep circulating in blood, irritate the nerves, kidneys, and often the bladder, causing inflammation especially to young women, who today are less resistant to bacterial attack.

In the presence of this degree of intoxication, the organism then tries to stimulate a detoxification process. It therefore activates the thyroid and lymphatic ganglion functions in charge of protecting us against toxins and microbes.

At first, in an attempt to accelerate detoxification in the circulating blood, the thyroid begins to work faster, it loses control, and begins to increase in volume, but in time this hyperactivity becomes ominous. After a certain amount of time, it reduces its rhythm and falls into hypo-activity. No longer managing to filter toxins, it becomes infected and degenerates. It transforms into a ball known as a goiter, which is characteristic in people who suffer from chronic constipation. When the goiter becomes troublesome, the path that follows is excision. Although its excision seems to be an inevitable solution, it is deceptive, as this organ is then missing from the body. In fact, the thyroid produces important hormones, such as thyroxin that controls the absorption of oxygen in the cells, with the aim of stimulating the metabolism. For the same reason, iodine is equally important in activating thyroid functions. However, it is not a decisive factor, as even many people who live in close proximity to the sea develop goiter.

The thyroid is equally responsible for regulating the level of blood sugar, promoting calcium homeostasis in the blood, regulating the temperature of the organism, and also, very important, enhancing the reaction of the nervous system when faced with stress. In these cases, the functions of the organism are diminished, unexplained fatigue appears, or there are pains in the bones. But above all, the organism continues to intoxicate itself faster without sounding any alarm. From here on, the organism begins to become unbalanced, leaving itself open to disease, although from a medical point of view we are considered to be in good health.

The Influence of Meat in the Organism's Intoxication

Meat is a food with a high protein value considered until some years ago by the medical community to be an essential food for adults and children. However abuse of cooked meat can become a real problem, since when cooked, it produces harmful toxic substances that first intoxicate the colon and then the blood, eventually poisoning the cells.

Eating an excess amount of meat during a meal, with a low intake of vegetables, first becomes a serious handicap for intestinal transit, since meat does not contain fibers and by not eating vegetables we reduce the need for vitamins, minerals, and enzymes that our body needs. This is the case of the U.S., leading the world with the highest consumption, 260 lbs. of meat per capita each year, and is also first in the world as far as death by cancer and cardiovascular diseases go. The U.S. comes in at the 27th position (the last) for health in industrialized countries, which has shown a real decline of health status among its population.

Worldwide, the Japanese eat the least amount of meat and dairy products. They also have the lowest percentage of cancer and cardiovascular diseases, followed by Cretans whose diet has recently been the object of various scientific studies.

We have come to a point where we should consider changing our eating habits, when meat becomes the main food on our plate. We need a revision of our ideas and concepts, many of which are erroneous, such as the theory of calories and the belief that meat is considered essential for life. Modern Western society is far from being a role model for physical and psychic health. But we are prisoners of a myth that considers and depicts us to be in a modern and developed society.

For a long time, I personally have wondered, similar to animals, if humans may also be considered to be carnivores. There are several physiological reasons against this concept. First, the human being does not possess the teeth, the physiology, or carnivore-like intestinal morphology to digest animal proteins. Man has flat molars for chewing food, whereas carnivores have pointed, well-developed canines as well as sharp molars. We must chew meat well for it to be correctly digested. Dogs, for example can grind meat quickly in their mouths and swallow it, without even chewing it. We are not able to do the same thing.

Our saliva is alkaline, but with carnivores their saliva is very acidic to efficiently digest animal proteins. In order to digest the ground-up muscles and bones, a carnivore's stomach contains ten times more acid salts than that of man. Finally, while our digestive tract is just over six meters long with folds and pleats, a carnivore's is short and straight to prevent putrefaction. When referencing meat, a wild animal can eat raw meat without falling ill, unlike humans. Chimpanzees are very similar to humans as far as Phylogenic evolution goes and possess 99.2% of similar human genes. In the wild they only eat raw food, and when captive in a laboratory or in a zoo, they can hardly tolerate cooked food.

Starting from this comparison, there is a high likelihood that the abuse of meat damages our digestive tract and transforms it into a real hotbed for disorders, putrefaction, and diseases. We have previously discussed colon cancer, which is really a problem linked with an excess of meat intake. Vegetarian people do not develop colon cancer and we should think about this. During the last world war (1939-1945) Holland, as well many other countries, were occupied by the German Army and people were subjected to major food restrictions, mainly meat. After three years, cancer disease started to really decrease, but few years after the war it began to increase again and here we are, back once again, when we have an excess consumption of meat and other foods as a cause of cancer. After the war many industries started to grow and develop and this was especially true for agriculture and raising bovines to increase the sale and consumption of meat that became an even important food in our diets.

We will see further that with lack of information and not knowing how to eat correctly, this can really be a factor leading to disease. Meat, especially when cooked and eaten in excess, leads to the production of toxic substances that we discussed in the book that are responsible for a number of organic disorders and symptoms that particularly overtax the liver and kidney function. This leads not only to auto-intoxication, which is one of the main causes of chronic and degenerative disease, but to kidney failure as well, relevant in today's contemporary society in epidemic proportion. However, becoming a vegetarian is often an option from a psychological standpoint, along with the desire to live healthier with a clean body. During the last two decades, I had influenced hundreds of patients, including young ones and those middle aged, to change their diet and avoid meat eating, which was a wonderful resolution.

Proteolytic Bacteria and Intestinal Poisons

We are going to analyze red meat intake in our daily diet including excess and cooked (particularly over-cooked) red meat, along with a lower vegetable intake which reduces nutrient and fiber intake. Such consumption can be responsible for a number of Health problems, and even kidney failure in the long term (or short term depending on hereditary status). Cooked red meat is badly digested, subject to inefficient mastication, often swallowed too quickly and remains longer in the large intestine causing putrefaction. Consequently intestinal feces also contain toxic compounds and worms. Furthermore, badly digested animal protein can enter the blood circulation through intestinal hyper- permeability and trigger immune response and auto-immune disease.

Through chemical transformation, these feces become an intentional source of poisonous substances for the body. These badly digested proteins are attacked by bacteria that decompose them and then subject them to a process known as decarboxylation, which is responsible for the formation of toxic amines.

Here is a known list of decarboxylation produced by amino acids, toxic amines:

Tryptophan	Indol and escatol
Cysteine	Mercaptan
Tyrosine	Tyramine
Lysine	Cadaverin
Arginine	Agmantinase
Ornithine	Putrescine
Histidine	Histamine

These substances, along with many others, were largely identified in England in 1912, by a group of seventy-five famous doctors considered at that time as the greatest surgical genius in England. During a meeting at the Royal Society of Medicine, they discussed the importance of colon hygiene and how a bad diet increased a condition of auto-intoxication in patients. According to Lane, when the tissues of the body have degenerated through an excess of poisons coming from the colon, a condition of auto-intoxication cancer can arise, being mistaken by patients as new disease symptoms. In his book called *The Treatment of Intestinal Chronic Stasis*, Lane wrote the following, "Hippocrates always spoke to the people of Athens that it was essential to have large bowel movement after each meal and to be sure it is necessary to eat little meat, good bread, fruits and vegetables." Where are we today in our beliefs and practices regarding this concept? I have already mentioned and emphasized that for most medical doctors, constipation is not important to our health status.

I have often asked myself: how can such important factors have escaped all interest from contemporary medicine? On the other hand, today we suffer from the consequences of a completely sterile intestinal flora, permeable to all pathogenic bacterial attacks. The discovery of antibiotics diverted a lot of new research subjects, since medicine at that time thought it could control all known bacteria with antibiotics, while the immune system remained totally neglected.

It would be impossible to specify all the toxic amines in detail. We will focus on the most important ones and their consequences on our state of health. We will see that not knowing how to eat correctly can be a factor leading to disease, because of an uncontrolled production of chemical substances can lead us to auto-intoxication. The reactions of these substances are often very severe on the organism.

Consequences of Amines in the Organism

Phenol, for example, is extremely toxic. This toxin is usually used as an antimicrobial agent. It acts as a corrosive, which can destroy the cover of the intestinal membrane and reach as far as the kidneys.

Generated in the intestine, Phenol is absorbed by the blood after having been transformed by the liver. In its toxic form, it must pass through the kidneys, and an excess of this substance can actually attack the kidneys. Therefore, we can see where overly carnivorous diets can lead us. That is, they can lead us to dialysis centers, which, as matter of fact, are overcrowded with patients of all ages.

Escatol produced by bacterial action on tryptophan, can cause serious disorders to the nervous and circulatory systems. I have always considered excessive meat consumption as being responsible for aggressiveness in adolescents. By modifying their diet, in particular reducing the consumption of meat for thirty or forty days, I have obtained a complete change in the personality of these youngsters.

Another factor linked to the excessive consumption of meat is bad breath about which so many people, particularly women complain. Often when receiving patients for the first time, I notice an unpleasant breath, without these people noticing it or being aware of this state. The general rule is that bad breath is always accompanied by unpleasant smelling feces, and then we can speak of intestinal putrefactions. These factors indicate a strong intestinal concentration of escatol and indol. It is a pity that little importance is given to this situation, as we have at least two diagnostic elements that show auto-intoxication.

With so many technical advances, and medicine being so positively superior, how is it that it is not able to explain the cause of a simple bad breath? A simple, traditional Chinese doctor understands the problem by examining the tongue of his patient. Do not be surprised, since the tongue reveals hepatic and intestinal problems.

Mercaptan is another substance, which comes from the decomposition of cysteine, causing an uncontrollable escape of intestinal gas that often has a nauseating smell, usually highly embarrassing in a social context. This gas signals bad protein digestion. As it accumulates in the intestine it enters the blood stream and can disturb the heart and cause migraines.

Tyramine is a substance putrefied by tyrosine. It causes the release of the norepinephrine hormone which disturbs the blood vessels, narrowing them and increasing blood hypertension.

Ammonia is another more common toxic substance formed in the intestine. The liver transforms ammonia in urea, which is eliminated by the kidneys. In cases of hepatic illnesses or cirrhosis, the level of ammonia in the blood system increases sometimes causing a coma or even death. Ammonia can infiltrate the organism in two ways, either by infiltrating the blood stream in large quantities, or by attacking the liver causing hepatitis or even cirrhosis. If ammonia infiltrates the spinal cord and cerebral fluids, it can cause serious nervous and mental problems.

An Experiment Carried Out by the National College of Chiropractic – Chicago

In an interesting experiment carried out some years ago by the National College of Chiropractic, Chicago, autopsies carried out on three hundred bodies enabled them to determine the condition of the colon in these deceased patients.

Some had only had an elimination every three or four days, which often occurs in many of the patients who come to see me. The results were incredible. A normal colon has a diameter of just over 2 inches, but in the bodies autopsied it reached nearly 5 inches in diameter. This is explained by the fact that the intestinal walls were encrusted with a layer of feces containing badly digested food and mucus about an inch and a half thick.

I was not overly surprised, as so many of the women who come to see me, have bloated abdomens, lazy intestines, and after detoxifying treatment, they eliminate enormous quantities of fecal matter, mucus, and intestinal parasites. The quantity of feces that accumulate in the colon is surprising and can be eliminated with a detox program as the one suggested in Chapter VI.

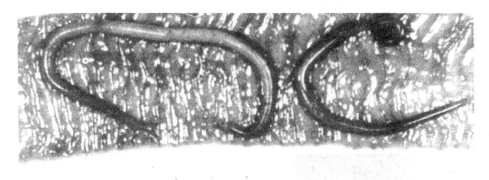

Ascaris Lumbricoides in the bowel (From Smith, A.L.:
Principles of microbiology, ed.8, St. Louis, 1977, The C.V. Mosby Co.)

In our modern society hospitals are still a necessity, but on the other hand, they become more like factories were patients lost their personality, where they were just bombarded with all kinds of medical drugs in excess. Food and nutrition were not considered an important factor, no matter who the patient, their age, the disease, or complaint, often making the patient's condition even worse, especially when interned for a couple of weeks or months and even longer in some cases I know about where the family has to bring some food and prepared vegetable juice to their relative.

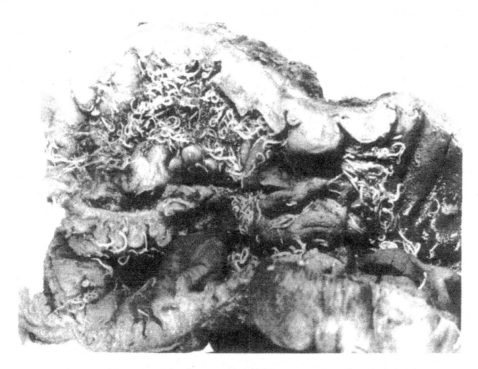

Trichuris trichiura, massive infestation in a child causing strong diarrhea and death.
A segment of the intestine was opened to show the number of parasites on mucous.
(From Anderson, W.A.D. and Kissane, J.M.: Pathology, ed.7, St. Louis, 1997, The C.V.Mosby Co.)

It would be good if hospitals, such as those found in Germany at the beginning of 1900, could again enjoy the popularity they once had. Dr. Bilz's Health Hospital managed to welcome up to one thousand patients per day, about the same as Louis Khune's sanatorium, where patients had undergone detoxification treatment and learned to maintain their health. At the time, Dr. Bilz published his two volume book set with over two thousand pages, *New Methods to Cure Diseases*, which sold over one million copies. I managed to find the French translation of this book in an old Paris library, a wealth of information and knowledge.

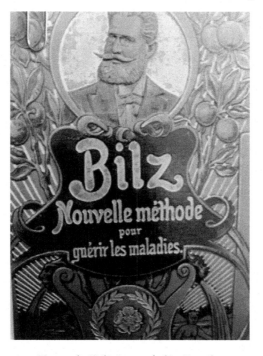

French Edition of the Book

At an earlier time toward the middle of the century in 1846 in France, P. V. Raspail, a well-known medical doctor, wrote a three volume book called *The Natural History of Health and Disease* where he spoke about hot baths, poultices, and enemas with aloes to clean up the colon and blood, and where he mentioned a diet based on vegetables. So, in passing, I learned from this pioneer's works how we may improve, but we really discovered nothing new.

Primitive Diet (Ancestral Nutrition)

The declining health of city dwellers, as well as country people, and the increase in degenerative diseases such as multiple sclerosis, Parkinson's, and cancer arose as a consequence from our bad dietary style and industrialization of food which lost most of its nutritional value, the lack of balance in important vitamins and minerals, such as vitamin C, calcium, potassium, and high sodium intake. Industrial foods lead to damaging the intestinal mucous membrane that becomes permeable and our physiological digestive system, which is not adapted to this type of transformed food. In truth, after the 1945 industrial and pharmaceutical era, the West subverted its eating habits and began to transform and modify food.

There are various stages which show the enormous change in our eating habits, the food proportions, and processed foods that our unprepared body has had to adjust to. Without going too far, or too in-depth into the subject of our ancestors, let us closely examine how Native Americans as well as European populations fed on food that nature offered them. The first Native Americans did not farm the land but limited themselves to gathering wild fruits, plants, and vegetables.

One of my concerns when I was studying in the United States was about learning the rules of health, understanding the healthiest populations, and comparing the various factors contributing to diseases.

One of my first works was to study a tribe of Native Americans called the Seminoles. At that time, they were very vigorous and only farmed vegetables as a sideline. They still fished and hunted, gathered wild edible plants and wild rice along the riverside. Today, due to the invasion of our industrialized and developed society, the Native Americans have become alcoholics, consuming frozen, sterilized, synthetic, preserved, or treated foods. They have joined the rest of the population in the race towards disease and cancer. But this is true for other unspoiled tribes or races in other parts of the world, even here in Portugal where physical, mental illness, and alcoholism have grown since the country was invaded by industrial food as part of the commercial exchange with the E.C.C. We call this modern civilization and progress.

Nowadays, science allows us to carry out highly precise observations. And according to the research and analysis of fossilized fecal matter, we know that during the Mesolithic era the human diet consisted of wild food that was rarely cooked. According to specialists, fire was invented more or less 400,000 years ago, being used above all as a means of protection against wild animals, with no evidence that it was used for cooking food until about 100,000 years ago.

We know that the human genome has only changed 0.5% in the past two million years, according to specialists in genetics. Our organism is still adapted to the original food, a term used by the Swiss physicist, G.C. Burger, and is not used to digest modified molecules (and industrialized food) which our enzymes are unable to metabolize. But, human beings always think they can improve on nature, modifying original food and changing its structure to make it better, but on the contrary it's made worse and responsible overall for the decline of the human health condition.

It is obvious that in a diet prescribed for treating a disease it is necessary to include a large proportion of raw vegetables, over cooked vegetables, and include fresh vegetable juice and fruit, being, "food for the gods." We can say this according to the law of the universe that rules our planet and keeps it working. Our body is directed under certain rules where only natural food may activate a body's functions, especially in the case of disease. It is only after returning to a natural food diet that your body reacts positively.

It is extraordinary to observe the benefits that a balanced nutritional diet, made from natural food has on an ailing body. One can appreciate the reaction it has by the way the patient begins to recover, feeling better both in spirit and body. As I have said, when I started to observe how well organic natural foods and vegetable juices could treat diseases over fifty years ago at Hidden Valley Health Ranch, I knew then it was possible to witness this miracle.

Unfortunately, instead of giving precedence to the quality of food, recent years have been catastrophic for our health. Indeed, we develop a modern, world-wide food fashion that affects all countries and all regions of each country. The classic burger and fries, ready-to-eat microwave food, hot dogs, and other similar meals, garnish the windows and counters of all cafes, even in the most remote areas. We find the same food, or similar food in Peru, Russia, or even in China. In Japan, the introduction of fast food has begun to change their typical morphology. In the same way, diseases affect all regions and countries without discrimination. Differences between the lowest and highest percentages, according to region, dietary habits and soils, tend to diminish. In the near future, we will likely all have the same levels of cancer diseases due to the consumption of processed food and to the abusive use of chemical fertilizers ever present in the soil.

Globally speaking, our food supply with the ever rising consumption of industrial foods, or artificial foods called "replacement foods," are now widely eaten by adults have become catastrophic for juveniles, even babies whose parents only buy food advertised by ad agencies on behalf of multinational companies. Food hygiene rules for infants do not exist; instead they are fed according to the dictates of TV ads, which influence parents and pediatricians.

Sometimes, this is why children and adolescents have intestinal problems, gas, diarrhea, repeated infection, and skin problems that are indicative signs raising alarm. Unfortunately, these symptoms are often combated by large doses of antibiotics, which stealthily intoxicate the organism. It is true that the organism is highly adaptable, adapting itself to processed food. These industrialized foods are not live, made with non-digestible macromolecules which the body cannot metabolize. Most likely they may be a threat to our health, associating with auto-immune disease. The economic news states that there is a large market for pickled, pasteurized, and sterilized ready-to-eat microwave vegetables. But just what exactly are we eating and what will the results be? Obviously this results in a rapid deterioration of our health.

If we compare the habits and customs of our ancestors with those of present-day society, the difference is enormous. The primitive diet was made up of 1/3 good meat (and not always cooked), 2/3 natural vegetables, wild fruits, seeds, wild sprouts, roots, nuts, wild cereals, honey and fish. At that time there were still no cultivated vegetables and cereals.

From the point of view of nutritional balance, our ancestors consumed five times more vitamin C, five times more fibers, half the calories and fats, two times more calcium, and ten times less sodium. With a dietary base of this kind, the remains and toxins are almost always nil. Wild vegetables and sprouts maintain a perfect balance of acidity for aerobic bacteria. The same occurs with fibers. All this balances the intestinal functions and maintains the liver in a perfect condition.

Then, for commercial reasons, ease, or gain, society began to exploit farming, abusing chemical fertilizers, producing and transforming food. One hundred years ago people only consumed 8% transformed food.

> 1900 – People consumed 8% transformed food. 1950 – People consumed 22% transformed food. 2003 – People consumed 75% transformed food.

Today we only consume 25% natural food instead of 100% required by the organism's physiology.

Over the past fifty years, this number has climbed from 22%, reaching 75% today. But personally I am convinced that many young people consume nearly 100% artificial food each day, especially in shopping malls and cinemas, where they gorge themselves on large quantities of popcorn which dangerously increases the risk of obesity and diabetes. This is a rapidly developed disease which doubles every five years and has become one of the main protection markets of the pharmaceutical cartel. Among so many examples I had cited was one day I was told the story of a fourteen-year-old girl who lives in a village and has to have four insulin shots a day, which is apparently considered normal and is accepted by everyone, including the medical establishment.

Nervous Diseases

Twenty years ago from frequent iris observation, I began to notice that as the nervous system degrades and degenerates, chronic and degenerative diseases increased at the same time. The liver becomes overloaded with toxins being unable to efficiently detoxify. The nervous system becomes weaker and more vulnerable to attack from an excess of neurotoxins and other fungus that includes bacterial toxins that irritate nerve ramifications and brain neurons.

While traveling in Switzerland I was lucky to buy from a library of old books, a two-volume set called *Analysis of the Function of the Nervous System* by Dr. M. De La Roche, published in Geneva in 1788. The author stressed that most diseases are simply associated with a bad nervous system (again, confirming my theory). At that time he was not wrong since today many researchers have dedicated themselves to this particular area which studies the causes and effects. Most organs are dependent on the condition of the nervous system like the liver, pancreas, ovaries, or spleen. More recently the condition of the nervous system has also been implicated with cancer disease, by preventing or limiting its development and growth. The nervous system is also associated with the immune system, thus the new science called "neuro-psycho-immunology," indeed associates a decreasing immune activity with nerve dysfunction, anxiety, and depression.

Through Iridology we can check the involvement of auto-intoxication in nervous and psychological problems. If we delve further into earlier works we can find publications that enforce this theory. For example, an American article that appeared in an old magazine published by the American Medical Association in 1917 shows an experiment carried out on 518 cases of nervous and mental disorders such as anxiety, irritability, depression, phobia, and idiocy. This experiment tried to relate these problems to colon intoxication, brought on by bad dietary habits. It is necessary to remember that, at that time, the United States had a large number of immigrants, farmers, and other workers whose diet was based on beans, meat, and potatoes, all swallowed too fast and badly digested. The report showed a reduction or even total elimination of symptoms after detoxification treatment according to a regimen from the Natura Medicatrix of that time.

Some twenty-five years ago, I carried out a special study on a group of 250 women between twenty-three and fifty years of age with the aim of verifying the relationship between chronic constipation and nervous disorders. Apart from an Iridology examination, I used special questionnaires designed to catalogue symptoms such as anxiety, amnesia, irritability, and loss of cognitive functions, in relation to the state of the colon. The result was worrying as it revealed that out of 250 cases 40% to 100% showed multiple symptoms, such as headache, vertigo, insomnia, and nervousness according to the degree of constipation.

Another alarming observation was that the age factor no longer depends or distances us from these symptoms, or even chronic diseases. We are currently witnessing the appearance of disorders of this kind in people of a much younger age. Disorders that range from loss of memory to Alzheimer's disease are appearing in younger generations ever more frequently. In fact, today we are aging before our chronological age, where the iridologist performing an iris observation, can reveal this condition. In 2000, during, The World Iridology Congress held in London where I lectured on Iridology and Aging, I developed and revealed to the audience an iris chart on aging; this being the first chart ever produced for Iridology showing how the iris signs associate with early aging. This aging chart is available in my Internet web site: www.sergejurasunas.com. Obviously, these are elements seen in the iris that make us think. How did we ever get to this situation, and what will the future hold?

A fifty year-old woman came to see me recently saying she felt a lot of confusion in her brain.

She could not remember which roads to use while driving in Lisbon, and she confused one road with another. On the beach she put solar protection on one arm and forgot about the other. At home it was even worse as she confused the lounge with the kitchen.

I suggested that these symptoms were signs attributed to Alzheimer's disease, but in hearing this she panicked rather than analyze how she got to this situation and learn how to fight it. She had heard doctors say that Alzheimer's is incurable and therefore nothing could be done. But recent studies have shown the importance of a diet rich in essential fatty acids and antioxidants as an answer to prevent this disease.

One continues to look for the illness only in the brain, forgetting that the origin can be found on the level of intestinal neurons, in one's erroneous eating habits, and an intoxicated colon. Lately some American researchers have expressed their convictions that intestinal putrefactions irritate the nerve endings in the colon walls. This irritation produces abnormal nervous impulses, triggering irregular sensorial reactions that communicate with the brain. Many of the intestinal factors are capable of acting on nerve endings that are linked to the brain. The neurotoxins disturb the neurons, reduce the potential redox, thereby reducing cerebral energy and give origin to neuro-psychological disorders.

Needless to say the brain is not the only organ capable of producing neurotransmitters such as dopamine. The intestine alone produces 70% of them; this is why we call our intestine our second brain.

I have often observed that a very toxic colon is usually associated with nerve dysfunction, bad memory, poor concentration, irritability, fatigue, or insomnia. This probably correlates with intestinal toxins that irritate the tiny nerves that reach the brain and provoke various symptoms. Intestinal bacteria circulating in blood produce toxins that may be responsible for brain inflammation and degenerative disease such Parkinson's. Although it is possible that intestinal bacteria is damaging first the intestinal neurons. Intestinal damage can decrease the production of local serotonin and dopamine and that further correlates with emotional behavior problems.

In traditional Chinese medicine the abdomen is regarded as a source of energy supplying the brain. One of the diagnostic methods of Oriental medicine is based upon the Qi or Ki that represents the potential energy of a patient. The methods of traditional Chinese medicine are highly valued, so much so that some faculties include them in their courses. This was the case at UCLA in California, which recently opened a school of Traditional Chinese Medicine. Maybe the theory of intestinal intoxication will once again be considered in more university programs.

Naturally, man has evolved, and in certain sectors of medicine, thanks to technology it is possible to prove facts that were only hypotheses in the past. For example, acupuncture had been severely criticized and its value denied, while today acupuncture is a technique widely used even in some hospitals in several countries of Europe as complementary treatments. We already have highly developed apparatus that show that the cell oscillates and vibrates. This is based on new technology that works by measuring oscillatory rhythms derived from physics developed for medical purposes that are simple and easy to use. At the extremity of long-chain of fatty acids in the membranes, these vibrations are very intense, in the order of approximately a thousand times per second. Electrodes or sensitive digital thermometry applied on the skin can detect any cellular disorders. These electromagnetic signs allow doctors to establish the biological profile of a patient's energy, verifying cellular disorders such as intoxication caused by toxins or heavy metals (which block oscillatory rhythms), inflammatory processes, brain function (either too low or too stimulated), or organic dysfunction.

The final result is given by computer and is similar to a complete cartography of the human body. This is one of the tests that I use, the results of which provide essential information on whole body function and how it reacts to a polluted environment. There is also a series of factors that are sure signs of the influence from the colon's auto-intoxication on the brain.

Schizophrenia, for example, is a psychological illness which does not escape the effect of intestinal neurotoxins. Some years ago an American researcher, Herbert Sprince, published a document entitled "Biochemical Aspects of Indol Metabolism in Normal Schizophrenia Subjects" in which he verified auto-intoxication of the colon in the cases studied. From this, he carried out urine tests on the patients and observed a high level of 6-hydroxi-escatol, a toxic substance resulting from the production of escatol that, as seen before, causes severe nervous disorders.

A famous Swiss homeopath, Dr. Dominique Seen, also carried out a curious experiment. He established the responsibility of intestinal toxins in the development of schizophrenia. In order to do so, he made a spider eat mosquitoes that had ingested some drops of blood from a schizophrenic patient. The web made by the spider, after this, was completely disorganized and unstructured. This is proof that blood transports toxins and bacteria that can disturb the brain.

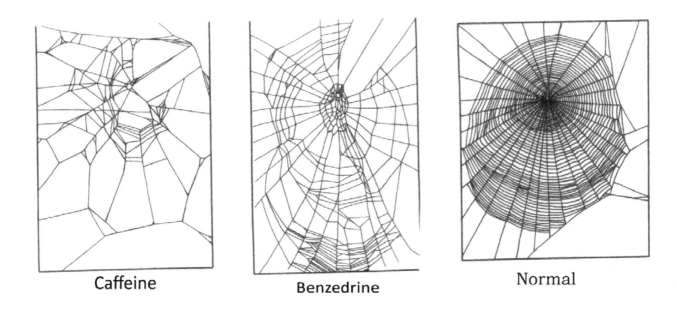

| Caffeine | Benzedrine | Normal |

Aspects of a Spider Web

Dr. Jean Seignalet's Experiment

Dr. Jean Seignalet is an immunologist in the Faculty of Medicine of Montpellier in France. He is a famous speaker, a renowned medical doctor and author of more than two hundred publications in medical journals in various languages. He is also the author of a highly original book on diet and health. The preface of the book is by Prof. Henri Joyeux, also an oncologist and author of a French best-seller entitled *Changing Your Diet–Prevention of Cancer*. Both doctors are currently highly respected because of their work and publications.

According to Dr. Jean Seignalet's theoretical and clinical experiments on patients from the University of Montpellier, he states that our way of eating greatly influences our health. Coming from a scientific personality, these ideas were highly publicized in the media, even though the idea was not original, since Naturopaths have always affirmed this. Dr. Jean Seignalet carried out medical research on the problem of the primitive or prehistoric diet that he learned from the Swiss Burger, whom I mentioned previously, also from the work and diet theory of Dr. Kousmine, according to him a mere reference from the jungle of so many diet-systems, more or less deserving minimal credit.

He studied the digestive and assimilative capacities, as well as the immune reaction from non-digested molecules crossing the intestinal mucosa, which according to him, when entering in blood circulation, was responsible for auto-immune diseases. His conclusions showed the danger of modern diet intoxicating tissue cells, and even the nervous system. According to Dr. Seignalet, cooking modifies the molecular structure of food molecules and can break, can shock each other, or can adhere to other structures to make new complex combinations called isomers. Vital enzymes were at the root of all the biological processes in our body including food digestion. Basically our body and digestive system can only absorb adapted foods, mainly raw vegetables, fruits, roots, mushrooms, fish, and some cereals except wheat and corn, but cooked food, especially red meat, is not so good for our digestive system. Industrial food, manipulated food, and cow's milk is a totally maladapted food, especially pasteurized milk, which our enzymes are not able to digest well. Furthermore, milk can be responsible for intestinal disorders, swelling of the abdomen, a ballooned colon, or excess gases. Even worse, new molecules, such as isomers, still with an unknown cause, can penetrate our blood circulation.

This is probably harmful to our good health as most wheat foods are very common in our daily eating habits. Bread, pastries, cookies, pizza, and pasta are considered as maladapted food. This is why often we remove cow's milk and foods containing wheat from the diet of MS patients. In the case of respiratory disease and allergy patients, it helps to improve their condition.

Dr. Seignalet observed how immune cells react against the body in the presence of unknown molecules from non-digested food. He worked with hundreds of patients including 297 cases of rheumatoid arthritis, 146 of MS, and more than 115 diseases. He also treated a considerable number of patients with only his diet, close as possible to the prehistoric food of our ancestors, with excellent results, although quite strict for a modern style, since most cereals as wheat, corn, and barley were eliminated. Some red meat was permitted, but raw, which was included in his book, *Food – or the Third Medicine*, updated four times, but unfortunately not translated from the original French into any other language.

According to Dr. Seignalet, psychiatric disorders are often evidence of intoxicated nerve cells because of our modern diet having chemicals, aluminum, excess endogenous toxins, badly digested animal proteins, and from being constantly irritated by industrial foods. It permits to non-digested foods and badly digested animal proteins to cross the intestinal barrier, which becomes permeable under stress and damaged from these industrial foods, to simultaneously penetrate into the blood circulation along with bacteria. In one way it correlates with our own work, especially with empirical observation of the iris, where often we observe the correlation between the intestine, nervous system, and psychiatric disorders. In addition, LBA permits an experienced doctor to observe the presence of intestinal bacteria, colonies of Candida overgrowth, and excess toxins circulating in blood. Dr. Seignalet's book has become a best seller, shortly after his unexpected death a few years ago. His method is now well divulgated, even on the French online "Medisite" along with many more articles beginning to emerge in serious publications.

Therefore, the related theory between intoxication and nervous disorders was justified and upheld in the works of a great specialist of our time. One should not be surprised if in the future it is proven that the colon is implicated in many more diseases.

Hypothesis of how modern food can promote disease and cancer

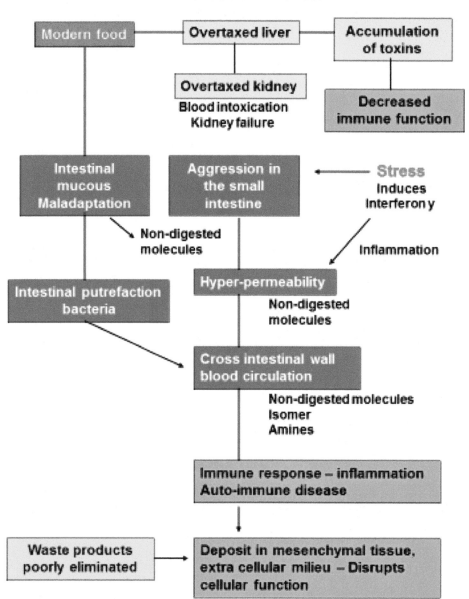

Consequences of the Auto-Intoxication of the Organism

It is increasingly rarer for patients to be informed by their doctors about the causes of the disease which affects them. In most cases, doctors are asking questions about symptoms, eventually send them to take some blood analysis and tests, and prescribed quick fix remedies without further explanation.

One day, a patient told me she had very strong pains in the spine and that her doctor had prescribed cortisone shots. She wanted to know why they prescribed these shots, but as yet she still does not know the reason. This silence and the lack of information largely explain why we still ignore the causes of disease and the consequences of auto-intoxication, along with its relationship to chronic and degenerative diseases.

Auto-intoxication can provide us with an obvious explanation as to why the organism weakens. Why it is that a person considered to be healthy, may gradually or rapidly become ill without any known reason?

Although the notion of intoxication is not yet completely understood, over the years enough proof has been accumulated to confirm the theory of intoxication in the genesis of illnesses and cellular poisoning. The most extraordinary thing is that the ancient works of the great physiologists who left their mark on eighteenth century medicine have been totally overlooked. One of the most noted of them was Rudolph Virchow, who, in his famous work entitled *Cellular Pathology*, in 1861 stated as follows: "Dear Sirs, let us summarize what I told you about blood. Sometimes, certain substances that penetrate the blood exert a harmful action on the cellular elements which become incapable of carrying out their functions. Other times, substances deriving from a precise point (outside or in the body) act harmfully on the other organs." One cannot be clearer! But medicine has erred in perpetuating the concept that an illness or lacuna is purely local and arises spontaneously. Medical paradigm favors the theory of local disease and neglects to study the causes and the condition of intoxicated blood. Medicine is really missing something, since at least we know that our cells are dependent on the quality of our blood.

More often research and tests are increasingly proving that, to the contrary, disease does not arise spontaneously, but rather develops itself inside of our body from excess toxins, nutritional deficiency, and inflammatory process while we are supposed to be healthy. We ourselves cause harm to our body from our wrong life style. The genetic theory is gaining momentum in the most recent works (*Science et Vie*, March 2003), which proves that even abnormal genes are not enough to trigger a disease as cancer since now it has demonstrated that it needs some harmful factors such as pollution or wrong dietary lifestyle. So, we stand between our genetic profile, our dietary style, and the polluted environment. We now have the possibility to act, even before the disease appears.

The first signs appear, but generally no particular attention is given to them. Urine becomes acidic, with a strong color, and sometimes with a strong smell. Feces can be dark, nauseating, the tongue can be white and intoxicated. These are actual signs of intoxication, which are also well known to Chinese doctors who watch them carefully. I had the case of a woman who had all these signs and even a thick and cracked tongue. After twenty days of detoxification she began to vomit viscous and dark tar-like substances. This was a case of severe intoxication.

But the appearance of disease can also be delayed. Despite everything the body constantly carries out magnificent work through auto-regulation of all the body's functions, transformation, and detox from excess toxins and chemicals, via a balanced homeostasis.

The Beginning of Intoxication

We must not think that we are indestructible, but even so, we have at our disposal a fantastic defense system. We have an extraordinary system of enzymatic detoxification and another less known one of compensation in case of intoxication. This is why, in the beginning, that intoxication of the organism is stealthy and not felt. Evidently, the organism becomes intoxicated, begins to struggle, and certain organs are maltreated. For example, an excess of toxins circulating in the blood may overload the skin causing scratching and eczema. The kidney will begin to accumulate strong acids, toxins, and dead microbes and will detoxify them during late night or early morning through the urine. An excess of uric acid shows that the kidneys are tired and that there is an excess of heavy foods, especially meat and beans. Basically, it is a sign of the beginning of intoxication.

But the human body will do everything to prevent the toxins from disturbing its numerous functions. Thanks to a subtle system, it will drain the excess toxins and dead microbes into specialized tissues, in other words, the mesenchymal tissue. This tissue has a similar role to that of a sponge storing acids, toxins, and dead microbes, both day and night.

> ## THE ORGANISM USUALLY DETOXIFIES DURING THE NIGHT

Urine is always more acidic during the night because of the elimination of acids accumulated during the day. In auto-intoxicated patients the urine is always acidic upon waking up. A good verification method is to test the pH. of the urine in the morning with a reactive paper, which can be bought in a pharmacy.

On the other hand, chronic intoxication with an increasing number of toxins and microbes begins to overcharge the mesenchymal tissue and blocks accumulation during the day. Eventually, the accumulation ends up becoming unbearable and the organism tries to find a way out. It then tries to create an internal or external repository. It can take different shapes affecting the weakened organs.

Iridology may be useful to define and detect these situations, observing the condition of the colon, liver, kidney, showing lymphatic circulation congestion, intoxicated tissues and which organs are weaker, as well as which could be most affected by accumulations of toxins, which appear in different zones of the iris structure. Alternatively, it may also be shown, depending on the degree of toxic accumulation, that there exists either an irritated nerve wreath (nervous system) or a lack of nerve supply in the affected tissues. This is why cancer patients feel no pain before the disease blows up having a total lack of nerve supply to the affected organ.

Through the observation of the iris I have managed to detect different conditions and levels of intoxication. If this intoxication settles in the blood and tissues, the color of the iris darkens. According to how chronic this intoxication is, the iris becomes covered in brown spots in brown irises and yellow or greenish-yellow blotches in blue irises. If the blood is charged with toxins, usually both irises appear with darker color in the area corresponding to blood circulation and other tissues area.

One can be surprised in LBA observation by the appearance of different colored crystals and even mucous colored red, green, blue, or violet, circulating in the blood with different origins, which for instance may indicate an excess of pharmaceutical drugs, chemicals from industrial food, or bad kidney elimination. This could modify the original color of irises, which I had observed since the beginning of my practice, but now I may know why; that this is an indication of where to start detoxification treatment.

In the same way, if chemical substances circulate, the colored spots and halos appear in different parts of the iris's structure, which are in fact related to auto-intoxication and accumulation of macromolecules circulating in blood from wrong diet. This also supports the theory of Dr. Jean Seignalet.

When the organism becomes unable to expel toxins and other residues, the emunctory reflex areas in the iris will be even darker, showing a slowing process in the outward elimination of toxins.

On the other hand, under the action of harmful substances, often resulting from an excess of animal proteins not being digested, they cross through the leaky gut and enter the blood stream as big macromolecules that the body is unable to metabolize. Thus these macromolecules activate the immune system that may overreact, attacking tissue and developing auto-immune disease. As an alternative, the body sends them to inert organs which can develop into breast nodules, uterine myomas, or even ovarian cysts.

Recently I had a real example in my clinic: a forty-nine-year-old woman came to me for consultation for a voluminous uterine myoma, along with asthma. She was using three different aerosols per day. She weighed 98Kg (216 lbs.) for a 1.56m (5' 1") woman. She ate meat twice a day and suffered from chronic constipation. One can understand very well the origin of her myoma from a deficient metabolism of animal-based food. In regard to breast nodules, experiments have proven that in many cases after surgery, they form again locally near the earlier ones or on the other breast.

This demonstrates that if nothing is done to change the diet, through detox or better internal hygiene to combat auto-intoxication, these manifestations may become chronic. These masses evolve because of blood and tissue intoxication and the incapacity of the mesenchymal tissues to absorb the excess of toxins circulating in the blood, including excess protein and non-digested macromolecules. Myomas of two kilos have been observed. How long does it take for a mass of these dimensions to form in the body? We may estimate that it takes over ten or even twenty years involving chronic constipation, accumulation of toxins, along with macromolecules not being absorbed.

This is not a new situation, as Hippocrates mentioned it in his works: "Any disease is caused by an accumulation of substances foreign to the body that remains more or less for a long period of time in this or that organ, more or less in a large quantity." Apparently, even after two thousand years we are still facing intoxication and our body still works in the same way. We have been created under the laws of universe and breaking them may dangerously harm the body with disease as a result.

THEORY OF DISEASE BY AUTO-INTOXICATION

First of all, it is necessary to understand that, whatever the disease, there is always a certain degree of intoxication and/or stage of inflammation which can be observed through the irises and also through other medical apparatus like the Vega or Mora system. Very rarely can a disease trigger, without first having chronic intoxication and oxidative stress, a condition ranging from mid to strong. In time, chronic intoxication can trigger serious problems and give rise to disease, some of which are still little known. Let us use fibromyalgia as an example. This is a fairly recent disease, the pathogenesis of which is not yet well understood. However, it is known that fibromyalgia is characterized by an inflammation of the connective tissue associated with damaged mitochondria components from excessive free radical activity and loss of ATP energy. Damaged mitochondria are unable to fully use oxygen, where we have the non-breakdown of pyruvate, an end product of glycolysis. As a consequence, it produces high levels of lactic acid responsible for muscle pains and fatigue, very similar to what athletes experience after an Olympic competition.

Let us talk further about this disease. This inflammation may be also largely a consequence of a diet rich in red meat, industrial foods, an excess of toxins, and free radical activity. It attacks muscles, tendons as well as neurons, where this excess consumption becomes another factor that may trigger an inflammatory process that in turn, generating more free radicals and increasing more inflammation in tissue, mainly within the extra cellular matrix.

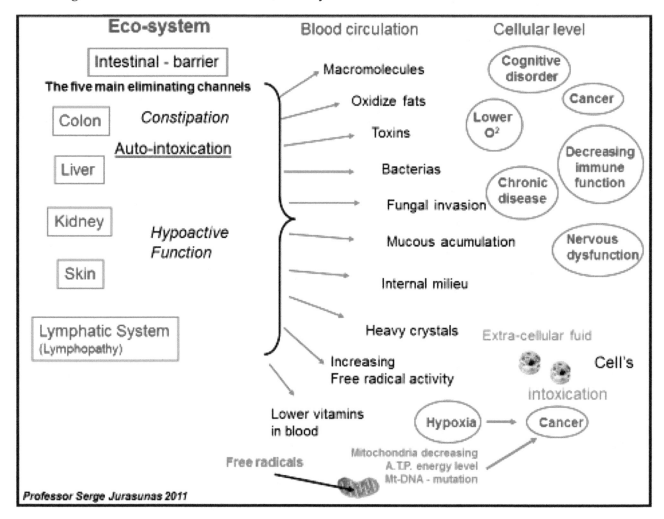

Professor Serge Jurasunas 2011

The patient with fibromyalgia feels very tired and has pains throughout their body. As the disease only appears in adulthood, it is apparent that an accumulation of a quantity of toxins is the logical cause of intoxication and inflammation of the tissues. Today, it is easier to carry out tests and analysis to check the condition of kidney elimination, liver detox, and intestinal permeability. At the same time, the function of mitochondria could be monitored to verify if it is working, accepting oxygen and producing ATP energy, whether at a high level or a lower output.

Therefore, we can say that, if patients are affected by fibromyalgia they do not suffer from one cause or condition of intoxication alone but also from social life style, nutrient deficiency and oxidative stress that also plays a key role in this syndrome. Mitochondrial dysfunction is usually associated with fibromyalgia, along with lower production of ATP energy and increasing lactic acid in the tissues. Mitochondria are essential to anaerobic life on this planet using oxygen as fuel to burn food and generating metabolic energy. ATP is absolutely necessary for all of the body's functions and for the regulatory systems.

Many diseases have an origin with damaged mitochondrial function from oxidative stress including diabetes, arthritis, asthma, chronic kidney disease, and cancer. We age through the mitochondria under free radical attack that damages their components leading to a dramatic decrease in ATP energy, cognitive disorders, and loss of vision, hearing, and muscles is associated with the loss of mitochondrial function.

This last decade's science has made important discoveries in the mechanism of how a normal cell can turn into cancer cell, although more recent research now points out the mitochondria are involved in the causation of cancer (see "Mitochondria, Oxygen and Cancer" – Townsend Letter – August/September 2006 – www.sergejurasunas .com). However, putting together and explaining the causes and the reasons remains a big challenge.

Cancer and Intoxication of the Tissues

Let us talk a bit more about this disease and try to explain, not from a cellular standpoint but from a different basis that implicates the environmental tissue known as the Extra Cellular Matrix that seems to have a major influence on the cell's behavior itself.

New lines of research show that the auto-intoxication and inflammation of the ECM is associated with tumorogenesis. Cancer initiation may have a link with the intoxication of the surrounding tissues, which now is supported by many researchers. For instance, according to Prof. W. Kostler, president of the Austrian Cancer Association, whom I had met several times during various congresses, there is no direct link between epithelial cells, blood vessels, or lymphatic vessels because of the inter-positioned connective tissue, the ECM. All nutrients, hormones, oxygen supply, enzymes, needed by the epithelial cells, including for detoxification, have to pass through this matrix.

Unfortunately, the accumulation of toxic waste, excess free radicals and lack of oxygen may have a negative effect on the components and consistency of the ECM. A state of auto-intoxication and high oxidative stress triggers a chronic inflammation that modifies the fluid consistency of the ECM, a semi gelatinous ground to become much stiffer, causing an edema. Consequently the edema leads to a total blockage of nearly all the exchange procedures between the body and the epithelial cells. This leads to an alteration of the epithelial cell metabolism, sending it on its way to gain a stepwise cancerous attitude, especially for a cell with a genomic instability. Malfunction of the connective tissue is responsible for nutritional deficiency and decreasing oxygen supply to epithelial cells, turning into an auto-intoxication of these cells from accumulations of waste produced from cellular metabolism. These wastes may have a negative impact on a cell's nutrient supply including electrolytes, trace elements, vitamins, hormones, and enzymes.

More recently a team of researchers from the University of California, Berkeley, discovered that the healthy influence from a normal breast extracellular matrix caused cancer cells to behave normally, even though they were genetically altered. Yet when the same cells were put into an artificial environment they again behaved like cancer cells. This shows that cancer cells are not isolated and that the ECM condition influences their capacity to thrive. Cancer cells that are stimulated by an abnormal environment, in fact, they cannot grow and expand without the angiogenic factors that the tumor attracts by launching signals that attract the blood vessels necessary to get nutrients and some oxygen into this tissue environment. Therefore, chronic inflammation and the modification of the ECM are often associated with tumorogenesis.

Furthermore, chronic hypoxia of epithelial cells caused by edema and mainly gel-like connective tissue consistency lead to a chronic deficiency of the mitochondrial oxygen supply, which is needed for the normal functioning of the respiratory chain and ATP synthesis. The lack of oxygen leads to an excess of disordered electrons, acting as free radicals since they cannot couple with oxygen and are damaging the mitochondria components, resulting in decreasing ATP production. The consequences can be dramatic on weak epithelial cells, since decreasing ATP energy may induce these cells to become less differentiated than normal healthy cells. ATP energy is needed to maintain the high degree of tissue differentiation, and also associates with apoptosis. Today we know, in cancer, different degrees of differentiation in cells can be found. For more information about cancer and the tissue environment, read my lecture that I delivered in Germany: "The Biological Approach to Breast Cancer." Deutscher Heilpraktikertag 2004. 27.28 März, Congress Center Dusseldorf Germany: www.sergejurasunas.com

ATP energy is also needed to activate a defined number of suppressor genes like the P53 tumor suppressor gene responsible for self-destruction of abnormal/cancer cells in our body. Furthermore, apoptosis is activated by the P53 gene where the self-destruct mechanism is triggered by the mitochondria and not the cells. This is why mitochondria play a central role in cancer. We then keep in mind several factors associated with a state of tumorogenesis, such as the auto-intoxication of the ECM induced by bad dietary style, oxidative stress, and low oxygen status.

Exaggerated red meat consumption is another concrete matter associated with the inflammation of the ECM. Meat is not only a source of proteins and fats, but it also contains other elements that can be harmful. Meat is rich in arachidonic acid, which is a fatty acid necessary for our cells in order to function properly. However, cells need only a very small quantity to be absorbed by the membranes. Excess meat consumption increases the level of arachidonic acid that cells cannot absorb and it starts to accumulate in the tissues, triggering an inflammatory process that can become chronic and responsible for inflammatory disease. A person's normal daily need for arachidonic acid is of about 1 milligram. In a modern diet with high meat intake, arachidonic acid can be elevated to 200mg and even in some cases reaches 1000mg per day.

Empirically, an accumulation of intracellular and extracellular toxic waste was always considered in Naturopathic medicine to be harmful to a cell's function, fatally leading to serious disorders and diseases. This fact is confirmed by the increasing number of chronic and degenerative diseases that are on the increase in all industrialized countries, because of increased consumption of industrial foods and junk foods that generate excess toxic waste.

We must not forget about menopause, which is one of the many conditions which can be affected by auto-intoxication. Menopause is, in most cases, accompanied by a series of unpleasant symptoms. Moreover, it affects an increasing number of women long before the normal age of acceptable hormonal change.

I met an eighteen-year-old girl who was suffering from menopause and was subject to hormonal substitutive treatment. I am convinced that auto-intoxication must be a determining factor in premature menopause, along with other factors, such as congestion in the lymphatic drainage system. Any of these situations can rapidly transform into a chronic intoxication of the extracellular matrix, in which the bioactivation and transmission of hormones takes place, strongly influencing a woman's menopause.

Currently, women are being affected more often and at an earlier age by menopausal problems, signifying an increasingly premature degradation of the female hormonal apparatus. Stress and bad colon function, gradual intoxication of the organism, and toxic substances such as xenobiotics are considered to be largely responsible for the alteration of hormonal mechanisms.

Recent research has shown that there is a relation between depression, the ovaries, and the early appearance of menopause (General Archives of Psychiatry, 2000 USA). It is the same as the changes that occur in the central nervous system influencing irregular menstrual cycles (Dept. of Physiology, College of Medicine – University of Kentucky, 2000 USA).

Obviously, being at the root of it, auto-intoxication plays a defining role in disturbing the central nervous system, especially if already weak from a hereditary status. While mitochondrial ATP production is necessary for the synthesis of hormones, decreasing ATP production may greatly affect female hormone production leading to premature menopause. Biological aging and brain deterioration can also have repercussions on the female hormonal apparatus which today has already been confirmed by researchers.

An Iridology examination could be most helpful to check on the level and degree of intoxication, the condition of the peripheral and central nervous system, the endocrine system, as well as the condition of the connective tissues. In this way we can prevent, delay, alleviate, or eliminate the symptoms of menopause.

In conclusion, it can be said that currently the tide is turning in defense of the ancient theory of auto-intoxication and its consequences on the functions of our organism.

Diagnosis of the Colon through the Tongue

All ancient schools of medicine, above all the Chinese, Indian, and Tibetan, make reference to the observation of the patient's tongue in order to determine health status as well as the function of various organs such as the colon, liver, spleen, and heart. According to historical documents, this type of examination has its origin in ancient Chinese medicine.

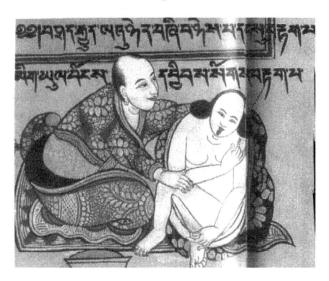

A Tibetan Doctor Observing a Patient's Tongue

Tibetan medicine stresses the importance of this method of evaluation. It is mentioned in various works I have had the chance to study. According to this and the theory of a modern Tibetan doctor, Dr. Yeshi Donden, the real diagnosis begins with the analysis of one's patient. Yet, according to him conventional diagnosis, only informs us about the local disease and abnormal blood parameters, but not on the real condition of the patient, or the link between disease and the colon.

This kind of observation is called "root diagnostics," of which Iridology is one of the primary pillars, serving as a diagnostic for the entire human body, along with indicating reflex disease condition.

According to Tibetan medicine, "Ignorance" is the first cause of suffering, and today I totally agree with them. People are becoming ill from ignorance. The cure begins by changing our mentality, envisioning the cause of illness and what we have done wrong. This is a logical statement that is highlighted in Western Naturopathy.

The simple observation of a tongue can sometimes be more useful in understanding the condition of the colon than many modern diagnostic tools. It is interesting to further notice that when an observation of the iris shows an auto-intoxication of the colon, the tongue of the patient always appears to be coated, intoxicated, or cracked.

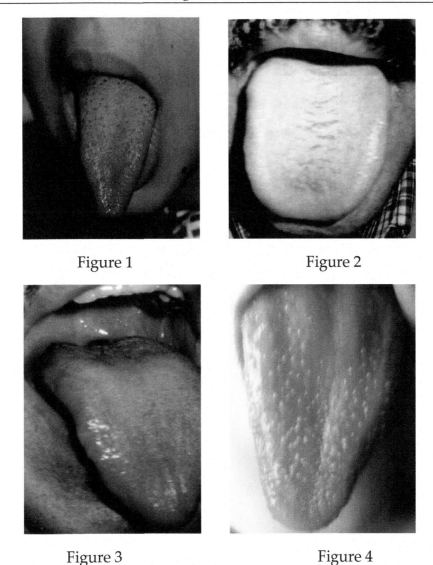

Figure 1   Figure 2

Figure 3   Figure 4

These four photos show various problems. The first three are tongues that show signs of intoxication, indicating intoxication of the liver and intestine as well. This is true even in younger people.

Figure 1 shows a tongue overcharged with mucous from an intoxicated liver and colon.

Figure 2 shows a cracked, whitened tongue, coated by mucus, which indicates stomach fermentation caused by deficient digestion. In turn, a bad digestion causes poor transformation of food in the intestine with gas and bloating.

Figure 3 is a tongue that shows signs of intoxication in the medial and internal part, definitely indicating disorders in the liver and spleen.

Figure 4 is that of a six-year-old child with a tongue infected by Candida, sign of an intestinal imbalance. The Candida penetrates the blood through the intestinal mucosa.

Diagnosis through the Tongue:

White tongue – toxins in the stomach and intestine;
Yellow tongue – hepatic problems;
Whitish tongue in the back area – large intestine problems;
Whitish tongue in the medial area – problems in the stomach and small intestine.

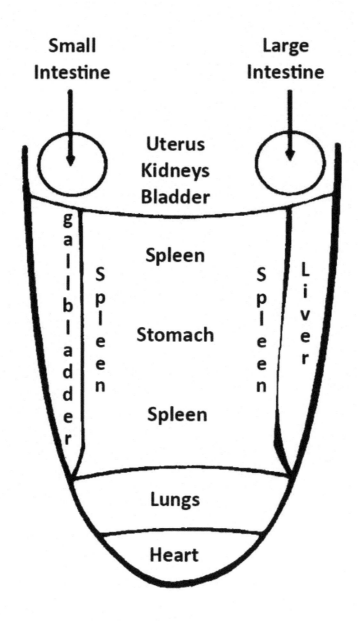

Part V

Iridology
Embryological Study of Organ Development
Interpretation of the Signs in the Iris
Practical Cases

Iridology

> *"It appears to me a most excellent thing for the Physician to cultivate Prognosis; for by foreseeing and foretelling, in the presence of the sick, the present, the past, and the future, and explaining the omissions which patients have been guilty of, he will be the more readily believed to be acquainted with the circumstances of the sick."*
>
> **Medical Works of Hippocrates**

Iridology is a system based on the analysis of the iris of the eyes which allows us to check on our health status, genetic background and organic dysfunction. The iris of eyes has always attracted doctors and priests in the past century since it could reflect not only our body, but our soul. Historically according to archeological records the practice of iris observation can be attributed to Chaldea, to Mesopotamia 1000 BC, but to Egyptians as well. A primitive iris chart was found in a cave in Israel dating to about 600 BC, of which I myself have a copy of a reproduction.

However, according to the German Iridologist Theodore Kriege, the first documented reference to iris analysis can be credited to the physician Philippus Meyens, who wrote a book, *Chromatica Medica*, published in 1670 and in 1786, Christian Haertels published a book in Germany titled, *The Eyes and its Signs*.

Modern Iridology in the nineteenth century was discovered by coincidence by the Hungarian medical doctor, Ignazt von Pecezely (1822-1911) who, in 1880, first published his research in a scientific journal and also wrote his only book, *Discoveries in the Realms of Nature and Art of Healing*.

Independently, about the same time, Neal Liljequist (1851-1936) a Swedish pastor claimed to have discovered Iridology and in 1893 published a first book on this new science. Just over a decade later, a German pastor, Leopold Erdmann Emanuel Felke (1856-1926), also published a book on Iridology in 1904, followed by many others such as Rudolf Schnabel (1882-1962), who was very well known in Germany.

This observation through the structure of the tissues of the iris, the most complex anatomy of the human body, points us to the innermost workings of the organism. Iridology is able to show any abnormal conditions and the changes that take place before a disease manifests itself or reveals its causes once it has been clinically detected. For example, the iris is capable of showing conditions of acute, chronic, or degenerative condition , linked with inflammatory process, whether genetic or constitutional deficiencies, nervous or endocrine disorders, circulatory, organic, and functional disorders.

One of the great advantages of Iridology is that we can amazingly detect any gastrointestinal disorders and above all the stages of colon auto-intoxication, liver and kidney disorders. It offers many advantages to doctors concerned with the health of their patients and looking to treat the cause of diseases, rather that only the symptoms.

Iridology is excellent as a basis of prevention and for identifying the various stages of inflammation associated with a disease, as well as theoretically, some improvement that we may observe in the ciliary zone of the iris, known as healing signs which usually appear in between lacunas after at least two or three months of treatment and changing diet. They indicate tissue regeneration and increasing nerve and blood supplies. However Iridology does not name diseases, even if it suggests some specific terrain for disease risk and profile, such for rheumatism, arthritis, allergy, diabetes, and even cancer risk to a certain extent, which indicates a further need for appropriate medical check-ups.

We may also appreciate and caution that in Iridology, however often practiced by doctors, if they have poor knowledge or lack of clinical experience. They may not always be in position to offer the most current diagnosis or may even offer the wrong interpretation, which I have seen and noticed both directly and indirectly. Iridology requires considerable knowledge, practice, and expertise.

For some, Iridology is not a precise science, yet I can affirm that it offers many advantages for the therapist. I have been practicing Iridology for nearly fifty years and it has always been an incredible help in understanding and in monitoring one or several causes associated with the disease.

It is a part of my normal routine that I associate with other diagnostic methods according to the case.

The most recent discoveries in embryology allow for a better understanding of Iridology, allowing the possibility to better understand the mechanism that links the body to the brain and in turn, to the eye and it's iris. This mechanism that embryologically has linked the colon to important organs such as the liver, pancreas, lung, and kidney, works while the body is entirely connected with the brain via the nervous system and in turn, to the iris of the eye. The iris is actually the only visible part of the brain, made from the same brain tissue. It reflects from a specific standpoint our nervous system, sympathetic and parasympathetic, and empirically our body's anatomy.

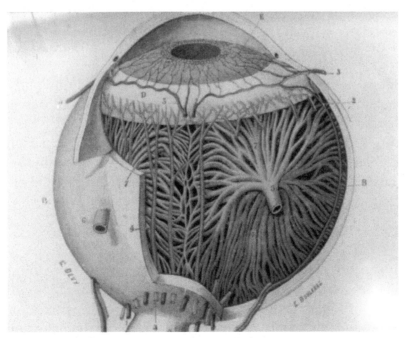

All new discoveries are subject to human criticism that merely delays or tries to prevent progress. Let us recall what happened when the stethoscope was discovered which was severely decried. Even more recently with the discovery of the "Water Memory" by the French researcher Jacques Benveniste, which explained so many things, but above all proof of the theory of Homeopathic Medicine regarding its dilution. Medical doctors and the media accused this researcher of sorcery. They wrote he should be burned at the stake, the same as if we were in the Middle Ages. He was obliged to hide his family because he received menacing threats against them. He was ready to leave France and go to other countries, where in fact, he had been invited to pursue his research.

There are numerous universities around the world that include studies on Iridology among their courses. For example, in Russia, an experiment was carried out on 80,000 patients, which was 85% accurate in detection. I can say that I am proud to have personally introduced to a certain point Iridology in the USSR around 1967 when I was meeting with Soviet medical doctors, in particular doctor Fiodor Romashow who apparently had never heard before about this science and was intriguing to realize that we can do diagnosis of the body through the irises. However, another story revealed that Dr. Evgeny Velkhover M.D., Dr. Sc., apparently introduced Iridology in Russia near the end of 1940 or in early 1950, though not very clear, but apparently Iridology was quite unknown in the USSR by the time had I met Dr. Romashow. He immediately showed an interest for this science and I gave him a book from Dr. Jensen, *The Science and Practice of Iridology*, that he then started to read. Years after Dr. Romashow was appointed as Dean of the Faculty of Medicine at Moscow University, he introduced Iridology as new diagnosis outside of the regular curriculum. Anyway, I even contributed by introducing Dr. Jensen in the USSR, where in fact he made a trip there to teach Iridology, where today this science is well developed.

In South Korea, the government organized clinical tests that were 78.25% accurate in detecting illnesses, with a 90.2% result in diagnosing gastrointestinal illnesses.

Fortunately we have entered an era in which new horizons of modern sciences allow one to appreciate and understand Iridology. For the first time Iridology seminars receive now credit, this is an enormous step which we owe to Dr. David Pesek, of the International Institute of Iridology. Ellen Tart Jensen Ph.D., D.Sc. is also teaching iridology, having learned from her father in law, Dr. Bernard Jensen. I believe that today we have more opportunity than ever to learn about iridology along with the support of new discoveries in the field of embryology, neurobiology and especially with the new discovery about the intestine as our second brain and the relationship that exists between the brain and the colon which Iridology can best show.

Modern biology offers a new extraordinary vision of the human body and of all its molecules. One of the books I recommend on this subject is by David S. Goodsell, assistant professor in the Department of Molecular Biology at the Scripps Research Institute (USA). The book is entitled *Our Molecular Nature – The Body's Motors, Machines and Messages*. It is a highly interesting book and is useful in understanding the fantastic mechanism that is life, although when confronted with disease we still feel limited, without a global and holistic vision of the human body.

Why the Iris?

Observation of the iris means discovering a marvelous concept not fully understood, and yet in a world of so many discoveries about the human body, the irises can be of great help in offering greater understanding our health status, especially our body as a whole. As I have said before, each iris is one of a kind, being the only cerebral tissue visible to the naked eye. The retina is also a visible cerebral tissue, which ophthalmologists can observe with their microscope. This allows detection of certain organic disorders such as diabetes.

Incredibly, the iris is the most enervated organ of the human body, and each iris cell and chromatophase contain more than 28,000 individual nerve fibers, demonstrating very sensitive reflex zone within the iris.

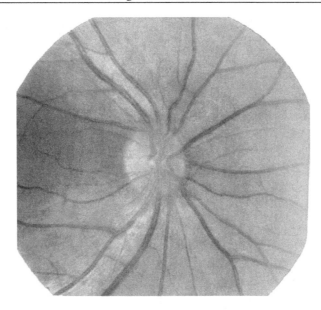

All the nerve cells of the iris are in direct contact with the optic nerve linked to the brain, which in turn is made up of an incredible number of nerves, filaments and nervous ramifications around the optic nerve. Today it is thought that 500,000 nerves connect the iris to the brain.

Since the eye is formed from embryonic brain tissue, it has a real neurological umbilical cord in which the data of the parental body's condition and nervous system are written. When we examine an iris, we are faced with an unimaginable and extremely complex world of information and knowledge.

But we can go even further into this outstanding technology as the iris is endowed with muscles and these in turn with nerves. The muscles are called the dilating muscle and sphincter muscle, which are the only two muscles in the organism that come from the nervous tissue during the development of the embryo. There is a nerve for every five or ten muscle cells, as compared to one nerve for every two hundred or three hundred muscle cells in the rest of the organism. This may explain the extreme sensitivity of all the functions and bonds between the eye and the brain. The brain is itself a super computer that contains billions of neurons specializing in transmitting electric impulses between them, or to any other part of the body. In the embryo as the brain develops, a lobe appears on either side from the inside of the brain towards the outside, forming the eyes.

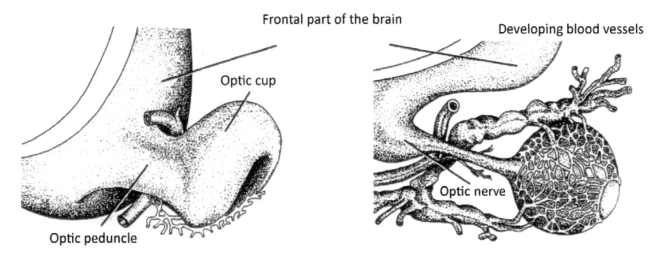

Eye and frontal part of the brain in a 6 mm long human embryo.

Eye and frontal part of the brain, in a 13 mm long human embryo.

The eye is formed by the cerebral tissues that literally drive the optic bulb towards the exterior. As these images show, the eye in the human embryo is anatomically linked to the brain by the optic nerve and its chains of millions of nerve and blood ramifications.

We can say that the iris of the eye is a window to our brain. The connection is created through nervous impulses from the hypothalamus and in particular the thalamus. This link to the spinal medulla records all the conditions of the organ tissues then retransmits them to the iris through the oculomotor nerve, then through the Edinger-Westphal cells.

The iris not only receives messages from the brain itself but also the recorded messages emanating from the entire organism, through a network of neurological communication. From here, the iris transforms itself into a map that must be observed and decoded.

For example, there are two autonomic nerve systems in the organism that control all the functions passing from the brain to the organism and vice-versa. These are the Sympathetic andParasympathetic nervous systems represented in the iris by the collarette, also known as the autonomic nerve wreath or minor arterial circle. Observed through an electron microscope, the collarette is formed by a dense network of extremely sensitive nerve fibers. The collarette not only correlates with heart rate variability, but it also indicates stress and condition of the heart.

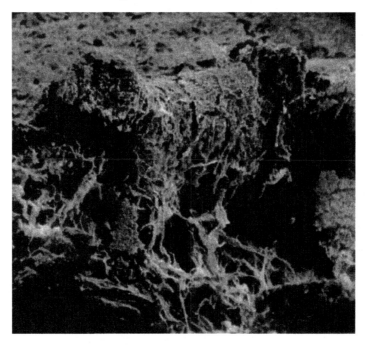

Note the granularity and density of the entwined nerve fibers of a section of the nerve collarette of the iris. (Electronic microscope 25x187)

During an examination of the iris, it is important to observe the collarette associated with the toxic condition of the colon, which by reflex can indicate which organ may be affected. This is a kind of neurogeneic reflex function which will be discussed in greater detail in the chapter on embryology.

Hypothalamus

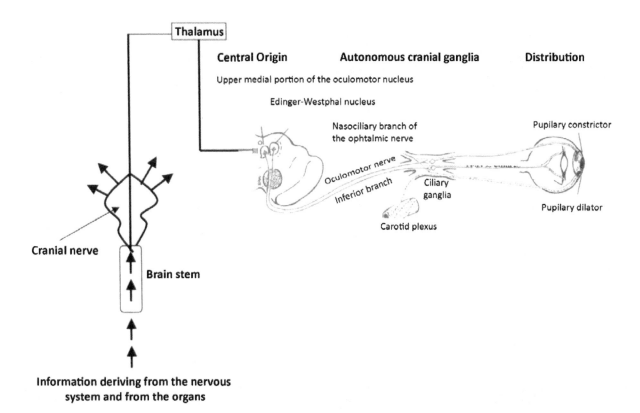

Image showing the relationship between the nervous impulses of the different organs of the body, with the ocular iris. The impulses to the front part of the thalamus which transmits them to the hypothalamus, which in turn sends them to the iris through the oculomotor nucleus and the Edinger-Westphal nucleus, change the muscular fibers of the iris.

The observation of the collarette, I repeat, is central since it is a membrane-like embryonic remnant that witnesses most of the embryological development. Observation of the entire body through the collarette can show which organ is affected. The collarette, introflexion, distension, absence, color, thickness and surrounding pigmentation can all be indicative of psychological or physical disease development. Let us say that there are two nervous systems. In this way, in the iris the nerves that control the interior of the collarette are the parasympathetic nerves, while the sympathetic nerves control the exterior zones of the collarette.

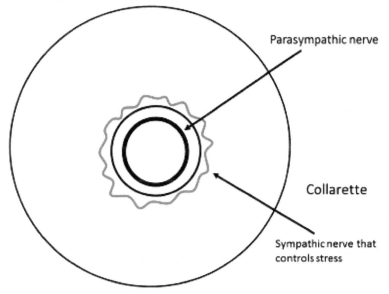

This observation allows one to verify the capacity of resistance, or deficiencies of the nervous system, showing also that certain organs are affected by and linked to this same nervous system. Let us take another example. The skin is an extremely enervated organ, the ramifications of which go throughout the nervous system to communicate with all the organs of the body. Thus through the skin we can also communicate with all of the internal organs. Today, it is already possible to establish a diagnosis or an energy test of the organs by placing electrodes on sensitive and anatomical parts of the skin. In the same way one can now treat the organ by applying electronic impulses on a reflex point of the skin.

An intoxicated colon irritates the thin nerve endings of the nervous system, sending an irritating impulse to the brain which in turn reacts negatively. In the iris the collarette or nerve wreath as called by Dr. Jensen may appear abnormal, jagged, dipping in close to the pupil, and will show the organs that suffer as a result. Here we have the case of a nervous reflex function.

Unfortunately the iris has been neglected where only a few studies have been carried out on it. But we know that the nervous system and the cerebral body are the first to be formed during the development of the fetus. The eye begins to form after the eighteenth day, at the same time as the brain.

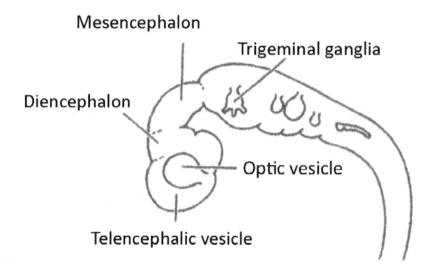

The eye (optic vesicle) begins to form after the eighteenth day, at the same time as the brain. All the genes are present in the mass of cells of the eye and are part of the genetic system.Unlike the other organs, this will only form later. In this way, the genes are obviously recognized in the iris and are intrinsic factors to the human body.

The epithelial tissue of the iris is made up of the same tissue which develops the nervous system, the neuroectoderm. Therefore, all the parental inheritance is formed right at the beginning of the embryonic development.

When we are born, all the data related to the tissues of the organism, the nervous system, the mechanical and psychological brain, the organs, the lymphatic system etc. etc. are all imprinted in the iris, just like a map or cartography. Overall, it is a hereditary condition known as terrain. First of all, the iris reflects the conditions of the tissues in the body, meaning the degree of inflammation, which is reflected through the fibers of the iris's stroma.

The body is formed by four kinds of tissues namely: epithelial, connective, muscular and nervous. Connective tissue connects the organs. These tissues determine and reflect the condition of the other kinds of tissues of the organism. In this way, the vitality and resistance of our organism can be observed with an irido-microscope that shows a highly magnified view of the iris detailing the density and alignment of the fibers composed of a network of fine and minute beams of connective elastic tissue of the stroma, which are formed by blood vessels and connective tissues.

Badly aligned, distorted tissues with visible spaces or formations of lacunas are signs of a general weakness and inflammation in specific organ tissues. The observation of these tissues and lacunas with an iridoscope that permits a high magnification and definition, such as the Pesek Clinical Iriscope shows a highly affected textural architecture, or sometimes empty and/or with several fissures.

These extraordinary Photos take us to the interior of existent lacunas in the stroma of the iris. One can observe an important structure of the fibers, some of which are apparently white, due to the inflammatory state.

Electronic microscope

9-x202   10-x507   11-x2028

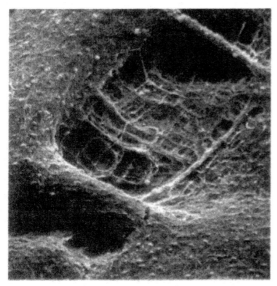

9— X202

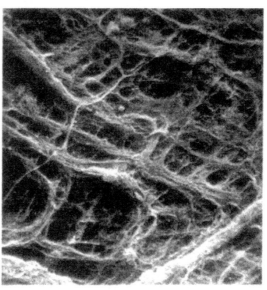

10— X507

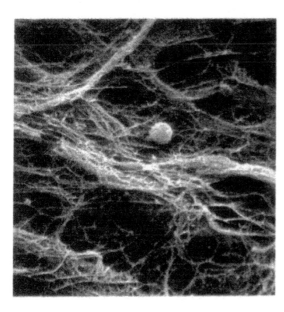

11— X2028

Photos from the book, "Iridology - The Science and Practice in the Healing Art", B. Jensen –USA

These Photographs were provided by a specialist in electronic microscopy. Thelma Carlysle – Department of Agriculture, Science and Education (Florida).

The organization of the human body and of the nervous system is the same throughout the body, the structure of the iris and of the collarette reflect the condition of an individual's state of health. Eventually other signs can appear on the surface of the iris, such as color of the pigment granulation, brown, dark lacunas, and crypts indicating some bad organic function, susceptibility or tendency in the future to develop chronic and degenerative disorders and disease. Your iris may tell you about which disease you are predisposed, which may develop (or not) according to your lifestyle, dietary habits, environment, and heredity.

Subsequently, over the years the iris is continually bombarded with chemical messages, vibratory impulses, particularly when under constant physical or social stress or alcohol. This builds excess acidity, where nerve tissue tension that can be observed through an iris examination. In this way the iris can change its color and even its initial structure.

SECTION OF THE IRIS

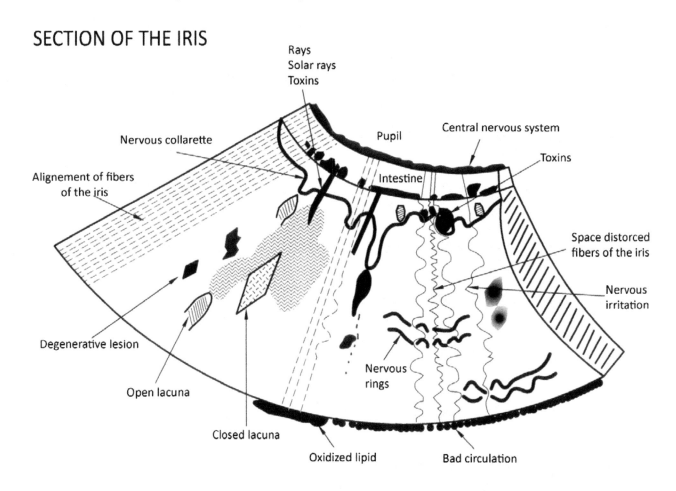

The iris has given us precious indications on the terrain and state of the organs but we are currently far from a total understanding and there is still much to be discovered.

Embryologic Study of the Development of the Organs

When I first discovered Iridology thanks to my encounter with Dr. Bernard Jensen around 1963, I had the clear impression that something important was happening in my life. I thought to myself, "How it is possible that the eyes can also reflect the health status of a person through the body's tissue anatomy reflected in specific areas of the iris?"

While reading Dr. Jensen's book, *The Science and Practice of Iridology*, taking some of his courses and listening to some of his seminars, I quickly understood the advantages of this science. It is important to say that I was in the presence of a great teacher who was highly eloquent. With Iridology, we first of all have the advantage of examining ourselves more thoroughly and maybe knowing ourselves better.

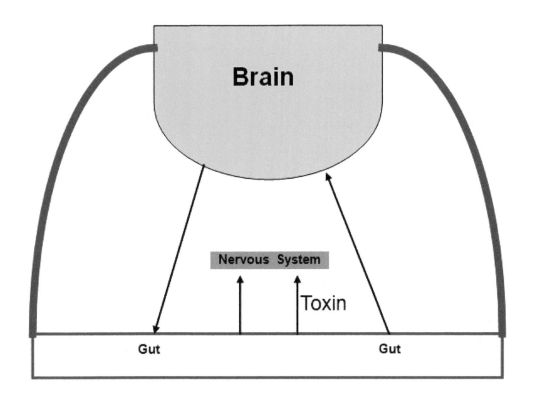

Interconnection between the Gut, Nervous System and Brain;
Between the Brain, Nervous System and Gut.
Prof. Serge Jurasunas 2011

The famous inscription of Delphos (Greece) reads, **"Man, Know Thyself First."** But in truth, after two thousand years, we are still fairly ignorant about ourselves, our health, and the reasons for diseases.

Could it be that this incredible organ, the eye along with the iris can be an extraordinary mechanism, maybe a rare system that is the reflection of our soul and of our health?

At the time I had a negative medical experience, which led me to reflect on the competence of medical checkups. From here, Iridology became a starting point for me, leading me to study and train in Naturopathic medicine. With Iridology I wanted to know all the secrets and answers. In spite of everything, my wish was not granted as fast as I wanted. Many, many years of study would lie ahead. It is true that we did not have the real answers as to what we could see in the iris, and this was a real handicap.

But with patience and various decades of study I finally began to understand why the organs of the body are reflected in a particular area of the iris. Fifteen years ago, and for some years following, I dedicated myself to a project destined to build up a more structured and complete anatomical iris chart, essentially based on my practical experience. The result was interesting, but the end project has yet to be realized, having been busy with other research. However, I may say that during those years, Dr. Bernard Jensen's chart of the iris was and continues to be a major reference for the entire world. Further on we will see that the organs are located with extreme precision. Later on several iris charts had been developed that were more or less precise, some totally useless and others of interest like the Holistic Iridology chart of Dr. David Pesek, focusing with more detail on the areas of the brain and endocrine system.

Certain professional situations led me to the study and research of biology, oxidative stress, neurobiology, and embryology. It is essential to master the knowledge of the human body in order to better understand the theories of alternative medicine, which are sometimes empirical. It is even more important when the subject is Iridology, as the challenge is substantial. In this way, I managed to gain a better understanding of the projection of the organs in the iris in order to have a perfect interpretation. Indeed, observing the signs located on specific areas of the iris are like examining the liver or the kidneys, yet proving the existence of this anatomical projection is something else.

Modern embryology has managed to supply answers and finally remove the empirical aspect, which deprecates Iridology and leads to negative criticisms. Embryology is an important step as it leads us to first of all understand from which germinal tissue this or that organ is formed and how, as we will see, it can indirectly associate one organ with another. Why it is that in the iris there is a place for each organ? And finally, why it is that after the embryonic organs are formed there is a special relationship between each one of them?

With Embryonic Iridology we are on the way to confirming a science that already had been in use more than a century ago. Over the years Iridology has been confirmed in many ways and has gained increasing acceptance as well. We know that in science nothing is finite and much remains to be discovered, an example being the intestine as our second brain and probably it is true for iridology.

Probably it had been known or used before without calling it Iridology. The first explicit description of iridology principles is found in *Chromatica Medica*, a famous work published in 1670 by Philippus Meyens in Dresden, Germany.

Note that there are likely to be more surprises and occurrences in store, since in science nothing is finite and much remains to be discovered. Modern biology is extraordinary and it shows us the body in depth. We are in the era of genes and molecules. Yet, we still return to discoveries and theories abandoned in the past and are shown later on. For now, it is important to know if there is really a relationship between the colon, the nervous system and the brain. Empirically, this relationship is proven daily through observing the iris of the patients, based on the topography of the iris.

Pointers on Evaluating Iris Signs and Constitutional Strength

1 – Constitutional Strength: Barometer of Hereditary Status

Our genetic heritage determines the overall strength of our body tissues and is the basis of our vitality, overall good health, longevity or weakness, the tendency to develop multiple symptoms, lack of resistance, or even disease. Five levels of overall constitutional health are represented in the iris by the characteristic quality and alignment of iris fibers and lacunas.

2 - Color

Abnormal blue, brown, or green color observable in several areas of the iris indicate drug residue, intoxication from xenobiotics or other negative chemical substances, new to us or transmitted by our parents.

Workers in chemically treated fields and those in chemical factories may exhibit abnormal yellowish to reddish or an orange-like color in their irises. They usually complain of various symptoms and over time may develop cancer and other diseases.

3 – Pigment Granulation

Look like brown or dark spots distributed in the iris, or in an iris area corresponding to a specific organ, reveal liver or pancreatic deficiencies and tissue build-up of toxins from inorganic drugs, known as pigment granulation. They may reflect the risk of chronic disease (brown) or degenerative disease (dark) such as cancer. If they are observed in specific zone organs such as the colon, lung, and breast areas they underline hereditary status and higher risk, which may develop a malignancy over the coming years. There might be other such markers in the colon, lung, liver, and breast areas.

4 - Scurf Rim

The Scurf rim is visible on the periphery of the iris, representing the skin area. It shows indications such as underactive skin, toxic, and acid build up in the body. When darker colorations appear over the lung, liver, or kidney area it indicates accumulation of toxins. A scurf rim is also observed in skin disease.

5 - Genetic Markings

Structures variously described as lacunae, crypts, and honeycombs are considered to be structural markers indicating acquired or inherited weakness in the body. The term "structural marking" is derived from the work of Joseph Deck (1954). Such structures represent about 80% of all defect markers. They may be recognized by their shapes and degree of dark coloring, all of which may suggest some tendency for chronic or degenerative disease.

A lacunae or crypt with a black interior is according to Joseph Deck frequently associated as a latent cancer making (constitutional factor with hereditary dispositions). (*Differentiation of Iris Markings* by Joseph Deck, 1980). It may also show an already formed tumor, which, however, should be confirmed, (B. Jensen, *The Science and Practice of Iridology in the Healing Arts*, pg105-1982).

Professor J. Deck and others, including myself, have also confirmed this correlation. I spent over forty-five years with Iridology practice and clinical practice with cancer disease which was an extraordinary source for observation and learning.

6 – Radial Furrows

Radial furrows originate from the colon area and radiate outward on the ciliary zone and to specific organs like the brain, legs, and arms. They indicate toxic materials from sluggish colon spread to the particular organs and usually more accentuated on the brain area, causing brain dysfunction such as bad memory, mental instability, fatigue etc. Radial furrows can look tiny or thick, very dark depending on the degree of intoxication. They indicate a mean for detoxification

7 – Contraction Furrows or Nerve Ring

They indicate the degree of nervous tension from acute to chronic condition. The number of contraction furrows and their localisation in some area of the iris or the whole periphery indicate some nerve and tissue tension. If visible in brain area they indicate mental stress, nervous tension, and irritability, lack of concentration and stress. They may originate in physical or mental areas.

Also called "neurovascular cramp rings," these structures appear in the iris as one or more segments of curved furrows, which follow the iris' circumference.

8 – Brushfield Spots

These are cloud like spots that are visible in the iris when the lymph system becomes sluggish and congested with toxic wastes, oxidize lipids and mucous. They are seen in the iris going all around the periphery in the 6th zone. They have color varying from white to yellow, such as in blue iris or brown in brown iris but also depending on the degree of intoxication and oxidation of the lymphatic system. Heavy yellow and light brown spots are always visible in intoxicated people with chronic disease and usually are visible in the irises of breast cancer patients.

Transversals

Transversals are anomalously formed capillary elements, which take a transverse course through the trabeculae. Transversals are genotyped with malignant tendency or other degenerative processes.

The irises of most of my published breast cancer cases contain a transversal crossing the breast area between the 8:00 and 9:00 in the right iris and between 3:00 and 4:00 in the left iris, but can also be visible on the liver, spleen, showing the implications of these organs in the disease.

The Intestine, Our Second Brain

Surprisingly science only discovered recently, or rather rediscovered that the intestine has a network of nerves that communicates with brain. Curiously, the first discovery took place around 1860 in France, but the Academy of Medicine considered the intestinal nervous system to be of little importance and simply an annex of a vagus nerve without much relevance.

About fifteen years ago, Dr. Michael Gershon, professor of molecular biology at Columbia University (USA), stated that our health depends on the relationship between the brain and the intestine, or better, the intestine and the brain. According to Dr. Gershon, there are two brains with the same chemical relationship between the same neurons of these two brains. When the one becomes irritated the other follows suit.

Two brains in one body ©**NewScientist**

The enteric nervous system in the gut, or "second brain", shares many features with the brain in your head.
It can act autonomously and even influences behaviour by sending messages up the vagus nerve to the brain

BRAIN	SECOND BRAIN
Glial cells support	Glial cells support
85 billion neurons	500 million neurons
100 neurotransmitters identified	40 neurotransmitters identified
Produces 50% of all dopamine	Produces 50% of all dopamine
Produces 5% of all serotonin	Produces 95% of all serotonin
Barrier restricts blood flow to brain	Barrier restricts blood flow to second brain

SPINAL CORD VAGUS NERVE

STOMACH

LARGE INTESTINE

SMALL INTESTINE

PELVIC NERVE

The enteric nervous system comprises a network of neurons spread throughout two layers of gut tissue, the submucosal plexus and the myenteric plexus

A new nervous system called the Enteric Nervous System (ENS) is now referred to as the "second brain". The E.N.S. consists of over 100 billion neurons embedded along the walls of the gut and is a part of the peripheral nervous system, being a division of the autonomic nervous system which controls the gastrointestinal tract. The neurons of the ENS may also greatly influence our emotions, considered as the origin of various nervous and degenerative diseases. The E.N.S. produces more than thirty neurotransmitters, just like the brain. The E.N.S. communicates with the Central Nervous System through the parasympathetic (via the vagus nerve) and the sympathetic via the prevertebral ganglia.

Is the Intestinal Brain Related to Alzheimer's and Parkinson's Disease?

This discovery leads one to think about the role that our "second brain" may play in the cause of certain diseases such as Parkinson's or Alzheimer's disease.

Since the 2009 publication of my book in the Portuguese language, along with my own discoveries based on the observation of thousands of irises, many articles have now been published in scientific magazines that have established the relationship between the intestinal second brain and diseases such as Parkinson's. Furthermore, new avenues of research are now pointing toward the role of intestinal bacteria circulating in the blood, being associated with nervous disease, depression, anxiety, and suicide. We had discovered this relationship about thirty years ago, when patients were observed with an Iridology examination together with Live Blood Analysis.

However, the important question is whether these lesions are formed primarily in the intestine before arising in the cerebral neurons? In my experience I can almost confirm that there cannot be any brain diseases such as Parkinson's or Alzheimer's if there were no prior intestinal lesions or chronic intestinal disorders, and intoxication. The many observations of the iris I have been able to carry out in patients affected by Alzheimer's and Parkinson's disease, systematically shows strong intestinal auto-intoxication and nervous disorders.

According to Professor Heiko Braak, a German anatomopathologist, Parkinson's disease may have its origin in the intestine's enteric nervous system, subsequently reaching the brain through existing central nervous system connections. Professor Braak has demonstrated the anomalies of the enteric nervous system that have shown the presence of Lewy bodies, observed in the brain of patients with Parkinson's Disease. A French team of neurologists and gastro-enterologists, under the direction of Professor Michel Neunlist, made some studies of the enteric nervous system neurons by utilizing biopsies during a colonoscopy. This confirmed various enteric nervous system anomalies through the presence of Lewy bodies. Importantly these anomalies correlate with the gravity of the Parkinson's disease. Some theories suggest that some toxic materials from the environment may cross the nasal mucous and the epithelial intestinal barriers, which provokes some lesions in the enteric nervous system, which itself is connected with the central nervous system through the vagus nerve and after reaching the brain.

If we perform an Iridology exam, it is wise to first look at the digestive tract, the position of the collarette, and then determine if there is a connection with the brain. Most of the time, we try to examine the brain, but forget that the root cause may be in the intestine. This is what I have done all my life. The iris reflects the disorders of the central nervous system perfectly, being its extension. The primary optical vesicular is lined with the same epithelial cells, which line the cavities of the central nervous system.

Embryonic Development of the Nervous System

In the embryo, the nervous system is developed right along the side of the gut, called the spinal nervous system or notochord. In an anatomical position, the nervous system is located behind the intestine. The spinal cord has little branches that go almost everywhere in the body and to the organs, maintaining a close relationship. In this way, the nervous system is already attached to the iris, right after the formation of the embryo. It develops and progresses according to genetic inheritance, having inherited half from the father and half from the mother. Therefore, when observing the nervous collarette and its morphology in the iris, these correspond to an embryonic reflection of our nervous system. In this way, we already have irrefutable evidence in favor of the interpretation of the nervous system through the iris.

The study of embryology leads us to discover how the organs are formed around the primitive intestine call the gut. Even more surprising is the way the organs that have a real embryonic position are located in the topography of the iris.

The first observations carried out in this field as well as the relationship between the position of the organs in the embryo and the topography of the iris, were also provided by Dr. Bernard Jensen.

The 2 weeks old embryo

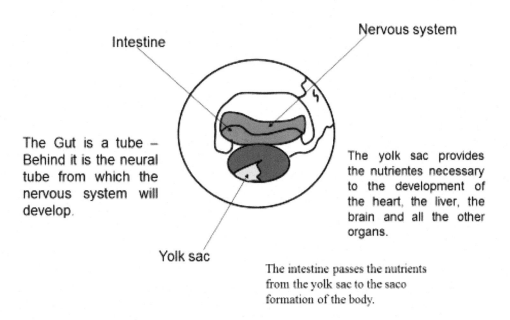

Intestine

Nervous system

The Gut is a tube – Behind it is the neural tube from which the nervous system will develop.

The yolk sac provides the nutrientes necessary to the development of the heart, the liver, the brain and all the other organs.

Yolk sac

The intestine passes the nutrients from the yolk sac to the saco formation of the body.

One can already guess the relationship between the brain, the nervous system, and the intestine. In the iris this generates what we call a "neuro-genetic arc reflex" that can equally occur in other organs with disease call neuro-genetic arc reflex syndrome. But the relationship between the brain, the nervous system and the intestine is already a known fact.

An 8 week old embryo (the organs are forming)

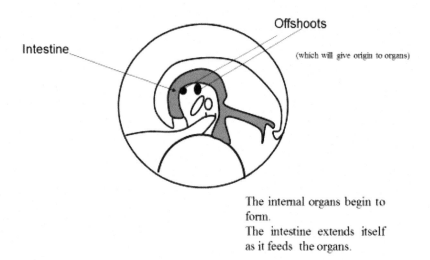

The internal organs begin to form.
The intestine extends itself as it feeds the organs.

In the embryo the ectoderm gives origin to the intestinal nervous system, while the endoderm gives origin to the intestine, the liver, the pancreas etc. In this way, there is a real correlation between the intestine, the liver, the pancreas and the ectoderm organs, which are the nervous system, the skin, the hair, mammary glands, liver and urogenital system.

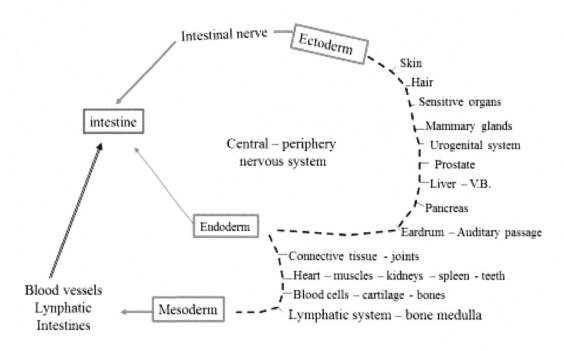

The **Arc Reflex** and the symptomatic relationship between the different organs

Prof. Serge Jurasunas. 2002

As shown in the image, there is a neural arc reflex between the intestines, linking the embryonic organs to one another. We therefore have the basic elements that lead us to understand and establish a relationship between one organ and any other which it might affect.

However, in order to understand the place of the organs in the topography of the iris we still have to explain how the organs are formed in the embryo.

From where and from what are they formed? We first explain all the elements, where moving forward the next ones upon which we will focus will serve to debunk the theory of disease being only local. Conventional medicine has taken a strong position on this theory for more than a century.

Formation of the Organs in the Embryo

Around the fourth week, according to the order of embryonic development, the intestinal gut begins to form offshoots from its wall that gives rise to organs such as the liver, pancreas, lung, and kidney. In order to better understand this phenomenon, we can give the example of a tree sprouting branches from the bark of the trunk. At this level of development, there seems to be a similarity between the plant and the animal worlds; this analogy of the tree being a good example.

Formation of the organs from the offshoots

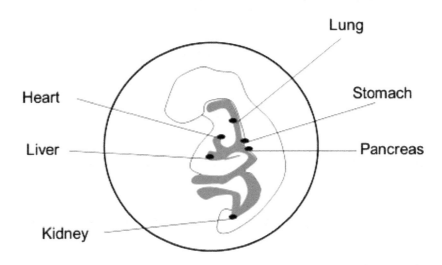

The beginning of the formation of each organ

A seed will grow into a small plant, then into a sapling that develops, grows, forms bark, with more bark forming in different areas giving life to its offshoots that, in turn, grow into branches. When the offshoots branch off the tree trunk they are in an embryonic state, with a growth factor and cellular division, all in all similar to embryonic organs. If we carefully observe a tree, we will see that the bark that covers the new branches is no less than the extension of the bark or of the original tree covering. In the human embryo we have a similar process with the intestine giving origin to division and development. The wonderful thing is that these offshoots will turn into organs such as the liver, heart, pancreas, and lungs. It is truly extraordinary yet very real.

By virtue of these extensive offshoots from the intestine, all the organs are literally embedded in tissue, which, at the beginning of development, was originally intestinal tissue. All these organs branching off from the intestinal tract, drag along with them the nerves that formed by the inside walls of the intestinal tract. In this way, they maintain a certain link of embryonic communication, first of all with the intestinal tract, but also obviously with the other organs.

This is how we can explain reflex disease coming from specific, as well as irritated parts of the colon that will subsequently affect the reflex to an adjacent organ.

Once the organs of our body are formed they are covered with tissue called the "peritoneum," which is itself generated from the intestine. All of our organs in the embryo are covered by this tissue, which originated from the walls of the colon. Therefore, each one of our organs has an embryonic relationship with the intestinal system. In the same way there is a relationship between the organs and the nervous system as they all primarily derive from the intestinal system. We can therefore understand why one organ can affect the other, especially realizing how wrong it is for modern medicine to disassociate the organs from each other.

Organs such as the heart, spleen, lungs, as well as the left arm, are formed above on the left by the colon. The liver, gallbladder, and pancreas are organs that are formed on the right. Well then! In the topography of the iris the position is exactly the same as the one in the embryo.

The primitive intestine, that is, in a certain way the basis of embryonic development seems to be well placed in the middle of the embryo, and therefore of the body. The organs are placed around this tract. The same thing takes place in the topography of the iris.

In this image we can verify the existence of an anatomical relationship between the position of the colon and the brain, both in the embryo and in the iris.

Relationship Between a Cut Section of the Human Embryo and the Iris

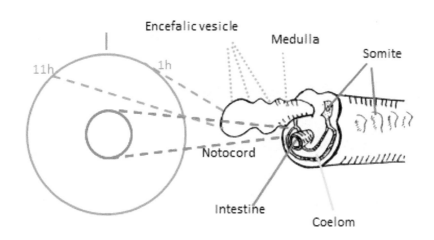

Organogenesis – brain, notocord and the neural plate are the first organs that will develope in the encefalic vesicle.

Serge Jurasunas 1999

Encephalic vesicle, medulla, notochord, mesodermal segment, coelom, intestine

Organogenesis – brain, notochord, and spinal medulla are amongst the first organs to develop in the encephalic vesicle.

Observing the anatomical framework of the nervous system the evidence shows that it projects itself throughout the body, but with a network of ramifications on the intestinal apparatus. Is there really an actual relationship between the colon, the nervous system, and a particular diseased organ? The answer is in the affirmative. Embryology proves it, and Iridology allows us to observe the relationship of this reflex syndrome.

166

1. The area included in the nervous collarette always shows taut and darker tissues than those located outside the collarette.
2. In various areas of the periphery of the collarette, one or various breaches and crypts can be observed extending in the direction of a specific organ.
3. Lacunas, crypts, and other markings are always located on the exterior part of the collarette, and therefore, of the colon.

This last characteristic shows very weak connective tissue, chronic inflammation because of an intoxicated colon, and lower nutritional supply meaning that tissues are not properly fed and become intoxicated from poor elimination by the emunctories. Iridology examination can therefore detect if tissues are intoxicated and the various inflammatory process from acute to degenerative, which may be associated with some abnormal condition or a disease yet to come, but not currently diagnosed.

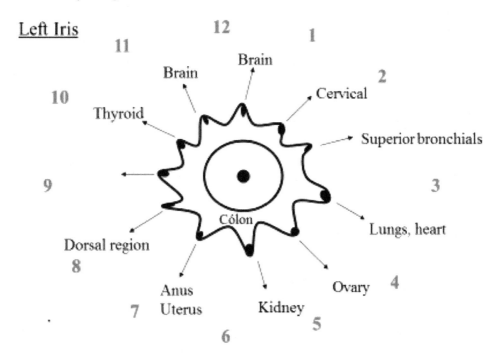

The schema represents the areas of the intestine and dilatated colon causing an irritation of the intestinal nerve endings by pressing on one or more organs of the body. They are usually reflex pains but also pathologies.

Generally, when people suffer from constipation, obviously the area of the colon, especially the descending colon appears darker than the other organs. Therefore, if in a certain area of the colon there is an accumulation of toxins or flatulence causing irritation of the nervous fibers, the same impulse is sent to the opposite organ which is nearest. Thus, we can be sure that we are faced with a reflex nervous syndrome between the colon, the nervous system, and the organ in question.

Sometimes there can be a deeper relationship also involving pathology. Let's remember that organs such as the liver and pancreas are formed from embryonic tissue, the endoderm, the same as the colon, and covered with a tissue called the peritoneum, actually from colon tissue. We can conclude that the colon is often involved in certain pathologies of these organs. When the iris shows an expansion of the intestinal tissues that cover the liver area, I have often observed a serious implication of the colon and the nervous system in irises of people affected by chronic hepatitis or cirrhosis. For example, Iridology can show some specific signs common to most people who have an intoxicated colon together with a neuro-genetic arc reflex that involves organs such as the liver, pancreas, ovary, or lungs leading to serious disorders including hepatitis, cirrhosis, and malignancy. The study of embryology has given me many insights that, at first, I had lacked.

In the chapter of illustrated examples with practical cases, there is the iris of a young thirteen-year-old girl with liver cirrhosis which shows an association with the colon and the nervous system. Hereditarily, this patient had a predisposition to this disease which is clearly visible in the iris. Although the pediatrician had always considered her to be in good health, he never paid any attention to her father and mother's health. At thirty six years of age, her father's cholesterol and triglycerides were extremely high. The liver and nervous system were in bad condition in both parents, as also observed in their irises.

At nine years of age she showed the first symptoms and was diagnosed with hepatitis. At thirteen her case had become very serious and her hepatitis turned into cirrhosis, yet she was considered as healthy before and had never received any dietary advice from the pediatric doctor after having been diagnosed. This situation could have been averted in order to prevent an eventual transplant.

Another example came from a thirty-eight-year-old patient. Three months before coming to see me he had suffered from gastrointestinal problems with severe pain, a bloated abdomen, and a feeling of extreme physical tiredness. During this period nobody had been able to determine what disease he was suffering from. No one paid attention to the problem of his intestinal disorder. An iris examination would have certainly been useful.

After three months, a CAT scan finally detected multiple metastases in the liver, but neglected the colon. After many other tests, a primary tumor was finally discovered in the upper part of the bronchials, already developed at an advanced stage.

In carrying out an iris examination I found the answer, in fact, shortly after which he showed me the medical report which he had forgotten in the car. In the right iris, the upper part of the descending colon literally submerged the upper part of the bronchials, implicating the nervous system. This man had a strong predisposition towards disease in one particular area. In this part of the colon a large quantity of toxins had accumulated negatively influencing the bronchials and also presenting a confirmed hereditary trait. It is understandable why the colon is so important above all when it is neglected, as in the case of this man who should have had a detoxification of the colon long before, in order to possibly prevent such a calamity.

Dr. Jensen cites the example of the famous actor, John Wayne, who died of cancer. He first developed lung cancer, then colon cancer, and in the end stomach cancer. The first time they removed a lung, secondly they removed part of the colon, and at the end, part of the stomach, but he did not survive. According to Dr. Jensen, the problem was almost certainly in the colon and the example I have given on bronchial cancer is proof of this theory. As Hippocrates so clearly stated, "The whole is more than a part, but the part belongs to the whole."

The lungs and the bronchials are linked to the colon, which embryology has now proven. By observing in the iris both the colon and lung areas, we may be able to detect the link and eventually prevent lung disease risk, or in case of disease, often including cancer. We can really observe that actually the disease started because of bad colon tissue. Therefore, we further know just where to first start treating the patient. Over the past twenty years, how many similar cases of lung cancer have I observed implicating the colon! Indeed, there were many cases where more attention should have been given to the colon when it comes to understanding how to begin treatment. Detox and colon regeneration make an overwhelming difference when you treat lung disease or lung cancer, based upon my decades of clinical experience.

Based upon my decades of observation and practice there is no doubt that first, Iridology is valuable to profile your patient, and secondly, to observe the association between the two organ's tissues, seeing how the lungs are associated with intestinal tissue. Then you will know where to start treating your patients.

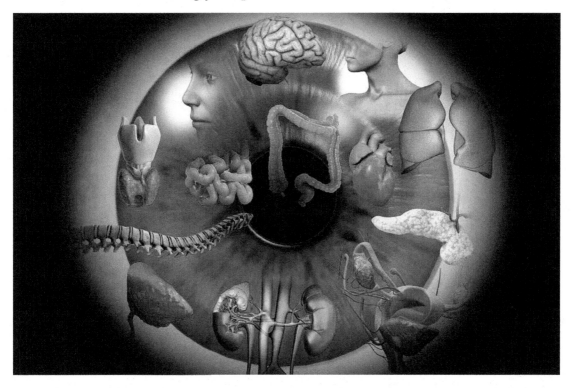

The iris is not only the window of our soul, but a true projection of all the organs of our body, with each one having been delimited in a specific area. Humans have been built in a total perfection, where the iris appears to be a way to examine directly the condition of our own development and hereditary profile.

Interpretation of the Signs in the Iris

The observation of the iris is carried out with the help of an iris chart in which the organs have an anatomical position.

The main organs such as the liver, pancreas, ovaries, and heart, have a special delimitation due to their importance in organic functions.

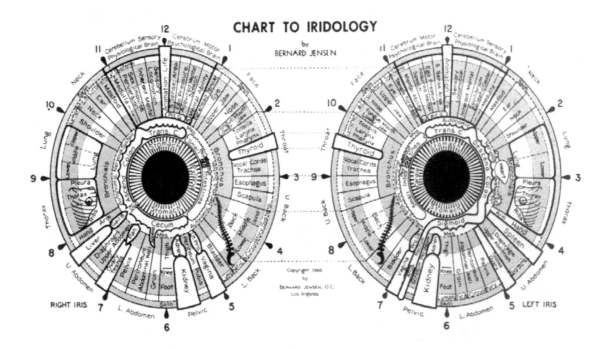

Iridology Chart Developed by Dr. Bernard Jensen, D.C.

These organs are located according to their embryological positioning and are read like the hands that read time on the face of a clock.

Iris Chart Zones

The iris chart is divided into Sectors (organs) and Zones (systems), being an important development in Iridology, where each system fits exactly, specifying an area which can be immediately observed. For example: skin, bone, muscles, intestinal area, and sensory nerves.

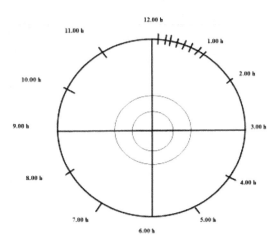

There are also definite areas in which various organs and systems are placed, for example skin, sensory nerves, bone, muscles, lymphatic system, stomach, and intestines.

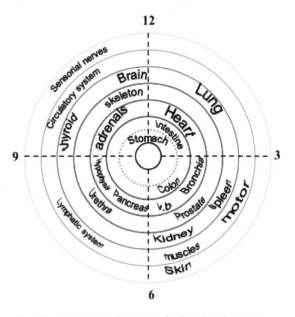

The 7 Iris areas: In the center is the digestive tract following embryonic development.

Besides the observation of the organs, the iris reading also interprets the abnormal colors, as well as other signs, crypts, lacunas, stains, or pigments.

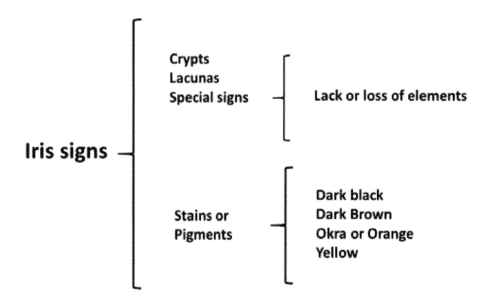

The alignment of the fibers in the iris are also the object of study, to determine whether they are tense, distorted, or deep, indicating the constitution of the connective tissue. This kind of observation shows the degree of an individual's constitution or the so-called density. The density shows the physiological constitution of a person, the quality of the connective tissues, as well as the ability to react and recuperate from a disease after a treatment.

Different Kinds of Constitutional Strength (Hereditary) Expressed by the Density of the Iris Fibers

Generally, a poor density corresponds to a weak constitution, usually with a fair or bad nervous and intestinal system and bowel function. The density ranges from a value that goes from 1 to 5. Today, it is rare to find a density with the value of 1.

Over the passing years, the constitution of our body has become weaker from inherited status, bad lifestyle, dietary style, nutrient deficiency, and an excess of pharmaceutical drugs. Most iris examinations provide us at first with the color of the iris from normal, to mixed or abnormal colors, along with poor constitution, with a density between 3 to 5, which shows how our bodies are degenerating. Patients with a bad constitution, as in a stage 4 for instance, have more difficulty to recover and are more subject to colds, change of weather, and nerve dysfunction. Improvement through detoxification, vitamins, supplementation, and nutrition seem more logical to improve health status and recuperation from a disease. Much too often, even with a patient's poor constitution, pharmaceutical drugs taken to treat symptoms or a disease should be prescribed with precaution since such a body is weak, but today we have an over abuse of drugs and forget about our body's constitution and what it means be healthy. We just accept disease too often and live with it. This is especially true in the USA but now in Europe as well.

As can be observed in the topography, there is a relationship between the colon and the other organs of the body. The area of the brain appears in the top of the iris chart at 11:00 and 1:00 dominating the rest of the organs. This reflects the same positioning as in the human body.

Moreover, the autonomic nervous system communicates with numerous plexuses of the body and can therefore influence the function of the specific organs. For example, the nerves in the transverse colon are linked to the brain. An intoxication of the transverse colon can irritate the nerve endings linked to the cervical nerves and then to the brain.

People who complain of cervical problems and, above all, have a stiff and sore neck are also, generally speaking, people who suffer from constipation and accumulation of toxins that irritate the nerve ramification and tissues.

As a consequence, the nerves affecting the solar plexus can cause disturbances in various organs, such as the heart, the rectum, the pancreas, the ovaries, or the abdomen. These nerves are often influenced by toxins from the descending colon that in turn affect the solar plexus, which controls the functions of these organs.

The observation of the iris can highlight the vast communication circuits, nervous, blood, and lymphatic, which are closely related to all our organs. It is a vast network of communication similar to a telephone exchange. Our body's equilibrium and correct functioning depends on the good performance of this enormous network of nerves that connect every organ, with 60 trillion cells, about 200 hectares of tissues that make up the human body, 300 to 400 square meters of intestine, and well-functioning elimination organs.

Physical build, parental inheritance, and our genetic condition are all distinctive factors which are already etched in the embryo, then in the iris, giving us a better understanding and direction for our way of life and our eating habits.

Colon Intoxication and Symptoms

From my own experience and observation, a large variety of symptoms, organic disorders, and indirectly, some diseases can be associated with chronic constipation. This had been advocated decades ago by pioneers both in USA and Europe. However, we must first give some serious explanation on how constipation and toxins can really be the cause of organic disorders and diseases. I, myself, for decades had come to the same conclusion; however, by observing irises, we can really understand better how the body is functioning and how it becomes intoxicated.

Constipation means that the colon is not eliminating feces daily, which then are stored and accumulate in the colon. This in turn intoxicates the body if the liver cannot itself detoxify, which is true, but do we have all the same colon, the same liver, and the same nervous system? Mostly not, where today we have to admit that the hereditary status, the quality of the colon, and the nervous system play a key role determining individual health.

From an Iridology standpoint what we actually see in the iris is that the autonomic nerve wreath (collarette) connects the bowel to the internal organs, which shows how our bodies are made. This connection emerges from the gut during the development of the embryo in the mother's womb. What we realize today from embryo study is that the organs as they appear in the iris chart are a genetic map of the make up or constitution of the body. Therefore, we also have to deal with colon constitutional weakness, localized in certain areas which appear darker than other parts of the colon. This has shown that specific areas of these tissues, which tend to pick up more toxins, may first have irritated the tissue and then developed inflammation. Furthermore, toxins may irritate the nerve ramification, and then by arc reflex, which may affect the nearest organs develop pain, providing this is not a pathological condition as I already have explained. From an Iridology standpoint, we observe that many organs are influenced by toxic build up in the part of the bowel that develops an irritation, but additionally one can develop a pathology of the colon itself.

We cannot just separate out the colon, that may accumulate toxins in some specific portion, creating a state of irritation, which by reflex action may affect other organs, developing pain for which we don't know the cause. Usually it also implicates the collarette (autonomic nerve wreath), when pointing toward an organ, and indicates the irritation and pain area in the specific organ.

Excess toxins and intestinal bacteria circulating in the blood may reach the brain causing inflammation, have a negative effect on our behavior, and may even be the basis of a disease such as Parkinson's, as demonstrated today by a number of university researchers. Some bacteria produce neuropeptides, which circulate through the blood and into the brain, disturbing neuron function. On the other hand, yeast Candida may cross the intestinal barrier, penetrate into the blood circulation, and be the cause of symptoms such as migraine, headaches, irritation, fatigue, and pains. In this case, an experienced practitioner can easily observe through a Live Blood Microscopy Analysis many yeast forms like Candida, often even colonies of Candida, visible in the case of chronic diseases, as well as cortisone intake, and weak immune defense. Often, this is seen in live blood observation. This is what I usually do after an iris examination showing toxic bowels, diverticulosis, and dark tissue. In this way you definitively prove what you observe in the irises of patients.

Some patients may complain about few symptoms that doctors cannot explain the origin while some patients, including juveniles twelve to fourteen years old, may complain daily about up to ten or, occasionally, even more symptoms. I have seen cases of juveniles affected by nearly fifteen different symptoms which we can easily associate to a bad colon constitution, modern food, poor bowel function, and poor nervous system as well.

I remember the case of an eight-year-old boy suffering from severe headaches, while doctors were unable to detect any particular problem or disease. They made a brain scan which showed everything was normal. I made a Live Blood Analysis observation, and what do you think I observed? Colonies of Candida, micro plaques composed of oxidized fats, and red blood cells in rouleaux. There was no need to complain further about the cause of these intense headaches, which disappeared after treating the boy.

From my experience multiple symptoms may manifest in two different ways:
   A – Some symptoms can demonstrate occasionally.
   B – Some symptoms can demonstrate frequently.

Possible disease and organic dysfunction indicated from iris observation include:
   - Vertigo
   - Pain in the back, neck, legs, arms
   - Headache
   - Migraine
   - Rheumatism, pains in articulation
   - Pains in the abdomen with flatulence
   - Pains in the muscle

Indications from behavior:
   - Insomnia
   - Fatigue
   - Agitation
   - Stress condition

Mental indication:
- Anxiety
- Worry
- Depression
- Bipolar behavior
- Cognitive disorder

Depression and cognitive disorders may have a cause with our intestinal neurons, intestinal bacteria, neurotoxins circulating in the blood, and chemicals such as phthalates that disturb the production of brain neurotransmitters and require detoxification, improvement of the intestinal micro-flora, increase bowel elimination, and adopting an appropriate nutritional program, including vitamin B complex, magnesium, taurine, GABA, lecithin, and zinc.

A bad constitution with a bad nervous system, which in the iris chart goes around the gastro intestinal system, makes a demarcation line between the digestive tract and the ciliary zone. Naturally, this can be viewed as a hypothesis, yet was well defined by all the pioneers in iridology like Dr. Bernard Jensen and J. Deck. The position of the colon, nervous system and the body's organs appear in the iris chart the same as they are positioned in the embryo. It becomes apparent only when you observe your patient's irises and ask questions about his lifestyle. Then you can make the connection, since it needs a great deal of experience and knowledge to be able to master Iridology observation.

List of Auto-Intoxication Symptoms

Rheumatism	High blood pressure
Eczema	Kidney disorders
Hepatitis	Fibromes of uterus
Circulatory disorder	Mammary cysts
Arthritis	Epilepsy
Meniere Syndrome	Parkinson's Disease
Depression	Lack of memory and concentration
Insomnia	Acne
Fibrocystic breast	Leg pains
Bladder infections	Kidney disorders
Ovarian cysts	Tumors

More recently I developed a new iris chart showing the relationship between the colon reflex points and body organs dysfunction. It really is a new approach to monitor reflex-disease or symptoms as well as a new avenue in complementary medicine, which serves to monitor not specifically the disease, but to associate its reflex cause. This chart is most useful to the Iridologist working with colon reflex disease and when looking to master the cause of certain pathologies.

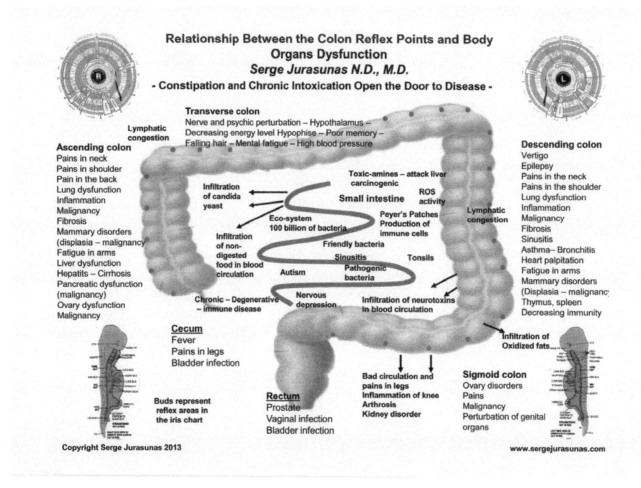

This iris chart is available in large format with iris photos that go along with reflex conditions.
Contact: sergejurasunas@hotmail.com

Practical Cases

This chapter illustrates some abnormal conditions of the colon as they are reflected in the iris and associated with reflex symptoms or diseases.

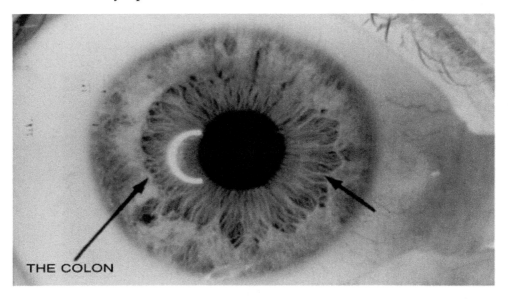

Figure 1

Abnormal morphology of the colon and the course of the nervous wreath (collarette) in intestinal disorders.

Nerve Wreath Collarette

Space occupied by the gastrointestinal system and collarette, indicating pathological conditions

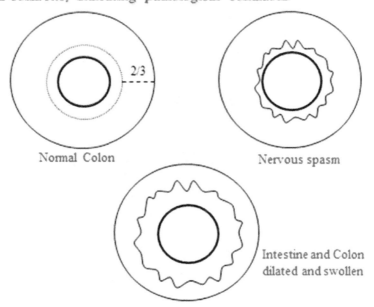

Normal Colon

Nervous spasm

Intestine and Colon dilated and swollen

As we can see in the images, the nervous system is highly involved in gastrointestinal disorders, according to the position of the collarette, depending on the distance from the pupil. We will also find out that there is a relationship between the colon and the other organs. Space occupied in the iris by the gastrointestinal system and collarette is associated with either a normal, healthy colon or colon dysfunction, not to mention pathological conditions and arc reflex syndrome. In the practical cases presented, there are various examples that show this reflex symptom. We can also verify that, according to the abnormal and zigzag route that the autonomic nervous system (collarette) forms, it can indicate a psychological profile, sensibility, anxiety, or other disorders that an Iridologist must carefully note. The collarette is a direct reflection of our genetics, as it is formed long before the differentiation of the organs. That is why its observation is always a valid trump card in the genetic examination of an individual.

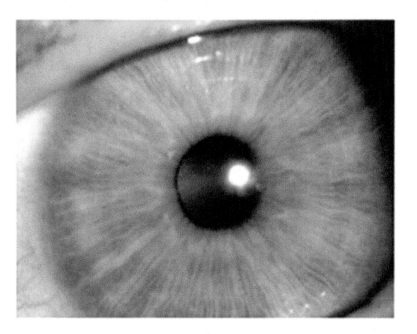

Figure 2

Iris: Typical example of an iris showing a very good physical constitution and gastrointestinal condition. It shows a case of good health status in an eighty-three-year-old man.

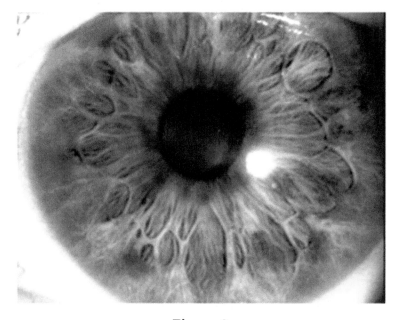

Figure 3

This iris, to the contrary, indicates a poor constitution and hereditary status. We observe an abnormal, ballooned colon, especially the descending colon, with strong pressure at 3:00 and 4:00 on heart, lung, and ovary (iris of a woman). We also observe an overwhelming expanded, enlarged collarette and the relationship between the colon and the nervous system. It also shows a tendency toward constipation, flatulence, and gas accumulation. The shape of the collarette is associated with low vitality, lowered function of the respiratory system, and emotional behavior. In this case, the patient has lost his energy level, always feels worried and tired, and has difficulty breathing. The condition of the descending colon with major inflammation also may show a cancer risk near 4:00, but not always; however, this is often observed in cases of colon cancer.

Collarette
Good versus Unbalanced

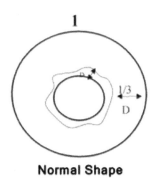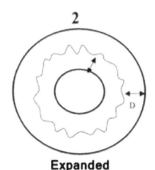

Normal Shape   **Expanded**

At birth we receive both physical and psychological hereditary baggage, transmitted through our parents, which will influence our state of health, as well as our behavior, which can also be influenced by the environment in which we live, as well as our eating habits. Our nervous system, represented in the iris by the shape of the collarette, its thickness or absence, determines at least three important interpretations. It represents the condition of the autonomic nervous system. It borders the intestinal area and is associated with bowel dysfunction, bad digestion, dysbiosis, spasms etc. It also represents the spinal vertebrae. (Bernard Jensen 1989; John Andrews 2015). However, the collarette determines not only the energy supply to the digestive organs, but the energy that feeds all our organs. It is linked to the central nervous system, is an indication of our physical inheritance, but also of the emotional behavior and psychosomatic state. It also influences our way of expressing ourselves. Some iridologists say they can detect a person's state of mind through the iris. Dr. David Pesek is one of the most advanced Iridologists in this particular area, having developed a brain-iris chart associated with our emotional behavior. Image 1 (above) shows a very good nervous system, good functioning, and a good quality of the gastrointestinal system. This indicates a good balanced nervous system and a person with good prospects for realizing their goals. In Image 2 we have a fairly extended imbalance in the collarette showing poor qualities inherited at the level of the nervous system, with colon problems.

Blocked energy and decreasing energy supply in certain organs and tiredness, are becoming more frequent and visible in the irises. As far as the psyche goes, note an increase in sensibility, difficulties in breathing, anxious and disturbed mind, and above all, difficulties in sleeping at night

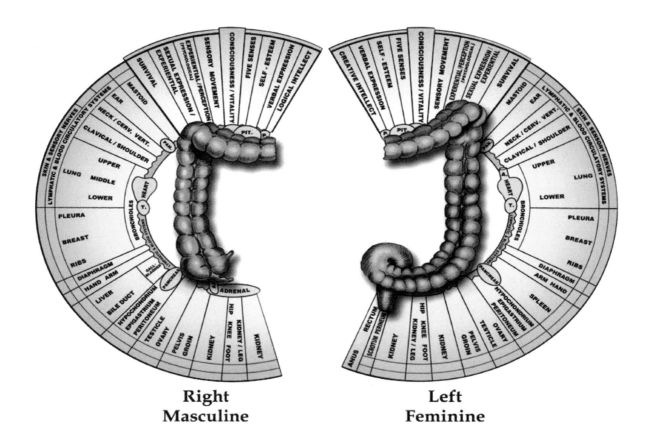

Right
Masculine

Left
Feminine

Relationship between the Colon and the Body's Organs

This image shows the relationship of the colon with each organ of the body and allows us to easily understand the reflex disorders that can appear in any organ, the cause of which is related to the colon.

Bloated/Swollen or Hypotonic Colon Descending Colon

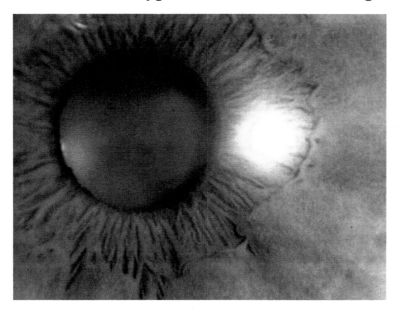

Figure 4

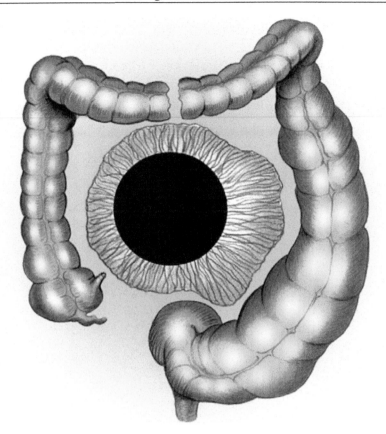

Figure 5

Left Iris

The left iris shows an extremely distended descending colon. Pressure at 2:00, just on the shoulder and neck, with reflex pain. Severe pressure at 3:00, heart, and thorax, palpitations, chest pain, and sometimes difficulty in breathing, constipation, gas, and pathogenic bacteria. At 6:50, note the small black lacunas in the anus area meaning strong gas pressure, fistulas and pain.

Prolapse of the Transverse Colon

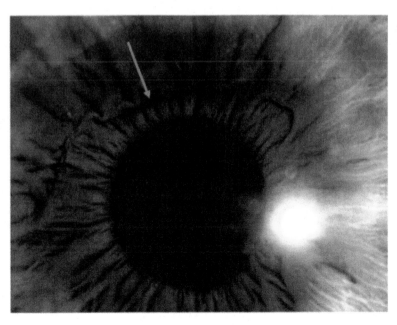

Figure 6

A prolapsed transverse colon can trigger unsuspected situations. The pressure exhorted affects the pelvic area influencing the ovaries in women and the prostate in men. This pressure interferes with the blood and lymphatic circulation of the lower limbs. Bad circulation in the legs is often caused by the consequences of a prolapsed transverse colon. An irregular menstrual cycle can also be caused by the consequences of this disorder.

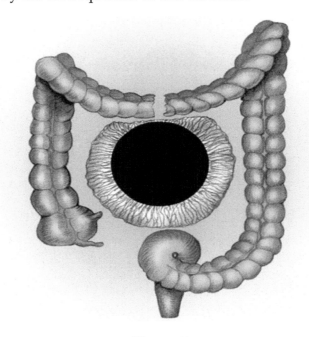

Figure 7

Prolapse of the Transverse Colon (Intestinal view)

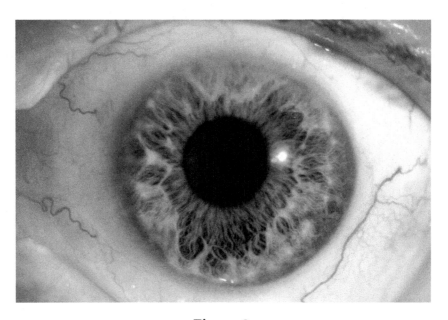

Figure 8

Prolapse of the Sigmoid Colon

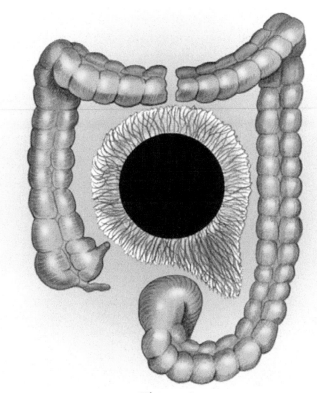

Figure 9

Prolapse of the Sigmoid Colon (Intestinal view)

In this case, the feces accumulated in this part of the colon cause a prolapse that further slows the elimination of feces.

Intoxication of the Descending Colon and Sigmoid

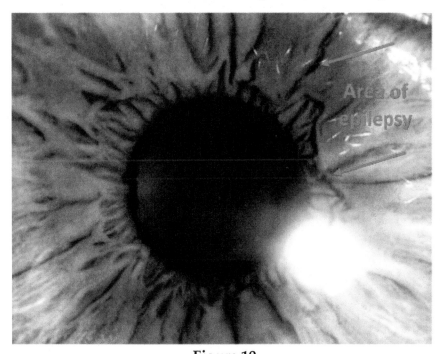

Figure 10

This is a bad inherited colon with chronic constipation and waste accumulation. The restricted collarette close to the edge of the pupil indicates an imbalance in nerve supply to the digestive system, poor food absorption, lack of digestive enzymes and spasms. It is often associated with migraines to epileptic situation, which is the case of the patient. Deep radial furrows are visible, especially on the brain area, an indication of toxin absorption and nerve dysfunction. In such case, appropriate detoxification, colon irrigation, changing diet, taking some supplementation such as probiotics, magnesium, taurine, glutathione, and lecithin, including SOD for a period of thirty to sixty days can start to improve the condition.

Case of a Man of 63 Years with Lung Cancer

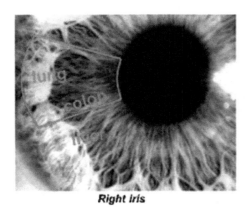

Right iris

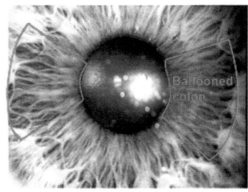

Left iris

Figure 11

The patient is a heavy smoker with bad dietary style, overeating, suffers from digestive disorders, having a very nervous and aggressive disposition. He complains about bad digestion and excess gases, an indication of flatulence, retention, poor assimilation of nutriments, confirming his bad food habits.

The right iris indicates a tendency toward respiratory problems, showing the existing relationship between the colon, the nervous system, and indication of the lung area where cancer is detected. There is a heavy acidity ground as seen by the white and inflamed tissue fibers. We notice some large, white, inflamed fibers coming from the border of the pupil crossing on the liver area at 9:00 to reach the collarette and the pancreas, a further indication of disturbances of the liver function which is the case.

Both irises show a very ballooned colon and exaggerated, distorted collarette, with many lacunas visible within going in a zig-zag pattern. This shows a weakness of tissue and indicates inflammation, underlining a disturbed nervous system and heavy stress. The stomach ring is a visible sign of gastric disorder. The right iris shows very well the colon that covers the lung area between 8:00 and 9:00, with a yellowish color where the tumor is localized further indicating drug settlement.

In Iridology, when we observe the embryonic association between the colon and the lungs, it provides an indication of where to start treating your patients. We must also never forget the microbiome and the intestinal immune system as part of our body's defense when it comes to establishing a holistic treatment. The reader needs to know that, first, it is an embryonic connection, and the microbiome then is one other thing.

Diverticula

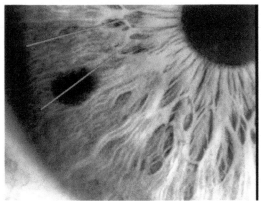

Figure 12

Diverticula in the ascending colon indicated by the arrows. They often contain toxic remains which have not been eliminated, as well as parasites.

Case with Diverticula in the Descending Colon

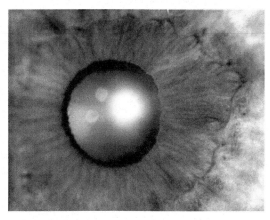

Figure 13

Left iris of a sixty-one-year-old man with an intestinal X-ray of the same case.

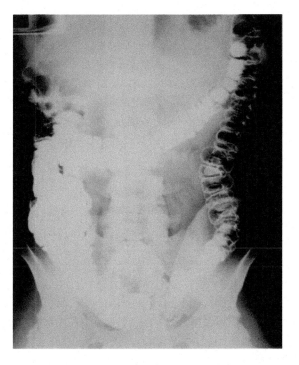

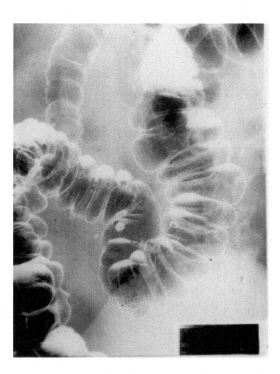

The X-ray revealed more than one hundred diverticula in the descending colon, which is extremely bloated because of the accumulation of gas. The iris shows the same characteristics in the descending colon (small sacs located on the edge of the collarette).

The state of tiredness, nervousness, and irritability that the patient suffered, are often the result of infections developed in the diverticula sacs that can irritate the nerve endings of the colon.

Male: Forty-eight-years old
Clinical story: Prostate-bladder cancer
Left iris color: Blue

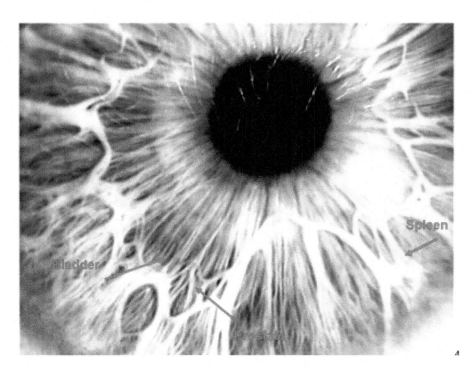

Figure 14

The iris shows an enlarged collarette, an indication of flatulence, tendency to bloating, lack of peristalsis, and prolapses. It also indicates speedy transit time of food passing through the digestive tract and poor assimilation of nutrients. Usually these subjects have a good appetite and eat very fast. Here we see the collarette going in zig zag, irritate and with major inflammation and more distended from 6:00 to 7:00 pushing the colon tissue over the prostate and bladder area. We observe irritated fibers coming from the pupil going to plexus area of the collarette showing strong nerve and tissue tension.

This iris clearly indicates the inflammation of the prostate and bladder associated with the colon and the nervous system. The ballooned sigmoid colon and pressure at 6:00 indicates an area of inflammation and feces retention.

The patient is a very nervous person, psychologically disturbed; having a very agitated life with high stress status, gets up every day at 3:00 or 4:00 a.m. to deliver merchandise, driving all morning. Basically, the iris perfectly shows a risk of developing problems of prostate and/or bladder. We have many similar irises, either blue or brown, with the same characteristics. Living a hasty life with so much nervous tension, no wonder the patient eats too fast and does not benefit from his food. Indeed, this is a very bad nervous system and inherited colon, getting worse from this wrong lifestyle. This is also a very acidic terrain that needs more alkaline food.

Ovarian Tumor, Very Intoxicated Bowel
Left Iris

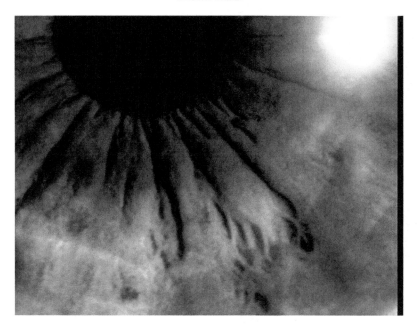

Figure 15

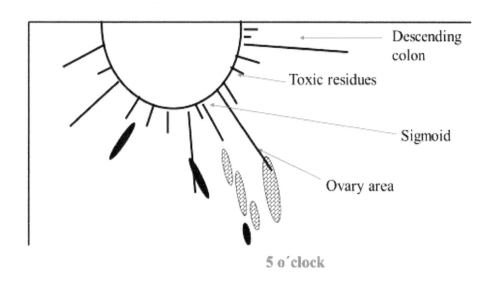

Figure 16

Very dark and toxic colon. Absent collarette. Poor nutrient absorption. Accumulation of toxins that by reflex affect the ovary area. Retraction of the descending colon.

Very Intoxicated Bowel

In this case, there is a strong connection between the ovary and the opposite part of the colon. At 5:00 we observe a large and deep radial furrow coming from the colon and crossing the ovary area with some visible open acute lacunas in the ciliary zone. The tissues of the colon are very dark showing a degenerative condition.

Bronchial Cancer
Male: Thirty-eight-years old

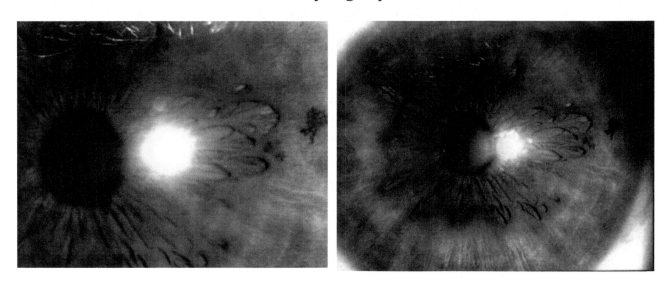

Thirty-eight-year old man / left iris –brown color

Figure 17

In this iris between 2:00 and 3:00 (bronchial area) several small, closed lacunas involving the colon tissue are pushing over the bronchial area, very close to each other seeming to turn towards the descending colon.

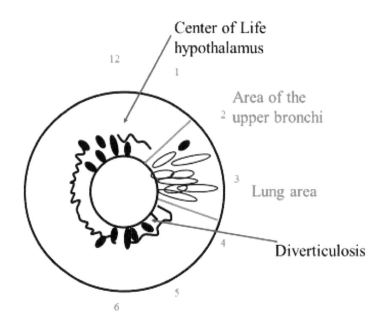

Figure 18

In this iris between 2:00 and 3:00 (bronchial area), we observe several closed lacunas that are coming from the colon tissue showing genetic weakness. The colon area is very dark accumulating a large quantity of toxins. Radial furrows are visible all around the colon and going into the brain area at 12:00 (center of life) that indicates toxins. The iris perfectly shows the links between the intoxicated colon, the collarette, and the bronchial area with the risk of disease, in this case a bronchial cancer.

Case of Cancer of the Rectum
Male: Sixty-six-years old
Left iris: light brown color - Density: 3
Clinical history: colon cancer

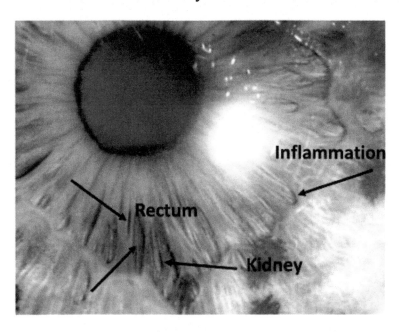

Figure 19

We can observe an enlarged collarette and a descending colon extremely ballooned with many inflammatory lacunas, an indication of acute activity of the tissues. The brown collarette and colon or a central heterochromia, indicates a disturbance of the intestinal tract and immune deficiency. At 6:00 and 7:00 notice two degenerative, small lacunas, one of which is located on the rectum area and the other at the end of the sigmoid where a tumor was diagnosed. Notice also the brown pigments, an indication of lower metabolism and bad liver function.

Chronic Hepatitis
Thirteen-year-old girl - Right Iris

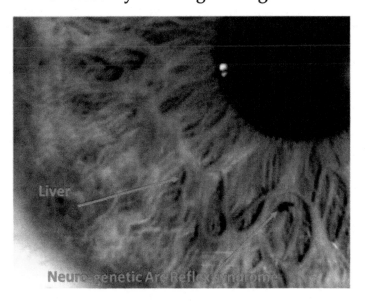

Figure 20

Clinical story: Chronic hepatitis detected at nine years of age turned into cirrhosis at twelve years of age. She came in for consultation at thirteen years of age.

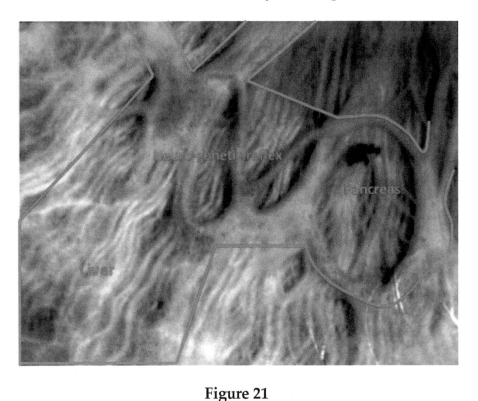

Figure 21

The red lines mark-down the area involving the neuro-genetic-arc-reflex syndrome

Right iris: This iris shows a neuro-genetic arc reflex syndrome involving the colon, the collarette, and the liver, while the pancreas seems also involved. We observe that the collarette becomes elevated, thickened and genetically multibridged. This is an indication of endocrine, immune, metabolic (blood sugar) inflammatory conditions. In his booklet on *Embryology in Iridology*, John Andrews, a famous Iridologist, mentioned, with good reason, that embryonic development can have a profound influence on the dynamic of the collarette itself, and therefore can carry the echoes of disease. We observe two lacunas at the outer border of the nerve wreath which connects with the colon and the liver, involving the pancreas, which always associates with weaker organs. This is an acidic ground with inflammation and high oxidative stress status. The iris of the mother and father indicate liver-nervous dysfunction that the young girl inherited during the embryonic development. If both the mother and father have a bad liver and colon, and then the child is likely to inherit a chronic/degenerative condition. However, from a medical standpoint she was classified as healthy.

Bad dietary style, excess vaccinations, and antibiotics may contribute to precipitate a dormant genetic problem. The first year is critical in establishing the health of a child.

Iris of the Mother
Right Iris

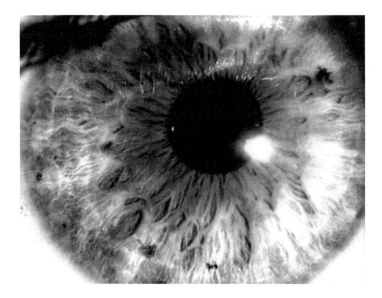

Figure 22

We observe an iris with abnormal color, dark and intoxicated colon, especially the ascending colon. Just before 8:00 on the liver area we observe a narrowing collarette and white fibers, a transversal indication of bad liver inherited by her daughter. At 7:00 a large lacuna is situated on the pancreas area. Observe the white irritated fibers visible on the ciliary zone, an indication of high oxidative stress. These are people working hard in the fields with bad eating habits and both with high cholesterol and triglyceride level. Notice transversals visible between 8:00 and 10:00 which indicate weakness in the connective tissues while the hepatic transversal shows a poor detoxification mechanism and a bad liver inherited by the daughter.

Iris of the Father
Right Iris

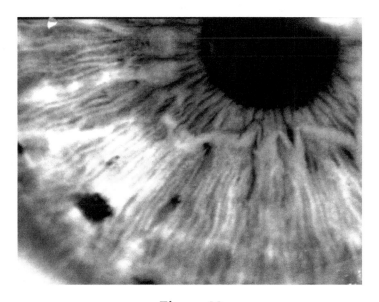

Figure 23

The iris shows a badly intoxicated colon, a collarette in zig-zag coming close to the pupil, being indication of poor food absorption and enzyme deficiency. At 8:00, on the liver area, the fibers are irritated, very white with a dark toxemic spot, an indication of bad liver function; same as his wife with cholesterol and triglycerides being very high.

Comment: Observing the iris of the father and mother we can perfectly understand the daughter's condition from a hereditary standpoint, having been born with the same organic disorders and weakness, which later turned into a degenerative process, as well as from being raised on the wrong foods.

Cancer of the Uterus
Female: Forty-five-years old
Left Iris
Height: 5.51 feet Weight: 206 pounds
Biological age: over 55 years
Mother died of colon cancer. Father suffers from intestinal disorders

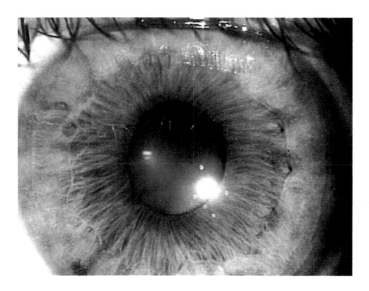

Figure 24

This iris shows a large, ballooned colon, distention and an irritated collarette, associated with gastrointestinal disturbances. We observe white fibers coming from the pupil border reaching the plexus of the collarette, then passing through the colon demonstrating the relationship between the colon and the brain. The enlarged pupil (mydrosis) can be a genetic, chronic or acute condition indicating a weak nervous system. The patient suffered from chronic constipation, up to eight days without evacuation, felt very tired, with pain in the legs (overweight and pressure from the colon), was very nervous, which probably associated with intestinal dysfunction, auto-intoxication, and insomnia (low serotonin). The colon is making strong pressure on the uterus at 7:00; plus, we observe darker tissue in the colon and outside the ciliary zone.

Before surgery, the patient agreed to follow a detoxification program to improve the bowel function. After two weeks of taking a mixture of enzyme yeast cells preparation, Sun Chlorella, probiotics, antioxidants, enzymes, and a cocktail of vegetable juice, she eliminated a large quantity of feces and over two pounds of worms. Afterward, she started to feel much better and was ready for surgery. After the surgery she started to follow a recommended diet, felt healthier, and lost fifty-eight pounds.

Female: Sixty-four years
Colon Cancer of the Descending Colon (Sigmoid)

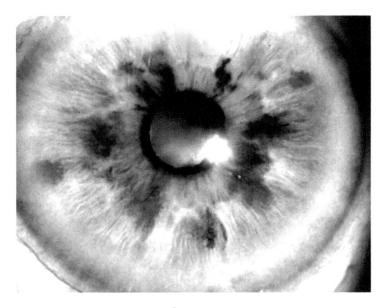

Figure 25

Left iris

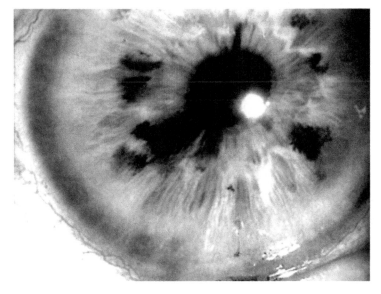

Figure 26

Right Iris

On the left iris (Fig. 25) two large brown metabolic pigments are visible in the sigmoid. On the right iris we observe several dark metabolic pigments (usually an indication of malignancy risk) including a larger one located on the liver area, an indication of poor liver function. Overall, this is a typical case of cancer risk and a profile that usually appears with age.

Male twenty-one-years old – Nervous Depression

Clinical story: Very nervous, depression, insomnia, intestinal gases, digestive disorder, acidosis
Family: Mother, father, grandmother suffer from liver disease and cardiovascular disorders

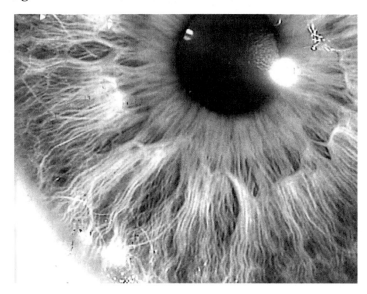

Figure 27

Right iris

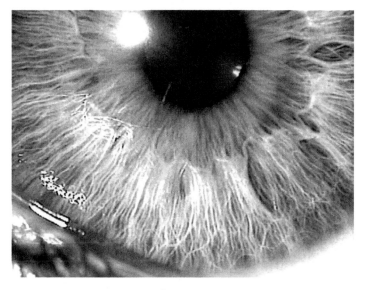

Figure 28

Left Iris

Iris signs. The irises show very white and irritated radials and especially the right iris at 8:00 on the liver area, showing a large concentration of irritated white radials together with visible transversals. It indicates a bad liver function from hereditary status as described above. This is a major condition of inflammation, oxidative stress, and acidosis. On the left iris we observe a distended collarette, ballooned colon with inflammation at about 3:00 to 3:20, an indication of bad digestion and gas retention. A lacuna is visible at 3:00 in the left iris, which may indicate heart dysfunction from family risk. This is a bad iris for a twenty-one-year old man with nervous and depressive condition and intestinal disorder, not only from bad hereditary status, but with wrong food intake. During her pregnancy, his mother was under stressful conditions,

195

which associates with other health problems in the family, which explains the constitution of the irises. Here we have a condition of nervous prevention, high oxidative stress, bad liver function that needs first to decrease oxidative stress, improve the nerve condition with some manganese, magnesium, phosphorus, taurine, vitamin B complex, lecithin, and GABA to detoxify the liver along with a better diet.

Case of Brain Cancer
Male: Twenty-six-years old

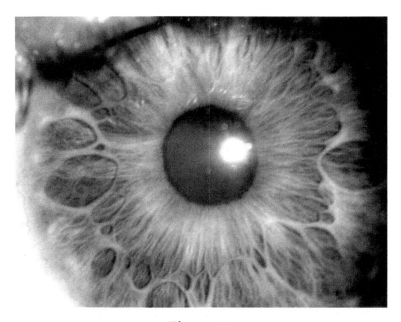

Figure 29

This is an iris with poor inherited constitution, tissue weakness shown by large lacunas, and a very bad nervous system, as visible with the abnormal and overwhelming (distended) collarette going in a zig-zag. We observe a ballooned colon from 1:00 to 4:00, an indication of digestive disorder, and flatulence, but also with a bad inherited colon from his father. We observe several lacunas and an inflammatory area (very white) near 12:00 which is the zone where the tumor was detected.

With the bad nervous system there is probably an association with the risk of brain tumor, which may have also been inherited as the iris shows a relationship with the brain/nervous system (collarette) and the white fibers (inflammation). We may be born with some genetic weakness and other deficiencies that may turn into disease according to our lifestyle and environment, as explained today by epigenetic science (see page 341).

Example of Breast Cancer Risk
Forty-four-year-old woman
Left Iris
Color of the iris: Blue
P53 testing

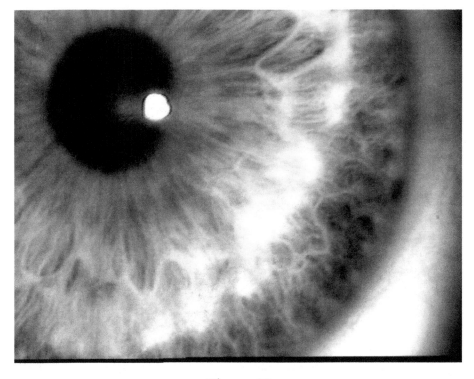

Figure 30

This iris is a typical case of breast cancer risk. The whiteness indicates extreme acidity, congestion of the lymphatic system especially at 3:00, along with a distorted collarette. A transversal is visible at 4:00 on the ovary area and may be implicated with a breast tumor. The scurf rim is dense showing considerable toxic accumulation. This being a case of high oxidative stress, we decided to perform a P53 tumor suppressor gene test to check if either there was an anti-cancer defense functioning or a P53 dysfunction. In this case the results of the test had shown a very high activity of P53 gene expression, with a high level of normal (WT) P53 protein level – 57.3 units of protein/ml of plasma – (normal range 0.10-1.00 units) and no detection of mutated protein.

Therefore, the test showed that there are many abnormal/damaged cells self-destructed by apoptosis from stress stimuli. In one side it is excellent as P53 acted as killer cells and the anti-cancer defense was functioning. However, over the long term, the P53 gene expression may decrease its activity and abnormal/damaged cells will not be destroyed and become cancer cells. The patient needs to reduce her oxidative load, decrease excess acidity that contributes to remove oxygen from the tissues, adapt to a better nutritional diet, take vegetable juices, and take some antioxidants supplementation. Perhaps an SGE bath would be beneficial.

Example of Chronic Auto-Intoxication as shown in the Iris
Sixty-year-old woman

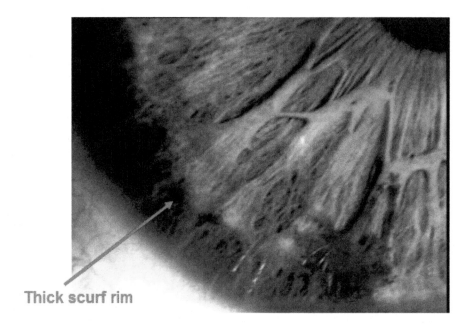

Thick scurf rim

Figure 31

In this sixty-year-old woman the iris shows a very heavy and dark scurf rim visible on the periphery of the iris in the seventh zone, representing the skin area with sensory nerves. It shows indications such as underactive skin function overload with toxins and acid build up in the body. When the skin area appears darker and wider over the lung or liver area or both in the iris it indicates an excess of toxins in the blood because liver is unable to detoxify. It also indicates some irritation of the nerves ramification. A skin and tactile sensory nerves may also be observed in skin disease such psoriasis. In such case, Dr. B. Jensen used to recommend a skin brushing every morning on all the body to open the pores and expulse toxins.

The lymphatic system whose duty is to detoxify cells is congested (orange stains) becoming gelatinous and unable to detoxify. The autonomic nervous system or the collarette is irregular, zig/zag and thickened with orange color double indication of nervous disturbance of the intestinal tract, digestive disorder, flatulence, congestion of the lymphatic system, disturbed peristalsis, etc.

The iris shows a thickened collarette that suggests nervous disorder, congestion of the intestinal lymph nodes, and poor immune cell activity. In this case the collarette is expanded almost stuck to the skin area and perfectly shows the connection between the nerves and the skin. The skin and the nervous system are generated by the same embryonic tissue the ectoderm. This is why skin disease is always worse when there is nervous tension.

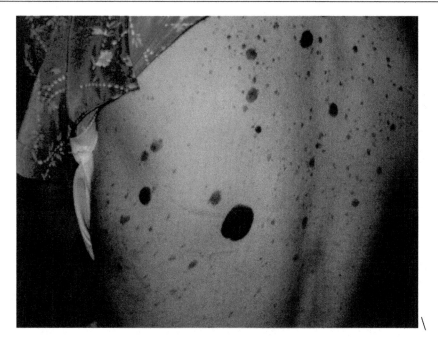

Figure 32

Here we observe on the back of the patient many cysts, dark spots, and plaques of oxidized lipid (also the chest) indication of poor metabolism, pancreatic deficiency, a sluggish liver, and accumulation of toxins wastes and macromolecules from non-digested proteins. Older persons have a decreased detoxification mechanism, but this also depends on the hereditary status, life style and dietary style that, along with our age and health status, usually declines.

Supplemental Iris Cases

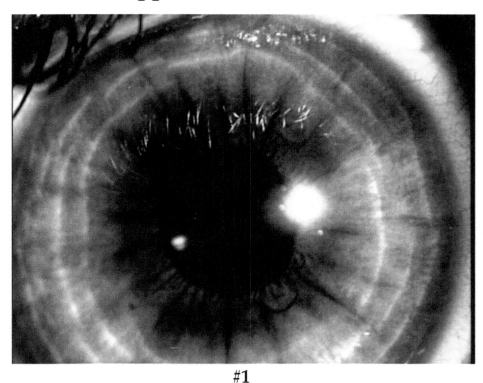

#1
Case #1
Female: thirty years old
Family Antecedents: Diabetes, Rheumatism, Tuberculosis
Left Iris:

This is a very toxic colon with dark radial furrows around the periphery of the intestine, including the brain, indication of brain dysfunction. The patient suffered from constipation since childhood. The absent collarette indicates diminished nerve activity and energy supply. She is depressed, with poor memory, experiencing cognitive disorders at her age, and feels tired; that can be attributed to the radial furrows coming from the colon, also visible going to brain showing cerebral dysfunction from an excess of toxins circulating to brain. White contraction furrows (nerve ring) going around the periphery shows an acute condition, an indication of nerve hyperactivity, irritation and from middle to high oxidative stress for which I often check. This shows strong nervous tension and lack of adaptation to stress, while the absent collarette indicates an inhibition in nutrient assimilation and deficiency of digestive enzymes. Usually chronic fatigue syndrome can often correlate with patients with an absent collarette. She also suffers from psoriasis and we may observe a scurf rim between 2:00 and 4:00 with a lipid ring. Often psoriasis is associated with a toxic colon and nervous disorder, a nervous sensitivity. There is an embryonic association between the skin and the nervous system where any approach to this disease needs to treat the nervous system as explained in this book, in addition to detoxifying the colon along with an anti-inflammatory food diet.

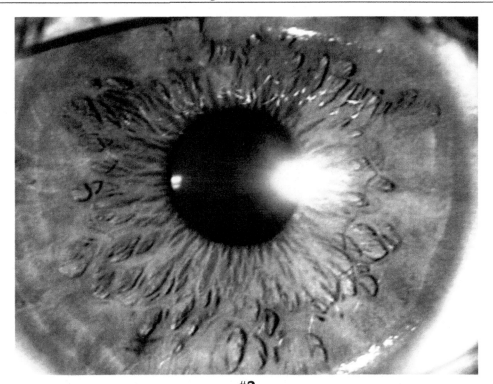

#2
Case #2
Male: Twenty-two-years old
Bad Inherited Colon
Right Iris

This iris shows a bad inherited colon, poor structure, many diverticulae, and bowel gas pockets. Indeed the hospital diagnosed a colon with weak tissue. We observe several closed lacunas inside the collarette just on liver area indication of weakness. The patient feels physically weak with intestinal pains, bad digestion, and much nervousness. From my point of view, this is an aged colon in a young body.

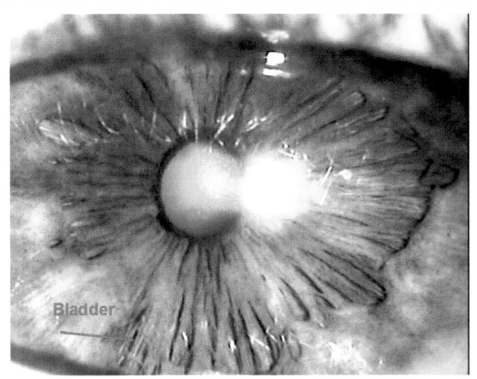

#3
Case #3
Male: Sixty-six-years old
Left iris
Color: brown
Density: 3
Cancer of the bladder

In this iris we observe an exaggerated distended collarette and extremely ballooned colon with flatulence, gases, and digestive disorder. At 3.00 we observe a highly inflammatory process and small dark lacunas in the sigmoid. It shows accumulation of toxic wastes and degenerative tissues. From 6:00 to 7:00 we notice several degenerative lacunas, one of which is situated on the bladder area where the tumor is detected. There is a lot of pressure and toxic accumulation includes feces retention on the terminal part of the sigmoid colon and rectum. This is a patient coming from the countryside working hard in the field all his life, eating wrong food, a meat eater who has a bad bowel function.

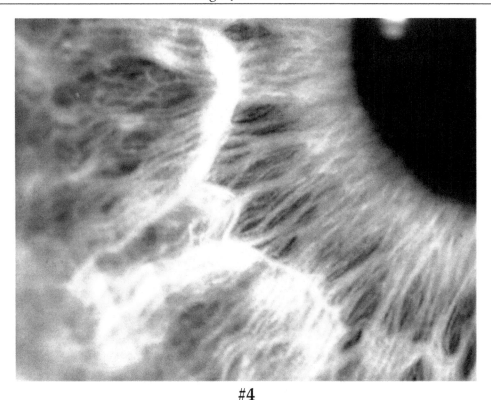

#4
Case #4
Male: Forty-eight-years old
Right iris
Color: blue
Liver Dysfunction

The iris shows a white thickened collarette going in a zig zag pattern, especially at 8:00 around the liver area with major inflammation. Many lacunas are visible inside the collarette, basically with the colon pushing into liver area.

The patient is a regular drinker of strong alcohol. No wonder the nervous wreath or collarette is irritated and associated with liver inflammation. The patient exhibited very high liver markers at the time of the consultation and was on the path to developing hepatitis and probably cirrhosis.

Case #5
Female: Twenty-six-years old
Depression Nervousness

Clinical story: Depression, nervousness, stress, pain in the legs, chronic constipation. Patient is under medical care with psychiatric medications. Restricted collarette associated with psycho-emotional imbalance affecting the hypothalamus. The patient inherited many characteristics from her mother as shown in the photo #B.

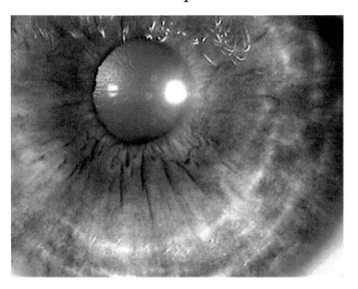

Case #5   Photo #A – Patient

Iris sign: Restricted collarette, an indication of constipation and sluggishness of the intestine – stagnation of the lymphatic fluid around the intestines – Bowel flora imbalance – It also disturbs the central nervous system and increase nervousness and psychological behavior – Deep contraction furrows are a visible indication of stress status and muscle contraction – Restricted collarette often formed embryologically or inherited in this case from her mother.

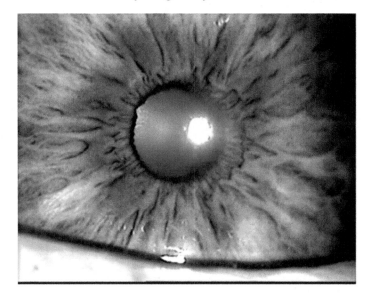

Case # 5 Photo #B – Mother

Photo shows central heterochromia indication of toxic colon, restricted collarette, intestinal pains, nervousness, and aging process.

Case # 6
Female: Forty-eight years-old
Cancer of the Ovary
Left Iris

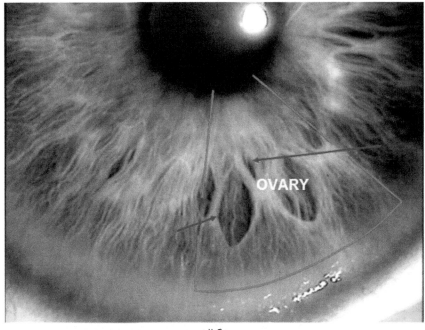

#6

We may observe a neuro-genetic arc reflex syndrome on the ovary with large lacunas (producing a butterfly like appearance) at inner and outer border of the collarette. It indicates a reflex condition between the toxic bowel area and associated organ weakness. An early Iridology checkup would have probably prevented cancer development on the ovary with detox and proper treatment.

Case # 7
Female: Twenty-six- years old
Toxic Colon
Left Iris

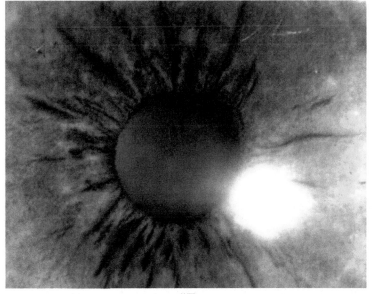

#7

This brown iris shows a very toxic colon with a state of chronic constipation, with deep radial furrows, some look like asparagus visible around the colon, especially going to the brain area, are often associated with cognitive disorders, migraines, poor memory, nervousness, and aggressivity, which was the case with this young woman. The collarette is absent or very hard to detect (smudged) indication of poor nerve supply, abdominal pains, stomach weakness, often poor appetite. It also indicates poor nutrient absorption, Emotivity and low physical resistance. This patient had a bad hereditary colon and weak intestinal tissue that picked up and accumulated more toxins.

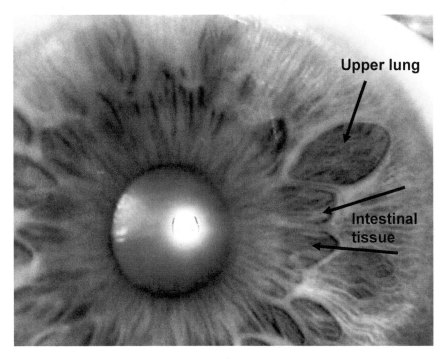

#8

Case #8
Male: Fifty-six-years old
Lung Cancer
Left Iris

From what we observe, this iris shows that the colon tissue overlaps the lung tissue, making it look like it was the same tissue as explained before. A large lacuna is visible on the upper part of the lung while below the colon, the collarette is pointing to the lower part of the lung making two lacunas. It definitively shows a very toxic ballooned colon and disturbed nervous system. It surely implicates the spleen located at 4:00 and also the thymus gland that should be below 3:00 (near the outer normal border of the collarette).

From an embryological standpoint, the colon in this case was associated with lung disease. Here again we can refer to the statement by Dr. Jensen concerning the movie star, John Wayne: "The disease starts in the colon."

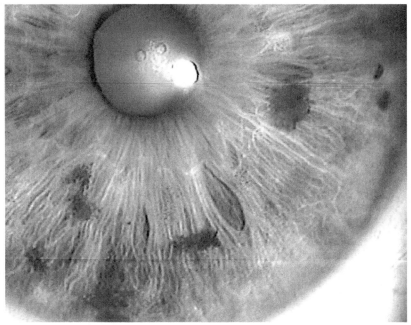

#9L

Case #9
Female: Fifty-six-years old
Color of the iris: abnormal blue
Breast cancer risk (mother died of breast cancer)

Left Iris:

We observe a large brown pigment granulation (formerly toxic spot) and some white radials at 3:00 – 3:20, on the mammary zone. Heavy lymphatic congestion is visible from 3:00 to 5:00, which is always involved in breast cancer profile. A transversal is visible at 3:30 just near the periphery of the iris. This indicates a genetic risk for cancer. The collarette just opposite to the mammary area is very thin, practically broken, and indicates inflammation and poor energy supply to the intestine.

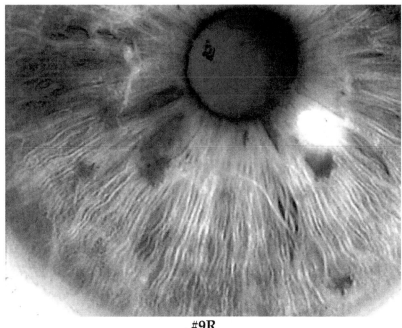

#9R

Right Iris:

Here we observe a large pigment granulation on liver and pancreas areas near 8.00, an indication of bad inherited liver function. This is a typical case of inflammation and irritation where the iris fibers are distorted.

Both irises show a typical breast cancer profile as shown on my breast cancer profile chart. See my iris breast cancer profile in color. (www.sergejurasunas.com)

P53 Tumor Suppressor Testing

The patient agreed to take a P53 test which is done through the intake of venous blood, which provides information relevant to P53 gene expression, P53 protein level and either a normal active P53 and normal or mutated protein. The result did not show mutant P53 yet but a very low expression of P53 and of P53 protein level. It showed that only a small fraction of abnormal, precancerous cells were destroyed by apoptosis leading to the accumulation of abnormal cells and their transformation after several mutations into cancer cells. Although in some other similar cases, P53 testing showed mutation. Therefore, the work I have developed associated with the iris signs, from my breast cancer profile, is confirmed by P53 tumor suppressor gene testing.

For more information see: "How to Understand and Treat Cancer with Molecular Markers" on Slideshare.com. Also read my article on the P53 Tumor Suppressor Gene: "Understanding P53 based Anti-cancer Therapies Utilizing Dietary Agents." *Townsend Letter*, August\September 2015.

Case # 10
Female: Fifty-three-years old
Left iris
Clinical story: Ovarian Tumor

In 2004 the patient complained from various symptoms: colon disorder, high blood pressure, heart palpitations, fatigue, and chronic constipation. (Elimination every 3-4 days)

The colon area is very dark, much toxins, and at 5.00, just on the ovary area, we observe a large dark pigment granulation that connects with the sigmoid. We may conclude to a relationship between the two organs.

This particular iris shows very well to me a risk of colon or ovary cancer and I warned the patient about it, but she didn't pay attention to my advice.

In 2011, six years later, the patient came back with a diagnostic of ovarian cancer taking chemotherapy that could have been prevented.

Case #10 below:

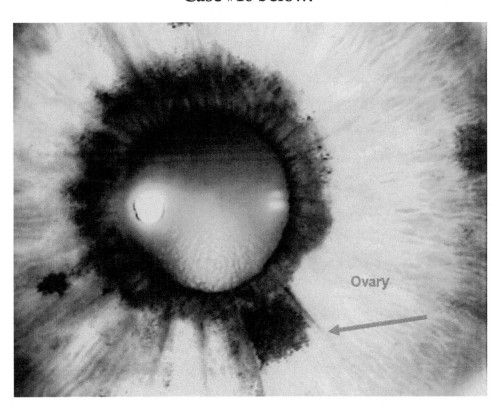

Case Notes and Questions:

Note down your case questions. This is a good opportunity for you, the reader, to review, jot down notes, gather thoughts, and reflect. Clinical cases begin on page 311. A listing of cases may be found on page 325.

Areas of further learning:

Special questions for Professor Jurasunas:

(Please note down case # and description with your questions)

Further learning and courses / Areas of Clinical Oncology and testing I would like to explore further in a webinar or course:

Part VI

Detoxification Program
Detoxification Crisis
Special Diet for Gastrointestinal Problems
Enemas and Colon Hydrotherapy
Changing Eating Habits

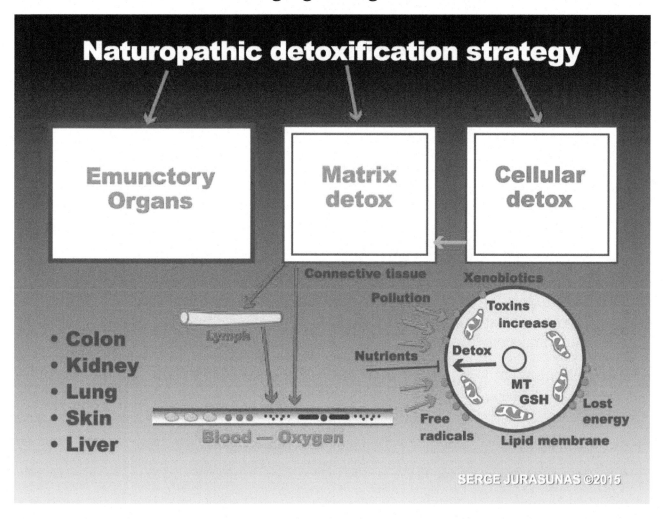

Detoxification Program

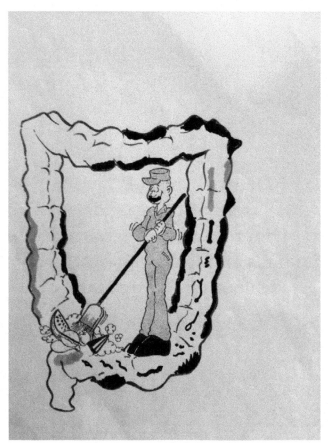

Clean-up of the colon

In this chapter I propose a complete detoxification program, also called "Naturopathic Detoxification Strategy" (see the figure on page 210), beneficial for everyone who is looking to clean up his body and be healthier. But above all for people with some intestinal problems and especially for cases of chronic constipation, patients with a bowel movement every two to three days or more and associate either with some symptoms or chronic diseases such as arthritis, rheumatism, multiple sclerosis, psoriasis, or dermatitis. When detoxifying the colon and the whole body, including the matrix, cellular detox provides overall relief from auto-intoxication, which in turn helps balance the auto-regulation system including inflammatory proteins, improve cellular function (less damage), and improve the immune defense.

Normally this program lasts one week, or even two, according to how chronic and auto-intoxicated the organism. People with acute colitis or intestinal hemorrhages must not follow this program without a doctor's advice, just as with any other treatment.

Follow the suggested diet but first, consult the list of foods necessary for the upcoming week.

Begin the detoxification program by:
- *One entire day of fruit and vegetable broths (only drink the broth) and cooked vegetables.*
- *Followed by seven days of vegetable juices, with one day of fruit juices (only eat fruit and vegetables that are in season).*

Important notes: drink at least four large glasses of vegetable or fruit juice.

In cases of persistent constipation, introduce the special Detoxification Formula into the program.

Before going to bed I suggest the following drink: one glass of lukewarm mineral water with one tablespoonful of cider vinegar and one spoonful of honey.

During this program a daily hot bath is recommended, especially before bed, in order to help detoxification and relax the muscles. Make sure that the bath is always taken after digestion of a meal.

If for personal reasons it is not possible to take a bath before bed, try to take it at about 5:00 p.m., making sure to rest for thirty minutes after the bath. For extremely busy people who cannot take a detoxification bath every day, try taking it at least on Fridays, Saturdays, and Sundays.

There are various kinds of baths. Experiment with a bath of fresh algae if possible, or dried (they are on sale in small doses). In France we have available a special combination of a bath with fresh algae mixed with essential oils developed by Dr. Jean Valnet, a former Army medical doctor who became famous for his research and studies in the field of aromatherapy. I met Dr. Valnet in Paris sometime in 1969, and at that time I suffered from a severe skin inflammation because of some heavy psychological stress upon my return to Europe. At the same time I met a very original person, Dr. Louis Sevelinges, who was not only a doctor of pharmacy but a pioneer in the field of essential oil research. He wrote his thesis while on the faculty of pharmacy about the antiseptic properties of lavender oil in 1929. Dr. Sevelinges also owned a pharmaceutical laboratory, Phytorama, engaged in research and manufacturing various medications made from essential oils. He was probably the first person to measure the biological value of essential oils using the Bioelectrometer of Professor L.C. Vincent, whom I later refer to in this book.

I was lucky to have met Dr. Sevelinges, who invited me to spend time with him in the laboratory located in a small country village near the city of Lyon, and learn about essential oils but also about the pH, oxido-reduction, and resistivity which are the three biological measures of all living things on earth and the science of Biolectronimeter from Professor Vincent.

After meeting Dr. Sevelinges, Dr. Valnet became interested in Aromatherapy and wrote several books on the subject of treating patients with various methods, but also his famous new bath made from essential oils and fresh seaweed that contained over one hundred minerals, especially rich in iodine, potassium, magnesium, cobalt, zinc, and boron. Thus, meeting him in Paris, he suggested I take this special bath, together with a mixture of essential oils developed by Dr. Sevelinges for liver cleansing to be taken orally. All the different essential oils in the bath have some properties as relaxing, antiseptic, bactericidal, anti-inflammatory, and detoxifying. Over the years, Dr. Jean Valnet wrote several interesting books about aromatherapy and how to treat disease with essential oils which today remain a reference.

Thanks to Dr. Valnet and Dr. Sevelinges, I since had learned a great deal of knowledge concerning essential oils and seaweed. France is one of the top countries for the production of special seaweed of high quality, especially from the Brittany coast, and for the manufacture of seaweed for external application especially in hotel spas on the sea cost. Aromatherapy is an important medicine in Europe, where essential oils have had since the time of antiquity, a confirmed medicinal value. The treatment of Dr. J. Valnet, both from fresh seaweed and essential oils together with the special enema from Mr. Xanty that I speak about later on in the book, this all definitely cured my skin problem and reinforced my belief in the necessity to detoxify the body and especially to treat disease with no harm to the body but, on the contrary, be gentle and helpful to restore normal function.

SGES (Super Growth Energy Stone)

Another kind of bath I strongly recommend is a bath with a powder extracted from a special stone discovered in 1978 on the island of Kyoto, Japan called Tenko-Seki in Japanese, meaning "Heaven Descending Stone." This stone activates cellular function and has the power to detoxify the body by eliminating heavy metals such as mercury or PCB. It is both a detoxifying and revitalizing bath.

This stone is called SGES (Super Growth Energy Stone) and is a special volcanic stone that produces a far-infrared ray with a wavelength of 4-14 microns, that energizes growth in humans, animals, and plants but also with a SOD activity, meaning it has antioxidant properties. This SGE treatment may be taken orally in tablets to treat some diseases, also in the form of a special bath with tiny ceramic balls containing SGE powder. This requires a special bath tub to contain a very large amount of ceramic balls, which I will now explain.

SGE has the property to decrease or eliminate accumulation of lipid peroxide through the skin, increase blood flow, improve mobility in case of rheumatoid arthritis, and increase energy level, while it really detoxifies the body. There are already many scientific treatises on the detoxifying effects of this bath, in particular some of these were carried out by the medical department at the University of Kyoto and by the College of Dermatology. It is recommended for cutaneous illnesses, obesity, chronic fatigue, and arthritic pain.

I spent many years investigating the therapeutic effects of SGE therapy. While not in position to purchase the special large bath tub equipped with a special heating process developed in Japan utilizing one ton of ceramic balls, I then decided, with the help of a Japanese company, to manufacture a power sand bath mixed with mineral salts. In 1999 I started to call it Energy Sand Bath (ESB), because it really increased the energy level in the body while it also detoxified and even inhibited tumor growth. After some success with the tablets and the ESB therapy, I started its promulgation.

In 1999 I wrote a full article published in *Townsend Letter*, "A Far Infrared Ray Emitting Stone to Treat Cancer and Degenerative Disease," available on the Internet. Another good article, available on the Internet is from Dr. Shigeyuki Hirose, director of Hirose clinic called, "SGE from the Viewpoint of Medicine." Today's major stress that people in certain professions are under, may require and largely benefit from this form of relaxation and detoxification, which these stone baths provide.

Bath therapy allows one to eliminate toxins, heavy metals, acids, and oxidized lipids through the skin and the kidneys. This can be completed through an oral therapy and eventually colon cleansing.

The detoxification obtained activates the functions of the organism, improving, amongst other functions the level of blood oxygen. Consequently the metabolism is stimulated and circulation and oxygen support to the brain are improved. An SGE bath also increases blood circulation, which has been shown, through thermography, to occur as quickly as ten minutes after a bath, producing a similar effect to that of detoxification through the skin. For example, it has been also proven that a fresh seaweed bath causes a vasodilatation of the arteries and capillaries, therefore improving the elimination of toxins and improving circulation. I believe that therapeutic bath is an essential part of our hygiene, in order to help the body recover when it comes to detoxification, increased energy level, and activating cellular growth, as seen with the SGE power bath. The bath and oral tablets are also efficient for cancer patients as I explain in my article.

The Romans were greatly fervent of baths and they were smart enough to use the medicinal power of water spas. Today an SGES bath is easily available through an Internet search. One can then realize that I am only at the beginning of this story in the Western world. Even Japanese doctors take note from the references to my work.

At the end of the detox program, I include a diet. After the bath it is wise to keep on with better quality food, vegetables, and fruits while continuing to keep regulating the intestine. It's always good to maintain some rules such as setting aside one day a week to eat only whole rice and cooked apples, or drinking only carrot juice. Apple juice also helps the body to rest and detox. On this special day, if necessary, I advise a laxative made from herbal extracts in tablets or to drink at night or an enema to help eliminate the waste, which has already been assisted and made easier by the special diet of fruit juice and whole rice.

A whole day of fasting is also good for people with stronger minds, although fasting during few days is recommended for patients with some chronic disorders. It stimulates the body's auto-regulation system and can concentrate energy to balance all the neurotransmitters, and inflammatory cytokines, thus creating better harmony in the body.

Fasting or detoxification of the colon, eating less food, treats the whole body, not just one organ, while the medical system treats a single organ and only one symptom, using drugs that indeed are not resolving the real problem. At the same time, the relationship between acid and alkaline must be balanced, as there is often a tendency towards acidity. This acid/alkaline theory of health has often been overlooked.

Acid-Base Balance

When we speak about the acid/alkaline balance we refer to the pH. value or the hydrating potential. In an aqueous solution, the body has the peculiarity of freeing two kinds of ions:

- *OH formed by oxygen and hydrogen*
- *H formed by hydrogen.*

When the OH ions prevail we call it an alkaline reaction.

When the H ions prevail we call it an acid reaction.

The pH. of any aqueous solution of a body indicates the degree of alkalinity or acidity of that body.

The pH. table was established in function of the concentration of H ions.

The acid-base neutral pH. is equal to 7.

Acidity is between 0 and 7.

Alkalinity is between 7 and 14.

Blood has a pH. of about 7.35.

Urine has a pH. of about 6 to 7.

As seen, the number 7 corresponds to neutrality, neither acid nor alkaline.

Any form of life requires an environment between pH. 5.5 and 8 in order for it to survive. The aerobe intestinal bacteria require an acid terrain to survive, the anaerobe bacteria develop in a clearly alkaline environment.

When we have a dietary regime with highly acidic foods, and when we eat the same food every day, such as meat, white rice, and white bread, our organism must use large quantities of potassium, sodium, calcium, and magnesium to neutralize the acids, to prevent cellular damage. The organism has some reserves of these minerals but must replenish them quickly, or else the tissues become deficient and the terrain becomes acidic. Nervous depression, arthritis, and insomnia always indicate too much acid and a deficiency of minerals.

On the other hand, certain eating habits tend to be alkalizing though rare, but can also be dangerous in the long run. Various medicines such as aspirin and antibiotics are highly alkaline and can be at the origin of certain chronic diseases. According to the research of L.C. Vincent from France and the biological terrain Assessment with the Bioelectrometer, an oxidized alkaline terrain is favorable to viruses and many diseases of civilization such as cardiovascular, multiple sclerosis, and post vaccination reactions. While good health is found in an acid reduction terrain, this optimizes the assimilation of vitamins, and minerals.

It is important to maintain a dietary balance, selecting medium alkaline foods that can balance the acid alkaline balance and a neutral pH.—which can be slightly acid or slightly alkaline. All green vegetables are rich in potassium, magnesium, and sodium with sea algae being perfect to prevent from excess acidity, the same as compounds such as chlorella and spirulina extract.

CHLORELLA AND DETOXIFICATION

About thirty years ago, when I was frequently traveling around the world to lecture and search out new medicines or new kinds of food to improve people's health status, treat diseases, and to also improve the detoxification process, I heard about a new substance developed in Japan, a kind of microscopic fresh water algae experimented upon since 1951 by Dr. Hirosahi Tarmya, of the Tokugawa Biological Institute, called chlorella. Through my Japanese colleagues I learned that chlorella is a strong body regenerator and also could detoxify the body from harmful toxins and heavy metals. It was interesting enough for me to investigate more deeply and see how it could help my own patients, the best course for me was to undergo a clinical trial and see the result directly with my patients.

First I learned that chlorella is a fresh water, green, microscopic algae the size of a red cell that originated on earth some 2.5 billion years ago (although new dating elements permit us to go back to 3.5 billion years or more) having remained unchanged.

What interested me was the story of Mr. Ryuseki Nakayama, who himself was a very sick person suffering from cancer, arthritis, a stomach ulcer etc. He was looking for something that could help him. Incidentally, he had heard about chlorella and started to treat himself with this substance and managed to cure himself. Later on we will come back to this story since Mr. Nakayama spent the rest of his life to investigate and develop chlorella in a way to make it available for the public.

Chlorella is a cell very much similar to our human cell. Inside there are a nucleus, a chloroplast and mitochondria necessary to promote cellular energy, the same as our cells, so that division and replication can occur at the fantastic rate of four new cells every 17- 24 hours. Now if we calculate the number of divisions and the survival of chlorella over the past billion years, we certainly reach an astronomical number and if chlorella has survived up to now. It is because of the strong walls that offer protection to the DNA cells. Only just over the past fifty years many herbs, plants, algae, and animal species have disappeared on our planet because of the deterioration of the environment by heavy toxicity. Here again I am coming back to the story of Mr. Ryuseki Nakayama because at the beginning he realized that chlorella was an assimilation problem for our digestive system because of this hard wall. But he managed to resolve the problem by inventing a special process with the help of researchers and engineers called the Dyno Mill process, patented by Sun Chlorella Corporation that disintegrated the chlorella's cell wall. You can see the whole story unfolding and the large manufacturing company in Japan. The Dyno Mill machine picture is in the book by Dr. Bernard Jensen, called *Chlorella, Gem of the Orient*, published by the author.

Today, contrary to the food we eat and grow in the soil with chemical fertilizers, pesticides, insecticides and other environmental pollution, chlorella grows in giant tankers with pure fresh water, much sun, and away from any source of pollution, in various Pacific Islands like Okinawa. Therefore, it may be considered as a unique non-polluted food.

NUTRITIONAL VALUE OF CHLORELLA

First of all during a detoxification program we may need to supply the body with important nutrients, vitamins, minerals, enzymes etc. and this is why chlorella plays a major role. Of the fifteen strains of chlorella found by scientists, the most nutritionally valuable is *chlorella pyrenoidosa* rich in minerals, vitamins, enzymes, trace elements, nucleic acid, and chlorophyll perfect to nourish the body and activate detoxification of the liver, colon and kidney, and improving the making of red cells. All green plants contain chlorophyll, but chlorella pyrenoidosa contains the highest level of chlorophyll (28.9g\Kg) of any other known plant on earth. It contains ten times that of spirulina and barley, about twenty times more than alfalfa. Thus we really have a very high level of chlorophyll that serves many purposes in the body such as preventing anemia, infection and radiation damage while helping to detoxify. All green leaves contain magnesium in which chlorella is very high. Magnesium activates bowel movement, balances the nervous system, helps the muscles, contributes to alkalize the body and combats hyperactivity, neurasthenia and fatigue. Chlorella is also very high in phosphorus 989.0mg\100g), almost three times the concentration of magnesium (315mg\100g) which further improves the entire nervous system and also the memory. This is the least patients report feeling after taking chlorella extract regularly for 30 days. Speaking of detoxification, chlorella is also rich in the peptide glutathione which together with methionine plays a crucial role to detoxify the liver and other organs.

Glutathione is a key molecule that activates the cellular detoxification of noxious compounds and activates the p450 cytochrome detoxification system where chemicals and toxic compounds are joined with the glutathione molecule to conjugate and increase the water solubility of chemical compounds to be later expelled.

Detoxification and activation of the colon is of course the subject of the book and chlorella extract has a strong capacity to activate bowel movements and expel toxins and this is why chlorella extract is included in my program.

THE CELLULAR MEMBRANE OF CHLORELLA

The cellular membrane of chlorella includes approximately 31% Hemicellulose, 27% protein, 15.4% alpha cellulose, and 3.3% of glucosamine which, together with the high percentage of magnesium, play a major role to increase bowel movement and expel toxic feces, not to forget about chlorophyll that purifies the colon.

CHLORELLA EXTRACT IS RICH IN NUCLEIC ACID (DNA\RNA)

One cannot speak about chlorella without explaining that it contains high levels of nucleic acids which, with other nutrients, not only increase detoxification but stimulates cell reproduction to rejuvenate the tissues and make new healthy cells. The nucleic acids found in the nucleus of pyrenoidosa are especially much more concentrated in the pure liquid chlorella than tablets. The extract contains a growth factor know as Chlorella Growth Factor (CGF), which is probably the most valuable component of the chlorella. CGF is not exactly a single substance, but a nucleotide peptide complex that contains glucose, mannose, arabinose, galactose, xylose, proteins and amino acids such glutamine, alanine, serine, glycine, proline and asparagine. It also contains vitamins, minerals like manganese important for bones, liver, pancreas, for the nervous system and the brain. Manganese is also important for the growth of Lactobacillus in the intestine. The structure of the CGF also contains five other active substances including sulphur, glutathione, and cysteine that all play a key role in detoxification as mentioned previously.

Now CGF contains 10% DNA, while the tablets and extract contain only 3%, which is about three times more DNA in the CGF. For years nucleic acids and nucleotides were not considered as essential nutrients, since it was thought that the body synthesized sufficient nucleotides to meet its physiological demands. However, we know today that exogenous nucleotides energize the endogenous nucleotide de Novo acid pathway. Exogenous nucleic acid (salvage synthesis) is essential to activate de novo pathways. A part of the exogenous nucleic acid is digested and used by the intestine to renew the fast turnover of intestinal mucosa cells, this is why food rich in nucleic acid is so important, required here to keep a healthy intestine. Cells need exogenous nucleic acids DNA and RNA, for the synthesis of new DNA\RNA, otherwise the body might be unable to make new healthy cells. This requirement that the body makes millions of new cells every minute relies on DNA and RNA synthesis. No wonder that CGF is considered as a perfect food to rejuvenate the whole body and also as we are going to explain stimulates detoxification.

For the past three decades, chlorella extract (Sun Chlorella) both in tablets and the liquid CGF have been some of my favorite compounds that we have used in our clinic acting as body and blood regenerators, even being very efficient to as support in several varieties of illness such diabetes, hepatitis, anemia, arthritis, and glioma; especially to combat chronic constipation, to stimulate detoxification process, expelling heavy metals as mercury, lead, and cadmium as demonstrated before and after with Hair Analysis and the Oxidative Dried Blood Test (See one example in the Chapter on Live Blood Analysis and the Oxidative Dried Blood Test).

Other actions of chlorella extract include the strong antioxidant activity since it contains SOD, glutathione, beta-Carotene, vitamin C, E, zinc, and copper (etc.), which today are important to counter the concentrated toxic effect of free radical activity especially these days with people living in polluted cities under physical and social stress. To protect our body against pollution and the genomic effect of free radicals, we have two main mechanisms, first the liver and second the antioxidants enzymatic defense system both endogenous and exogenous. Chronic constipation is also responsible for the large quantities of toxins and bacteria that penetrate into blood circulation but lucky we also have the liver that plays a key role to filter, detoxify and kill bad bacteria. The liver is built with a battery of cellular enzymes known as cytochromes of which up to now, around five hundred varieties have been identified. These enzymes serve to activate the biotransformation of chemical compounds to a less reactive one, into water soluble forms for excretion and elimination by the urine. However, this enzymatic system, known as Liver P450 cytochrome, requires a battery of vitamins, minerals, and extra enzymes to support the conversion of chemical compounds.

First, the liver constantly needs iron, sulphur, zinc, and potassium (etc.) in order to function 24 hours per day and 365 days per year. But to support this detoxification process the liver also requires vitamins A, C, E, selenium, zinc, some glutathione, methionine, cysteine, sulphur and some oxygen of course to maintain a high level of ATP production in the liver's mitochondria to boost the detoxification process. While cells in most organs in the body contain from 300 to 2000 mitochondria, liver cells contain about 4000 mitochondria to show you the fabulous energy needed by the liver to accomplish all the necessary functions.

Therefore, first we cannot separate the colon from the liver which can be damaged by toxins from sluggish colon and not expulsed. Now chlorella contains all the nutrients necessary to activate detoxification including, not to forget, a high level of chlorophyll and especially iron, zinc and potassium to support the liver function and the detoxification process.

My clinical work includes taking of care of thousands of patients who, each year, come to our clinic. The bedrock of my method is based on detoxification and rejuvenation of the body no matter the problem or the disease, and both chlorella extract in tablets and liquid CGF has been an important part of our success.

HOW CHLORELLA EXTRACT SUPPORTS YOUR BODY

1. Cleans up the blood, improves the manufacture of red cells, increases the oxygen level in the blood circulation
2. Improves the immune function
3. Stimulation of colon elimination
4. Detoxification of the liver
5. Increasing energy level by stimulation of ATP production
6. Helping the turnover of new healthy cells
7. Increasing resistance to infection

A DETOXIFICATION PROGRAM WITH CHLORELLA EXTRACT AND CGF

Some years ago I decided to develop a detoxification program based only on chlorella extract and CGF together with a healthy diet. Of course it can be used with peoples who have limited time or do not wish to take many supplements as suggested in the book. However, this program is not recommended for patients with diarrhea or intestinal colitis who need medical care and advice. However most people can take this program that also rejuvenates the body.

1st week:

5 tablets of chlorella extract 3 times per day
20 ml of CGF

2nd week:

10 tablets of chlorella extract 3 times per day
30ml of CGF

3rd week

15 tablets of chlorella extract 3 times per day
40 ml of CGF

According to each person's reaction, the dosage (posology) can be reduced for instance by taking 10 tablets of chlorella 3 times per day instead of 15 tablets. You can also stay with 10 tablets after the second week and taking the CGF. Don't forget to drink some fresh vegetable or fruit juice that helps to absorb the chlorella tablets. Vegetable broth between meals is useful to increase the excretion of toxins via the kidneys.

Of course, this is only a short introduction about chlorella and not a full presentation since my idea is just to show how this chlorella extract is so important in detoxification process having used both the tablets and the liquid CGF for so many years it probably demonstrates some great efficacy even as mentioned with some other diseases including kidney dysfunction, even using only the liquid CGF.

In order to properly control a good pH. balance and prevent acidity, there are already tests on reactive paper that allow us to control these contents. For convenience, reactive pH. salivary paper, which is sold in drug stores or in some health food stores, is useful.

> ***Ideal pH. Values**
> Saliva – 6.5
> Urine – 6.8
> Venous blood – 7.35 –7.45*

Classification of Foods

Acidifying Foods	Alkalizing Foods
Animal products: meats, fish	Vegetables
Alcohol: wine, beer, cider, etc.	Potatoes, Jerusalem , yam
Refined cereals, pastas, toasts, cakes, etc.	Beetroot, carrots, turnips, radishes
Saturated fats	Celery
Refined sugar	Garlic, onion, leek
Seasonings and spices	Artichokes, asparagus, eggplant
Eggs	Pumpkin, cucumber, zucchini, chard
Dairy products: milk, cheeses	Endive
Coffee, chocolate, tea, cocoa	Mushrooms, ripe tomatoes
	Ripe fruit
	Acid fruit or fruits like oranges, tangerines, lemons, grapefruit, pineapple (although containing organic acids they have a final and alkalizing reaction)
	Strawberries, apples, pears, peaches, grapes, and
	cherries
	Dried fruits, dates, raisins, and figs

Rules to Complement Detoxification Treatment

In order to obtain the best results from this treatment, it is necessary to follow some rules in order to balance the varieties and proportions of food, among which vegetable juices rich in potassium, magnesium, sodium, and calcium must be included.

But apart from the diet and in order to increase the detoxification process, some food supplements must be included along with the detoxification program, each day. Of the natural supplement I use for several decades the famous Zell enzyme yeast cells preparation, Sun Chlorella, and CGF have been my favorite products.

List of Food Supplements for a 7-Day Treatment

1 pack Sun-Chlorella –252 tablets
1 pack Vitamin C 1000mg – 42 tablets
1 pack Papaya – enzyme – 84 tablets
1 pack Kelp – 21 tablets
1 pack cod liver oil – 14 capsules
1 bottle of Osteocare liquid or similar (calcium supplement)
1 bottle of liquid Aloe/Papaya mixture
1 bottle of enzyme yeast cells preparation (Zell-Oxygen)

This may seem to be an excessive quantity of supplements to ingest, but it is the most effective way to simultaneously counterbalance the body and trigger a detoxification process, eliminate feces that accumulate in the colon and encrusted matter in the intestinal wall, stimulate the liver, digestive system, and the immune system as well.

Distribution of Food in the Daily Diet

> ## 60% of Alkaline Food

60% raw vegetables
20% cooked food
20% fruits
For a healing therapy we can add to these percentages by including even more raw vegetable juice cocktails.
40% acidifying foods
20% animal products: meat, fish, dairy products
20% plant products: cereals, legumes

Food Proportion

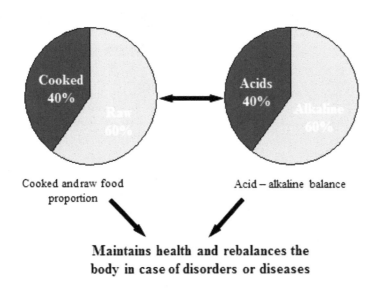

Cooked and raw food proportion

Acid – alkaline balance

Maintains health and rebalances the body in case of disorders or diseases

Maintains health or rebalances the organism in case of organic disorders or illness.

7-Day Detoxifying Treatment Program

Upon waking up:
Drink 1 glass lukewarm mineral water with 1 tablespoon of cider vinegar, and 1 teaspoon of honey.

15 minutes later:
Mix the following: 1 glass carrot juice, 4 oz. linseed juice.
 1 tablespoon live enzyme yeast cells (Zell-Oxygen).
 1 cup of pineapple juice.
 1 cup of mineral water.

Please Note: Enzyme yeast cells are mostly advised to achieve a total detoxification of the body. You can also alternate enzyme yeast cells with some Aloe Papaya concentrate in liquid.

Mix the ingredients well and drink slowly, very slowly, as if you were chewing. At the same time take:

- - 6 tablets Sun Chlorella
- - 2 tablets papaya enzyme

Mix 2 tablespoons linseed with 2 liters water. Boil very slowly until it has reduced to about half the initial quantity. Once it has cooled, place in the refrigerator and serve daily.

Breakfast:
See suggestion in special diet of the detoxification program.

After breakfast:
1 capsule cod liver oil
1 tablet of kelp
2 tablets vitamin C (1000 mg)

Mid-Morning:
One cup vegetable broth 6 tablets Sun- Chlorella
2 tablets papaya enzyme

Lunch:
See suggestion in special diet of the detoxification program.

After Lunch:
1 capsule cod liver oil
1 tablet of kelp
1 tablespoon Osteocare

Mid-Afternoon:
A glass of carrot juice: 60% carrot, 40% Apple
1 tablespoon of Live Enzyme yeast cells
6 tablets of Sun-Chlorella
2 tablets of Papaya enzyme

Around 7 pm:
Either a hot bath with SGE, algae, or essential oils of pine needles, lavender, juniper etc.

The bath should last more or less for twenty minutes and should be followed by a 15 to 20 minute rest.

After a period of rest, take an enema made with herbs and clay. Then immediately rest again for a short while.

Dinner:
See suggestion in special diet of the detoxification program.

After dinner:
1 tablespoon Osteocare 6 tablets Sun Chlorella
2 tablets Papaya enzyme

Bedtime:

1 glass lukewarm water with 2 teaspoons of cider vinegar, and 1 teaspoon of honey
2 tablets plant-based laxatives
1 tablespoon Aloe Papaya

JUICES - the vegetable or fruit juices should vary from day to day, according to the season and the kinds available (Carrot can be mixed with turnip, watercress, beetroot, etc. Apple can be substituted by grapes, watermelon, pear, etc.).

RECIPE FOR VEGETABLE BROTH

In a suitable soup pot, place one liter of water on the fire with 2 carrots cut in slices, 3 organic potatoes (use only the skin with 1 cm), 2 organic apples (use only the skin), 4 stalks of organic celery (you can use a handful of celery leaf). Boil the water, add the vegetables. Simmer slowly for 30 minutes. Season with vegetable salt, strain, and serve. Use the broth to drink during the day. The remaining vegetables can be used to make a puree or soup. This is an alkaline broth that detoxifies the blood and kidney.

Suggested Vegetables for Cooking:

Artichokes	Zucchini	Onions
Broccoli	Leek	Asparagus
Carrots	Peas	Vegetable shoots
Cauliflower	Green beans	Sprouts
Savoy cabbage	Turnips	Beetroot
Eggplant	Spinach	

Important note: In certain cases of colitis there are people who do not tolerate certain vegetables such as kale, cauliflower, or turnips. If so, these people should avoid them.

Suggestions for Salads:

Grated carrots	Radishes	Spring onions
Soy sprouts	Lettuce	Parsley
Alfalfa	Chicory	Coriander
Water cress	Endive	Avocado
Azuki beans	Grated zucchini	Onion
Grated apple		

Suggested Drinks:

Fruit juices (apple, grape, pineapple etc.)	Vegetable broth
Digestive herbal teas	Fruit and protein smoothies
Papaya tea	Pure Water

Drink digestive herbal teas or vegetable broths. Liquids tend to drown out the digestive enzymes impeding good digestion.

List of Foods for the Detoxification Week: (Preferably organic fruits or vegetables)

Fruits - according to season, choose ripe fruit, but not overly ripe. Apples, bananas, pears, apricots, oranges, clementines, tangerines, grapes, peaches, pineapples, and papaya.

Vegetables – carrots, turnips, spinach, cabbage, beetroot, potatoes, sweet potatoes, watercress, parsley, tomatoes (only in season, avoid greenhouse vegetables especially tomatoes), green beans, peas.

__Important note:__ Always buy a variety of fruits and vegetables depending on the quantity and available choice of each one. However, it is important to make a list according to established menus and keep everything on hand at home. In this way, there will be no excuse for quitting the program.

Dairy Products – natural organic yogurt, Kefir.

Cereals and other ingredients:

1 packet oat flakes
1 packet of bulgur
1 packet of whole rice
250g linseed
250g raisins
100g ground or whole sesame 100g wheat or oat bran
1 bottle cider vinegar
1 jar honey
6 bottles distilled mineral water (1 Ounce = 28.3495231 grams)

Obviously, the flakes or other ingredients can be varied, but attention should be paid that you are consuming whole or organic food, rice flakes, barley flakes, ground corn, (but make sure this is not GMO corn responsible for severe long term allergies, which may damage the liver and kidneys with long term use) couscous, oatmeal porridge, barley, or wheat.

Vegetable and fruit juices should be made at home using a juicer. It is best to drink them immediately but fresh juice can be kept in the refrigerator during the day to follow the detox program. Fresh organic vegetables contain all the vitamins, minerals, fibers, and enzymes ready to be absorbed to perform detox and healing the body. However, sometimes it is difficult to make fresh juices at home; however, other varieties of organic juices can be obtained in health food stores, especially lacto-fermented vegetable juices, which are also appropriate in this program. In this case you can buy beetroot, sauerkraut, potato, and celery juice as an example.

Sauerkraut juice is excellent to protect the digestive tract from bad bacteria as it contains the beneficial bacteria, *lactobacillus plantarum*, that inhibits the growth of cancer cells. It also contains compounds called isothiocyanate and sulphoraphane that inhibit the expression of carcinogens and the formation of cancerous tumors. The lactic acid it contains is also important to keep a healthy intestinal flora. In fact, all lacto-fermented vegetable juices enhance digestibility, increase vitamin levels, and boost detoxification.

Germany and Austria have produced, for over fifty years, high quality fermented vegetable juices. These are excellent to detoxify or restore many body functions such as for the liver. I recommend carrot, sauerkraut, and red beet mixed together for colon-liver cleansing and even as support, in the case of colon cancer treatment. The Romans, and especially the Greeks, knew about the value of lacto-fermented foods and their therapeutic effects to treat many diseases. Lacto-fermented juices are highly appropriate in this program.

Examples: Cocktail of vegetable juice
- carrot
- beetroot
- celery
- sauerkraut juice (very beneficial for the intestines)

Cocktail of fruit juice
- pineapple
- grapes
- blueberries

Special Diet for the Detoxification Program

During this 7-day diet 21 meals are prepared which should be varied, pleasant and appetizing as possible. Throughout this book you will find various suggestions and ideas that might be helpful.

Important:
It is always best to consume the fruits of season such as cherries, apricots in spring, then peaches, pears etc. In winter there is less choice. You can first get organic fruit juice in some health food stores and alternate with dried fruits soaked overnight (prunes, figs, raisins, apricots, etc.)

During the summer months, watermelon is wonderful and can be introduced in the program as it helps to detoxify the kidneys and gallbladder and helps to eliminate excess liquid accumulation in the tissues. You can make wonderful drink with watermelon juice alone or best mixed with pineapple juice.

Breakfast:
Fruit in season: Especially plums, peaches, apricots, watermelon, grapes; and in winter, we can alternate with dried fruits soaked overnight (prunes, figs, raisins, damsons, apricots)

Carbohydrates:

A bowl of oats, where whole rice, muesli, barley, millet, and banana can also be used for variety. The following can be added to cereals: wheat germ, ground linseeds, sesame seed, etc.... A teaspoon of each ingredient is sufficient. For variety, some ripe banana slices can be added to the cereal.

Sesame, hazelnut, or almond puree can be mixed with chopped fruits and eaten at breakfast.

Also mix in, according to your taste, yogurt, kefir (which is a kind of fermented milk), or buttermilk to be added your list of foods required for your diet.

Drink herbal tea, coffee substitute made from cereal (usually Swiss brand or bamboo) green tea, chicory extract, etc. If it is too difficult to forego coffee, simply try a very weak coffee.

Drink plenty of spring water in between meals since it is important to clean up the kidneys, but also note that good water serves to help vitamins and minerals to cross cellular membranes.

226

Water is the basis of our life on our planet. However, only spring water can be utilized by your body at a cellular level.

Lunch:

A plate of mixed salads, with a variety of grated raw vegetables such as carrot, broccoli, cauliflower, young turnip, red cabbage, squash, onion and green onion. We may add chopped walnuts, hazelnuts, sesame purée, cottage cheese, tofu, or vegetable pate. That makes a nice complete dish.

For seasoning, it is recommended to use 100% cold pressed virgin olive oil, nut oil, grape seed oil, cider vinegar, fresh garlic, vegetable salt and chopped parsley or a variety of sprouts such as broccoli, alfalfa, mung beans, etc.

A choice of one carbohydrate:
> Millet
> Wild rice
> Red Quinoa
> Whole bran rice
> Barley
> Lentils
> Bulgur
> Baked potatoes in jackets

For seasoning we may want to use tamari, soy sauce, sesame oil, lemon.

Dinner:

A dish of mixed salads, or a bowl of vegetable soup

Proteins
Fish, tofu, soy product, eggs, and mushrooms.
Meat is not advisable during a program of detoxification.
A dish of steamed vegetables.

Dessert:

1 portion of soy yogurt, goat milk yogurt that you can flavor with some strawberry jam, (best without sugar) or one serving of natural yogurt or one cooked apple.
A slice of pineapple with some cottage cheese.
Apple purée mixed with some jams or sesame.

Important: These menus should be changed according to the season using available fruits and vegetables. Suggestions for lunch and dinner can be varied according to individual taste.

Raw vegetable (or fruit) juice must be taken 15 minutes before each meal and/or in between.

It is not recommended to drink during a meal, but we may have a digestive herbal tea or vegetable broth as healthy drink afterwards. Drink vegetable cocktails between meals to increase detoxification.

During detoxification it is suggested to drink large quantities of vegetable and/or fruit juices during the morning and in the afternoon is recommended. Drink at least three or four 16-ounce glasses per day, along with adequate water.

How to Use and Prepare Vegetables at Home (with a Juicer)

Normally the vegetable juices should be consumed at breaks or between meals.
Drink a glassful ten minutes before breakfast and main meals.
Drink slowly, as if you were chewing and salivating properly as this is an actual food.
During detoxification one drinks larger quantities during the morning and in the afternoon.
Preparation – use a brush or your hand to scrub the vegetables in water to which a tablespoon of cider vinegar has been added, in this way the traces of pesticides and fertilizers are eliminated (if not organically grown).

If they are organic vegetables, it is not necessary to clean them as thoroughly. Vegetables farmed organically have a high nutritional content and a much more pleasant taste than commercially produced vegetables.

Practical Advice on Juicing

I suggest that you buy a very good vegetable juicer since it is a good investment in your health. The Champion juicer, for example, is excellent and you can also make some nut purées or other healthy dishes.

- Raw vegetable juices tend to oxidize; therefore, it is best to drink them as soon as they have been prepared.
- Apple juice, for example, oxidizes very quickly, and it is definitely not a good idea to leave it standing. To avoid oxidation, immediately add the juice from ½ lemon and mix it in with the apple juice.
- You can prepare one liter of mixed vegetable juice and store it in the refrigerator to drink during the day. But don't leave vegetable juice to sit until the next day, since it will start to lose vitamins.
- When you prepare vegetable juice, in order to give it a more pleasant flavor, use some lemon, apple, or some strawberry juice, especially for those not used to drinking vegetable juices.

It is always better to use organic vegetables to make fresh juices at home. First, they are free from pesticides and chemical fertilizers, contain more vitamins, and taste much better. Overall, we get more benefit and healing property, but if not, clean well your vegetables in water with a little added vinegar and brush well to remove pesticides. However, as mentioned, you can also buy organic lacto-fermented vegetables juices to offer as an alternative when you have no time to prepare your own fresh vegetable juice at home or work.

Recipes for Cocktails and Juices:

Constipation:
This drink that I formulated helps very much to combat constipation and increase bowel elimination.
Carrot
Spinach (can be alternated with beetroot or potato)
Radish

Diarrhea:
Cabbage

Beetroot (may be alternated with carrot or a little blueberry juice)
Papaya

Colitis and gas:
Carrot
Potato (can be alternated with a little coconut milk)
Papaya

Hemorrhoids:
Turnip leaves
Watercress
Spinach
Potato

Flatulence:
Carrot
Papaya
Potato

Detoxification:
Carrot
Beetroot
Watercress
Asparagus

Revitalizing Cocktail for the Intestine:
1 glass carrot juice
1/2 glass black grapes 1/2 glass pineapple
1 teaspoon ground dried seaweed
1 teaspoon ground sesame seeds
2 tablespoons of alfalfa or sesame sprouts

Alkaline Cocktail:
This mixture is rich in antioxidants and is also good for intestinal disturbances.
Carrot juice
Pineapple juice
Apple juice
Some spinach leaves
2 tablespoons of alfalfa or sesame sprouts

Mix the ingredients for one minute in a blender or mixer. Drink slowly.

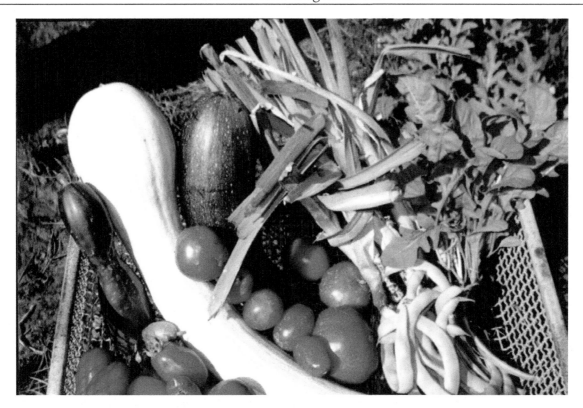

Revitalizing Drink for the Intestines:

Juice
    1 carrot
    1 large apple
    1 kiwi
    1 orange
    100g fresh pineapple

Transfer the juice into your blender and add the following ingredients:
    1 teaspoon flaxseed
    1 teaspoon sesame seeds
    1 teaspoon oat bran

Place all the ingredients in a blender and mix for about two minutes. Drink slowly throughout the day. This is one of my favorite cocktails that I developed over the years in my clinic. Not only does it stimulates intestinal function and detoxifies, but it increases energy because of high levels of vitamin C from kiwi, orange and apple. I recommend this cocktail juice for my patients, and of course, if we can get organic carrot, apple and kiwi, these contain higher nutritional value, better taste and are free of pesticides. This revitalizing drink is best taken at breakfast. It also helps to combat constipation.

Cocktails to Relieve Constipation and Detox the Liver:

    1\2 pineapple
    2 small apples
    1\3 cup alfalfa sprouts
    1\4 mug watercress
    1\3 cup parsley
    1\3 cup broccoli
    10ml chlorella growth factor

Mix the ingredients in a blender or mixer for one minute and drink slowly.

2 apples
1\4 pineapple
1\4 cucumber
1\2 avocado
30gr of green wheat or barley
1 coffee spoon of ground chlorella tablets (or in powder form)
2 capsules (powder) of acidophilus

Mix the ingredients in a blender or mixer for one minute and then drink slowly.

As a suggestion for people undergoing detoxification with chronic constipation who only eliminate feces every few days, this cocktail juice can be taken as one glass every three hours starting at 8:00 or 9:00 a.m., so it requires about six glasses per day, but of course for people away from their home they can drink three glasses or more per day. You can always carry cocktail juice in a thermos.

The Healing Properties of Vegetable Juices

Raw vegetable juice is like fresh blood, it contains all minerals, vitamins, enzymes, antioxidants and especially chlorophyll from green leaves. Chlorophyll is very efficient against infection and to detoxify the blood, liver and colon. Additionally these recipes of mixed vegetable juices increase the oxygen supply circulating in your blood, since all green leaves contain oxygen molecules. Dr. Jensen knew what he was doing fifty years ago when he start to use liquid chlorophyll manufactured by his company, Dr. Jensen Products. Today most of the original products such as the liquid chlorophyll, grape concentrate, dulse, whey, and apple concentrate that I knew when I first met him and used later on for my patients in Montreal, Canada, are still available at Dr. Bernard Jensen International.

Generally speaking, green leafy vegetables are very rich in chlorophyll, vitamin C, potassium, and when consumed in the form of juices offer real protection against infections, are detoxifying, and stimulating for the liver and intestines, protecting them against pollution. Vegetable juice also allows for a larger consumption of raw vegetables since it is generally advised to eat 4 to 6 different vegetables per day, which sometimes is difficult. Thus juices are an excellent alternative. Besides, raw vegetables keep their enzymes intact while the temperature used during cooking partially or totally destroys these precious nutrients.

Vegetable juices are used as therapeutic support in the treatment of various illnesses. Since the beginning of the last century, vegetable juices have been widely used in numerous clinics, many of which I personally had visited in Germany, Switzerland, Austria, and England. The Swiss, Germans, and the Swedish were pioneers in the use of vegetable juices as a LIVING FOOD, but I had also seen fresh juices used in the United States and Canada.

In the beginning of this past century, the Swiss doctor, Dr. Bircher-Benner of the Bircher Benner Clinic was one of the first to use vegetable juices as a natural therapy. His name is famous for having created the well-known Bircher-Muesli cereal and has also been one of the first to pioneer raw food (instead of cooked food) to treat patients with chronic disease, weak digestive systems, and even for degenerative diseases such as multiple sclerosis.

Alfred Vogel (1902-1996), also from Switzerland, was a real pioneer in Swiss popular medicine who I had met several times, but especially during the World Congress that we organized, such the one in Aix-en-Provence (France) in 1973 together with Dr. Bernard Jensen, Ann Wigmore, and K. Asai. He founded the world famous Bioforce Laboratory, and contributed significantly to the medicinal value of fresh herbs (not dried), and developed a wide range of fresh herbal specialties. He also contributed to increasing the popularity of raw organic vegetable juice.

He was an innovator in manufacturing fresh extract of herbs to treat disease and recommended vegetable juices, indeed offering them to patients in his own clinic. Dr. Vogel recommended potato juice for stomach ulcers and gastric disturbances that he manufactured in small bottle. However, you can prepare this at home using one tablespoon of organic potato juice mixed with carrot juice. After all it is such a simple food source with so many healing properties.

In the United States, Dr. H.E. Kirchner, became famous for writing a book called *Live Food Juice*, which was the basis of treatment and cure for thousands of people. As a young man Kirchner was very ill, and sent to countryside to stay with relatives and family, who owned a farm, where he started eating more natural food, breathing fresh air and observing life, all around. He was the one who, by coincidence, started to make carrot juice, a fact which not many people today are aware. Dr. Bernard Jensen, with whom I studied and worked at his Health Ranch, in Escondido, California, had created his own organic garden, growing vegetables and fruits on only a few acres producing vegetables of high quality and nutritional value for the need of his patients. He used only manure, compost, worms, and ground stone such dolomite rich in magnesium and seaweed to make the soil richer. The juices produced by these special vegetables not only were tasty, but high in therapeutic value. I saw patients improving, with the benefit from the daily diet. These were mixtures of fresh organic vegetable juices, not to mention those patients only on vegetable juice during a period of several days.

While I had been staying at Hidden Valley Health Ranch, both studying and observing, I saw some patients benefit from the daily diet and these juices, not mentioning patients on only vegetable juice during several days. I really witnessed many cases and it made no doubt in my mind that food is our best medicine, as proclaimed by Hippocrates.

I was often able to observe patients drinking their organic vegetable juices at different hours of the day. It was really quite an experience for me since I saw many patients improving the condition of their health and feeling much better. This included arthritis, anemia, asthma, and a few cases of cancer. However, at that time, it was a crime to treat cancer patients with food and vegetable juices, where one could be arrested. Dr. Jensen suggested a drink of carrot juice with fresh goat milk for some cancer patients, probably beneficial to help their condition.

One of the best examples I witnessed was the case of an asthmatic man that I personally brought from Canada, after I moved from Los Angeles with a group of patients, to the Ranch, whose suffering had made him suicidal. Upon arrival in Los Angeles by plane from Montreal, the man had a severe crisis and we were obliged to take him to hospital. The next day, arriving at the Ranch by bus, the man could barely walk, only for a very short distance from his room to Dr. Jensen's Office, treatment rooms, or to the restaurant. His diet included a large quantity of organic vegetable juices, such as carrot, turnip with green turnip leaves, beetroot and celery, together with colonic irrigation to clean up the colon, diapulse short wave therapy, along with some supplementation and a healthy food diet. Soon he recuperated in an incredibly rapid manner, and was able to walk up to the main Ranch entrance, which was quite far from the facility rooms. I remember the man used to say, "I don't understand I take so much medication and I get worse, now I take no medication and I am improving". One can easily understand how impressed I was to have observed such a good result, while all the drugs prescribed previously by his doctors could not help him.

Today, few people are aware of the great nutritional value and therapeutic effects that organic vegetable juices can offer. It would be quite interesting for doctors to acquire this knowledge instead of constantly prescribing drugs that only intoxicate the patient and often make them worse from multiple side effects listed on the insert sheet. How can you expect to improve your patient? As previously mentioned, the use of vegetable juices began at the end of the last century but has been gradually overlooked. We have also lost the notion of live food, in considering only the caloric value of foods, whichever kind and whatever way was used to cook them. Now, we know perfectly well that certain forms of cooking are completely wrong and destroy a large part of the nutritional value of food.

Much can be said about the nutritional value of organic vegetables and fruits to keep our body healthy, but we need to understand that in addition to vitamins, minerals, and enzymes, raw vegetable juice contains electrical potential that they have absorbed from the sun. Indeed vegetables are the energy store of the sun, ready for us to absorb in our bodies.

Each cell of our body vibrates constantly since the cellular membranes have their own electrical potential, necessary for controlling the ions + pump (entrance and exit of electrolytes in the cells). At the University of Vienna, researchers have shown that (raw) live foods, and especially vegetable juice, increases the electrical potential of cell's membrane and tissues. It also improves the capacity of the capillary vessels to regulate the transportation of nutritive elements and improve detoxification.

Oxido-Reduction

Vegetables juices help to keep a good ratio of the acid/alkaline balance but also possess the same as all living and raw food, a biological factor called oxido-reduction (RH2) or redox, which defines the electron's potential in a cell and enzymatic activity, critical to the physiological and pathological process, as to balance the extra and intracellular exchange through a cell's membrane. Oxido-reduction balance is necessary to create high cellular energy in the form of ATP. This process which is part of the so-called Biological Terrain, as developed in Europe by Professor Louis Claude Vincent, is the basis of life, well-known to biologists.

The three main important biological factors are:
pH-magnetic
RH2-oxido-reduction electric
RHO- electro resistivity

The RH2 value defines an oxido-reduction balance
Oxidation – refers to a molecule that has lost its electron.
Reduction – refers to a molecule that has gained an electron.

If a substance oxidizes, it means that the molecule loses one electron, which is stolen by radical oxygen that gained this electron.

> *An RH2 value from 0 to 28 = Reductive terrain*
> **Is Favorable for Life**
> *An RH2 value from 28 to 42 = Oxidizing terrain*
> **Is Harmful for Life**

We can compare this to the activity of free radicals that have lost one electron and attack other molecule to steal one extra electron. This chain reaction leads to a process of oxidation. One simple example is the process of oxidation by oxygen on iron.

Today, in Europe and USA the biological terrain can be measured from an intake of urine, blood, saliva, and analyzed with a computerized device called a BTA-1000 (available in USA) or Mora (Germany). The obtained pH. value, RH2 and RHO allows for a better picture of the patient's metabolic condition, especially about the value of the pH. and oxido-reduction. If we use this measurement together with the LBA (and Iridology) we get the real health condition of a person concerning the terrain and any potential risks of upcoming disease. This offers a really complete picture of your patient either during a pathological condition or as prevention from a precancerous terrain.

Everything is not so simple in biology when explaining how our body functions. We derived the term oxido-reduction because cells need to be protected from excessive free radical activity (oxidation), but need a little oxidation to activate the cellular signaling pathway. The enzyme SOD converts the superoxide radical into radical hydrogen peroxide, which in turn is converted into water by catalase and glutathione enzymes. A small amount of radical hydrogen peroxide is required to activate the cellular signaling pathway. However, cellular repair of damaged membranes by endogenous enzymes requires a reduced terrain. In other words to activate this process, a small amount of oxidation is necessary, but for repair it must take place in this reduced terrain. This is called oxido-reduction, since both are necessary, explaining why a true antioxidant compound should also have some oxido/reduction or redox property, the purpose of which is to activate the electron chain transport in the mitochondria to synthesize high cellular ATP energy. Oxidation is necessary to burn up food in the mitochondria, but also reduction in order to reduce the unnecessary oxidation from free radical activity. It is also important to oxidize invading pollutants and xenobiotics, so that they are further eliminated. Oxido/reduction is beneficial to all the biological functions in our body.

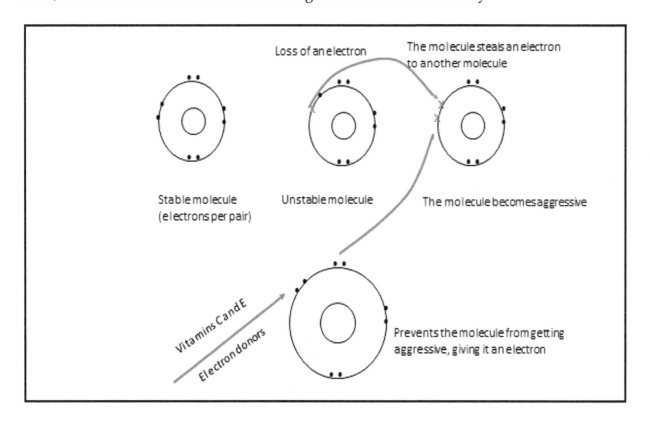

A molecule contains four pairs of electrons that give it stability. When subjected to aggression (ultraviolet, X-ray, stress, etc.) the molecule loses an electron and becomes unstable. It will then attack another molecule, and try to steal an electron starting a chain reaction, which is harmful to the cells. The antioxidants (vitamins C, E, and other substances) provide an electron to an unstable molecule, preventing it from becoming a toxic free-radical.

Live foods, mainly fresh organic vegetables (and fruits) possess certain bioelectronic properties meaning pH., RH2, RHO, while industrial food is either too acidic or too alkaline with no RH2 and RHO properties and thus does not have any preventive or healing properties. For instance, if we compare organic carrots and industrial carrots, here is the difference:

<u>**Organic carrots:**</u>
   pH.: 5.6
   RH2: 9.5
   RHO: 500 ohms

<u>**Industrial carrots:**</u>
   pH.: 6.5
   RH2: 26.2 (high)
   RHO: 152 ohms (low)

<u>**Organic Strawberry:**</u>
   pH.: 5.5
   RH2: 16.8
   RHO: 1150 ohms

<u>**Industrial Strawberry:**</u>
   pH.: 4.0 low and acid
   RH2: 23
   RHO: 210 (very low)

We can observe how an industrial strawberry is acidic with high RH2 and low RHO compared to an organic strawberry that can also boost energy levels. This is only a small example where we can better understand how we can drive our ground to become too acidic or too alkaline, depending on our food choices, which in turn may open the door to disease and infection.

Acid/Alkaline Food Chart:

Highly Alkaline:
Grasses
Cucumber
Kale
Kelp
Broccoli sprouts
Moderately Alkaline:
Beetroot
Garlic
Onion
Radish
Tomatoes

Mildly Alkaline:
Asparagus
Artichokes
Brussels sprouts
Pumpkin
Tofu
Buckwheat

Highly Acidic:
Honey
Soy sauce
Beef
Cheese
Dairy
Eggs
Shellfish
Dried fruits
Pork meat
White bread
White rice

Moderately Acidic:
Blackberry Grapes
Pineapple Peaches
Guava
Fish
Wild rice
Rye bread

It also associates with industrial food, highly acidic food, decreasing mineral levels and bad kidney function. Most disease first develops in a toxic and acidic ground, with low redox properties and excessive free radical activity. Refined food, industrial food, pasta, and white bread are considered acidic food and burn up our reserve of minerals in the body that in turn increase acidity in tissue and cellular milieu. We have several ways to monitor the biological terrain of patients, verify the level of oxidative stress, and excess toxins. The LBA and the MBT, to which I refer in this book is helpful if someone doesn't have a BTA-1000 device.

Excessive oxidation creates an unfavorable terrain and is responsible for a number of organic diseases, inflammatory processes, and even pathological diseases from Parkinson's to diabetes, or cancer. We understood all along just how to decrease excessive oxidation from high free-radical activity and wrong diet. We knew how to correct the terrain to by reducing oxidation with vegetable juices not only rich in antioxidants, but more alkaline, so as to balance or correct this terrain with diet, detox, and vegetable juice. However, one thing needs to be understood, that disease cannot develop in a healthy body with a well-balanced terrain. You have to work with patients and diet, detoxification, to understand how you can change a body over a period of 3-6 months. This is not prescribing pills for pains or to control some abnormal mechanism, but you build up new tissues and make the body stronger, but of course this needs further investigation and research.

Remember that microbes and bacteria start to grow and become aggressive if the ground becomes too acid or too alkaline. The vitamins contained in these juices have a reductive value.

They provide electrons to unstable molecules that have lost an electron (oxygen radical) and hence prevent the attack and deterioration of cellular membranes through an oxidizing process. Claude Bernard made it clear when he said that the microbe is nothing, the terrain is everything.

Raw vegetable juices also allow for a better absorption and use of oxygen by muscular and cardiac cells. Obviously green vegetables, but also any vegetable contains oxygen molecules and enzymes that may help both to increase blood oxygen level and to activate the chain of cellular respiration in the mitochondria. All green leaves are rich in chlorophyll and oxygen molecules, but we are most ignorant about its benefits. Chlorophyll increases the oxygen intake to a blood level of 25%.

Oxygen is crucial for many functions in our body for detoxification but especially necessary to our mitochondrial function in order to break down food into electrons so that a steady level of ATP energy is kept in production, necessary to activate all the physiological functions of our body. Did you know that 90% of the oxygen you breathe is used by the mitochondria while your brain need ten times more oxygen that any other organ at rest in the body! This is something to think about.

Many degenerative diseases have a direct correlation with damaged mitochondria components, DNA mutation, and decreasing ATP synthesis. Melas Syndrome is one typical example of a degenerative disease involving mutation of COX 2 in the electron transport chain of the mitochondria, and usually fatal for the patient. However, I have obtained considerable success with such a case, that I will present at the end of this book. This case was published in *Townsend Letter*, the journal of Integrative Medicine, on June, 2015.

For example, we can appreciate what happened some years ago at California's San Diego Zoo. Fledgling birds, born in cages did not manage to survive and started to die. The diet of these birds consisted of a variety of lettuce common in the United States which has a very light green, almost white color, and was farmed commercially with the help of chemical fertilizers and a large amount of hormones. Lettuce, farmed in this way was very poor in chlorophyll, vitamin C, and iron. After having studied various foods suitable for these fledgling birds, the zoo specialists turned to sprouted alfalfa seeds rich in chlorophyll, minerals, and enzymes.

They carried out an experiment using this kind of food and the baby birds became more disease resistant and healthier. Unfortunately, not many mothers connect their children's health to the kind of food they consume. More the pity, since they could avoid many health problems for their children.

In the United States, Dr. Virginia Livingstone (Livingstone Medical Center), who was a well-known immunologist treating cancer patients, consulted with me as a professional contact. We exchanged ideas and protocols. It was interesting to note that she advised her patients to drink fresh vegetable juice, recommending one liter of carrot juice a day for her cancer patients. The use of cocktails of vegetable juice in particular with carrot juice, red beet juice, and celery juice, is an excellent means to balance the redox level, detoxify the body, and for stimulating the immune defense. Carrots are highly rich in beta-Carotene, a potential preventative substance for degenerative diseases. Laboratory studies have shown that Beta-Carotene can inhibit the development of tumors in animals. Vitamin C, also present in carrots and in many green-leaved vegetables, blocks the formation of nitrosamines, which are carcinogenic substances.

In his book entitled *Cancer - Future Strategies*, Dr. Lucien Israel, world renowned Oncologist suggests that cancer patients could get more benefit by drinking carrot juice, eating more fruits, and vegetables rich in beta-Carotene, vitamin C, magnesium, and potassium, during chemotherapy treatment, as well as daily fiber intake that has a beneficial effect on the intestinal tract in order to reduce the contact time of carcinogenic substances with the intestinal mucosa.

On average carrots contain about 2 gr. of fiber, while a glass of carrot juice contains approximately six carrots and therefore about 12 gr. of fiber, which is beneficial to prevent constipation. Carrots also may have a good effect on the heart since it needs potassium to keep its muscles in good condition. Potassium is also important for good nerve and brain function, reducing acidity and increasing alkalinity. Generally speaking, green leaves are rich in potassium but it is obvious that today people are eating much less vegetables (mostly overcooked) and an excess of industrial foods high in sodium, such as cured meats, canned foods and soups, shakes, salami, roasted peanuts, hot dogs, and other fast foods, resulting in a total imbalance between potassium and sodium. This dangerously increases sodium levels that disturb the ion pump of the cells. Since the day I had observed how patients react to a carrot juice cure at Dr. Jensen's Health ranch, I have always believed that carrot juice is probably not a panacea, but may certainly keep our body young and healthy.

A large glass of organic carrot juice contains 3100 u of beta-Carotene, which is immediately absorbed. Beta-Carotene is a good antioxidant, good for the eyes, skin, reduces inflammation, and prevents from some cancers such as breast cancer by inhibition of the early stages of carcinogenesis. Carrot is one of the best vegetables to use in raw juice cocktails offering great therapeutic value, with one exception, in cases of diabetes, as carrots contain large quantities of sugar.

I refer again to my past experience in Los Angeles over fifty years ago, when I discovered for the first time the existence of raw vegetable juices, when indeed it was carrot and green leaf juices that saved me from wearing glasses, increased my nerve strength, and were instrumental in recovering from a nervous breakdown. I confess that I mixed in some lecithin granules with the juices as suggested to me by Dr. Jensen.

Carrot juice combines well with green leaves, being very rich not only in potassium but calcium, being a very good way to strengthen the bones and combat osteoporosis. It is always best to combine several varieties of vegetables to make a vegetable juice cocktail for detoxification or for other nutritional purposes.

Nature offers a large variety of vegetables and fruits for us to combine so that we may keep healthy. Green leaves for instance are very rich in calcium and magnesium, like kale, spinach, cabbage, and carrots. While milk is promoted to combat osteoporosis, vegetable juice is a good alternative, milk not being so healthy. Ironically, about 40-50 years ago osteoporosis was practically unknown among middle-age women, but today with poor diet style, osteoporosis increasingly appears at a younger age, while dairy food seems not to have done that much to prevent osteoporosis.

Vegetables	Mg/100g
Spinach	483
Parsley	330
Watercress	222

Do not hesitate to create your own combinations and variations of green vegetables and fruit when making juices. I, myself, am still making my daily mixture of vegetable and fruit juices that I take between meals or even substitute for my lunch, often three times per week. Here is one of my favorite juicing combinations:

Carrot	Apple
Celery	Parsley
Red beet	Lemon

Advantages of vegetable and fruit juice cocktails:

- Excellent source of vitamins and minerals.
- Detoxifies the body and eliminate toxins.
- Clean up and stimulate the liver.
- Detoxify and increase blood circulation.
- Revitalize the vascular system.
- Support the elimination of catarrh, improve cases of asthma.
- Decrease excess of acidity in tissue.
- Revitalize the body with extra vitamins, minerals, and enzymes.
- Decreases inflammation.
- Improves bowel function, alleviates hemorrhoids

100g of Vegetables contain an average of:	Cauliflower	Broccoli	Chinese cabbage	Portuguese cabbage	Brussels sprouts	Purple cabbage	Cabbage	Savoy cabbage	Kale	Rhubarb	Asparagus	Chard
Proteids	2.4	3.5	1.2	6	4.9	1.7	1.3	1.5	206	0.6	2.2	2.1
Lipid	0.2	0.2	0.3	0.9	0.6	0.2	0.2	0.3	0.4	0.1	0.2	0.3
Carbohydra	4	4.3	2	6.1	6.7	5.3	4.6	4	4.1	3.7	3.8	2.9
Calories	27	33	16	57	52	30	25	25	30	18	26	23
Joules	113	138	67	238	218	126	105	103	126	75	109	96
Sodium	16	14	7	44	7	4	13	355	9	2	4	90
Potassium	311	410	202	436	390	267	233	288	257	270	220	375
Calcium	22	113	40	230	36	38	49	48	57	52	22	103
Magnesium	7	24	11	34	22	16	20	-	12	13	20	65
Phosphorus	72	78	30	90	80	32	29	43	55	24	46	39
Iron	1.1	1.3	0.6	2.7	1.5	0.5	0.4	0.6	0.9	0.5	1	2.7
Chlorine	30	76	-	122	40	100	37	-	-	53	53	-
Manganese	0.17	0.15	-	2.2	0.27	0.1	0.4	-	-	0.15	0.19	0.3
Copper	0.14	0.14	-	0.09	0.1	0.06	0.06	0.1	-	0.05	0.14	0.11
Sulfur	29	137	15	115	-	-	-	-	-	8	46	-
Vitamin A	21	316	13	833	55	5	10	20	12	12	50	583
Vitamin B1	0.1	0.1	0.03	0.2	0.1	0.07	0.05	0.03	0.05	0.02	0.14	0.1
Vitamin B2	0.11	0.2	0.04	0.2	0.16	0.05	0.05	0.05	0.07	0.03	0.16	0.2
Vitamin PP	0.6	1.1	0.4	2.1	0.9	0.4	0.3	0.2	0.3	0.2	1	0.6
(Niacin)	0.2	0.17	-	0.19	0.16	0.15	0.11	-	0.2	0.035	0.6	-
Vitamin B6	1.1	1.3	1.3	1.4	0.7	0.32	0.26	0.08	-	0.08	0.62	0.17
Vitamin B5	69	110	36	140	102	50	47	20	50	10	28	39
Vitamin C	0.15	0.27	-	4	1	0.2	0.7	-	-	0.2	2.5	1.5
Vitamin E	3.6	-	-	-	3	-	+	-	-	-	-	-
Vitamin K												

Nutritional Value of Vegetables

Vegetables Have Nutritional and Healing Properties According to Their Active Nutrients

Properties and Use of Vegetable Juices

Vegetable	Vegetable Juice	Observations
Beetroot	Is one of the best vegetables to increase red blood cell levels and hemoglobin in cases of anemia. It's very rich in potassium as well. One cup of red beet provides 442 mg of this mineral. Red beets contain a pigment called glucosin-betanin that substitutes critical enzymes for cellular repair, increasing cellular respiration itself, ATP production and protecting against a number of diseases including cancer. It also drives apoptosis. Because of its high level of beta-Carotene, iron, potassium, vitamin C, magnesium, sodium, Phosphorus. Red beet juice increases detoxification, cleans up the liver, kidney and gallbladder. Red beets and red beet juice are considered in Europe by many doctors as an anti-cancer food. In his famous book *A Cancer Therapy – The Result of Fifty Cases*, Max Gerson spoke highly of red beet juice as a support in cancer treatment. I, myself, have included red beet juice in my cancer protocol for the past forty years, especially for patients developing anemia during chemotherapy. Red beet can be consumed raw in salad or baked in the oven and flavored with cold-pressed olive oil; however, red beet juice is highly recommended.	It is a very strong juice when taken by itself and should be mixed with carrot juice. Apple juice. when combined, provides more vitamins, plenty of vitamin A, beta-Carotene, potassium etc. Our intestines need plenty of potassium, magnesium, and manganese for a better function, which can be better provided with fresh organic vegetable juices rather than supplementation. We may need more vitamin supplementation during the winter, but not in summer, the best way to get all the nutrients we need is from natural sources.
Carrot	Is a juice with many properties. Being tonic, it helps digestion, is good for vision, and cleanses the organism. Improves the condition of the skin and helps combat infections and any type of inflammation and ulcers. It gives vitality and well-being. It is rich in vitamin A. Carrot juice is recommended as an introduction to any juice	One can drink carrot juice in large quantities during a detoxification cure and revitalization and to strengthen the immune system, being the ideal base for mixtures of vegetable juices.

Celery	Celery is rich in organic sodium that, along with organic potassium, is essential for maintaining the organism's fluids. It also contains calcium and other minerals that help to strengthen the nervous system. It is an important juice to aid in eliminating waste and toxins accumulated in the intestine and kidney, which can cause arthritis, diabetes, kidney stones, and even coronary diseases.	Is pleasant when mixed with carrot juice. Celery contains minerals that balance and strengthen the nervous system and is recommended for depression, and helps to remove excess acidity in the joints. Celery leaves should also be used.
Cucumber	Excellent natural diuretic, thanks to its strong content of sulfur and silica. It favors the growth and strengthening of hair. Eliminates uric acid from the organism. Helps to balance arterial pressure due to its rich potassium content.	Mix well with apple and carrot juice. It is quickly absorbed and rapidly increases detoxification in the body. Cucumber juice is good during the Summer to supply more mineral salts and cools off the blood.
Kale	Kale juice helps treat stomach ulcers and combat constipation. It is excellent for cleaning the intestinal mucosa and combat gut infections. This juice can cause gas because it frees putrefied matter in the intestine (which is a great quality).	Is a juice with a very strong flavor. It can be drunk alone but is better mixed with other juices. The reason this juice can cause flatulence is because it releases putrefied matter accumulated in the colon, which then needs to be expulsed.
Lettuce	Lettuce is a natural tranquilizer, and is a light diuretic. It calms stomach aches. Any lettuce or green leaved vegetable can be juiced. Most are rich in iron and chlorophyll.	Lettuce is a natural tranquilizer and is highly diuretic. Lettuce can be combined with any other vegetable. Most green vegetables are rich in chlorophyll and iron.
Parsley	Although it is considered to be an aromatic herb and not a vegetable, its juice has a very beneficial effect. It is good for the thyroid and the adrenal glands. Parsley is a very rich source of nutrients. It contains several times, the vitamin C of citrus and very high source of vitamin A, chlorophyll, calcium, sodium, magnesium, and iron. Parsley promotes a healthy uro-genital function, and is recommended in the treatment of stones in the bladder and kidney or gall bladder. It calms kidney pain and treats eye problems. Parsley further strengthens the adrenal glands and is benefits brain nerves and vision.	To be taken in small quantities (2 tablespoons at a time with some carrot, red beet juice). It has a very strong taste. Parsley is antiseptic and was used by the Romans and Greeks thousands of years ago for women with ovary pain. Parsley is beneficial for the uro-genital system, kidney pains and some eye problems. Parsley is rich in chlorophyll, vitamin C, iron and potassium and used as a mild antiseptic.

Soups for Health and Detox

In Europe, over the past centuries soups have been a popular way to adapt vegetables, often mixed with meat, bread, and cheese to become the evening meal of poor and middle class families. Soup recipes are probably some of the oldest ones. The word "soup" comes from a Germanic origin with the word *suppa* meaning "to dip," and soon became a popular meal.

Until the middle of the last century, vegetable broth was prescribed by medical doctors for their patients in bed with fever or from a liver crisis since it really cleans up the body and detoxes the liver and kidneys. Born in France before WWII, I was raised by having vegetable soup for dinner, as a starter, or even as a whole meal. As a result, I always keep attention inside of my mind about how soups and vegetable broth is important for patients. Over the past decades I always prescribe some special vegetable broth or soup for my patients for various purposes such as rheumatism, arthrosis, or intestinal disorders. We even prescribed nettle soup (urtiga) that patients get from fields during spring, being rich in calcium both to nourish and to detoxify the body. Of course some of the vegetable soups I have been using over the past decades were there simply to detoxify the body, which is nothing new, while it is true that I was also influenced by some great pioneers like Dr. A.Vogel of Switzerland who manufactured an organic vegetable broth in powder as a healthy drink. However, I use vegetable broth as a basis to cook regular vegetables instead of using plain water; it makes for a much richer and tasty soup for therapeutic purpose.

In preparing soup recipes you can use, beside vegetables, whole rice, quinoa, lentils, barley, or oats that contain vitamins, minerals, proteins, and fibers, and it is also a way to consume more vegetables in the diet. Such soups serve to supply more nutrients to our body, combat fatigue, remineralize the bones, balance the nervous system, balance the acid basic pH, are anti-cholesterol, and even combat constipation. The extra fibers contained in many vegetables help the intestinal transit and impair the stagnation of wastes; therefore, being important to keep a clean colon.

The main purpose of my book is based upon detoxification, especially activating the two main emunctories: the liver and the kidney. The liver is usually overtaxed from an excess of fats, sugar, and alcohol, not to mention cooked red meat and pharmaceutical drugs. The kidneys suffer from an excess of red meat, beans, alcohol and pharmaceutical drugs. All green vegetables help the liver to detoxify, but some boosters include garlic, onions, ginger, curcumin, cucumber, sweet potatoes, black radish, artichoke, and apple that can be used in soups or added to juices.

For a detoxification program you can have a very good soup as diner if, for instance, it's made from mixed vegetables, lentils, or quinoa and some cottage cheese, and one apple for dessert.

Soup Cleansing Recipes

First for any soup you need a vegetable broth as a basis that you can make yourself with leeks, onions, carrots, garlic, parsley, celery, and spring water and you keep in the refrigerator. As an alternative, you can buy in health food stores some vegetable both in powder, but make sure it is natural.

Radish Soup
This is mainly a detox and slimming soup, good for the liver and gall bladder. It also purifies the skin.

Ingredients for 4 persons:

    2 bunches of red radish
    2 potatoes
    2 onions
    1 liter of vegetable broth
    2 tablespoons of cold pressed virgin olive oil
    2 tablespoons of soya cream

A pinch of vegetable salt

Peel and cut the onions into tiny slices and cook them rapidly in a pot with the olive oil. Then add the radishes, cut into slices. Peel the potatoes and cut them into cubes and put them in the pot with the onions and radishes. Cover with the vegetable broth and the salt.

Cook the soup for 10 to 15 minutes, then blend it rapidly and serve with the soya cream, cold or hot according to your taste. You can also add a tablespoon of sesame puree for better taste and to increase your Omega-3 intake.

Red Beet Soup
This is a real detoxing and delicious soup.

Ingredients for 4 persons:

    4 raw small red beets
    3 carrots cut in small cubes
    2 chopped onions
    2 heads of garlic crushed
    1 leek chopped
    2 tablespoons of sunflower oil
    2 pinches of vegetable salt
    1 tablespoon of cold pressed virgin oil olive
    1 liter of vegetable broth
    1 tablespoon of sunflower or pumpkin seeds
    2 tablespoons of soya cream

First use the root of the red beets, cover with water in a pot and cook for 30 minutes to make a broth. Let it cool off and filter the liquid.

Heat the oil in a pan and add the onions, garlic, leeks, and carrots, then let it cook slowly for 10 minutes. Afterwards, add 1 liter of vegetable broth and continue cooking for few more minutes. Peel the red beets and cut them into cubes and blend them together with the vegetable broth and the water of the cooked red beets. Mix well in the blender until you obtain a cream. Flavor with soya cream or olive oil and add the sunflower or pumpkin seeds. To have more detoxing and a richer broth, you can add some spirulina or even chlorella powder in the blender.

Watercress, Lettuce, and Tofu Soup
This is a green soup rich in vitamins, fibers, and minerals. Watercress is high in iron, potassium and sulphur for detox.

Ingredients for 4 persons:

    150g of watercress
    150g of green lettuce
    2 small potatoes
    150g of tofu
    600 ml of vegetable broth
    A pinch of vegetable salt
    1 tablespoon of cold pressed virgin olive oil
    1\2 sheet of nori algae

Peel the potatoes and cut them in cubes. Carefully wash the watercress and lettuce.

In a pot heat the olive oil and add the potatoes and cook them slowly for 5 minutes. Add the watercress and lettuce and cook them while mixing well the ingredients for 5 more minutes Add in the vegetable broth and cook the soup for an additional 15 minutes

In meantime, cut the tofu into small pieces and mix well. Blend all the ingredients include the tofu and season to your taste with the vegetable salt. Serve the soup with the nori.

You can use other types of algae and substitute the lettuce with spinach. This soup is rich in Omega-3 and iodine.

White Soup (Cauliflower)

This is an excellent soup for detox, rich in fibers and minerals such as magnesium, calcium, potassium, and also an anti-cancer soup.

Ingredients for 4 persons:

 1 small cauliflower
 2 onions
 1 leek
 2 small potatoes
 3 or 4 branches of parsley
 1 liter of vegetable broth
 2 tablespoons of cold pressed virgin oil olive
 A pinch of vegetable salt.

Pour the vegetable broth into the pot under high heat and bring it to broil, then reduce to a simmer. Slice the onions and cut the potatoes, chop the leeks, detach the clumps of cauliflower, all well washed. Heat the olive oil in a pan and add first the onions, then the potatoes and the leeks for color; this also extracts the flavor. Then add in all the ingredients to the pot with the vegetable salt and chopped parsley. Cover and let slowly simmer for 30 minutes. To serve, add a tablespoon of soya cream or some grated cheddar cheese or Swiss gruyere. You can do the same but replace the cauliflower with broccoli, a cruciferous vegetable with anti-cancer properties, especially to reduce risk of colon cancer.

Spinach, Asparagus, and Fennel Soup

This is a very good soup that you can best prepare when you can buy fresh asparagus (otherwise frozen or in can). This soup detoxes the body especially with the fennel and asparagus. This is a healthy detox soup.

Ingredients for 4 persons:

 300g of green* asparagus (*best otherwise use white asparagus)
 3 small onions
 2 heads of garlic
 2 tablespoon of cold pressed virgin oil olive
 1 bunch of fennel
 120g of spinach sprouts (otherwise broccoli)
 1 liter of vegetable broth

1 tablespoon of cider vinegar
A small quantity of parsley
2 tablespoon of grilled pumpkin seeds
1 tablespoon of chia seed
A pinch of vegetable salt
1/2 leaf of nori

Remove the hard extremity of the fresh asparagus, wash well and cut them in small pieces. Heat the olive oil in a large pot. Chop finely the onions, garlic and fennel and put it in the pot and cook them for 5 minutes.

Then add the asparagus and mix them well on low heat for one minute then add the spinach sprouts, vegetable broth, the cider vinegar, some vegetable salt, and pepper if you wish. Bring the mixture to a boil and then reduce the fire and cook the soup for 10-15 minutes. Put all the ingredients in the cooled liquid in a blender and mix well. According to your taste you may add little vegetable salt if necessary. In each serving plate, add some chopped parsley and the grilled pumpkin seed and chia seed. You can always substitute the asparagus with turnip as alternative.

Artichoke Soup

This is a really excellent soup to detox the liver and good for the skin. In season you use the bottom (heart) of fresh artichoke, or in a can, even frozen bottom artichoke if available. If fresh, remove all the leaves, the hair and use only the bottom.

Ingredients for 4 persons:

4 bottoms of artichoke
4 leeks (only the white part)
500 ml of vegetable broth
Pinch of vegetable salt

First cut the bottom of the artichoke into four quarters, carefully wash and then cut up the leeks. Cook the two vegetables in the broth for 20 minutes. Add a pinch of vegetable salt and to make the soup richer; to detoxify add a full tablespoon of spirulina or chlorella powder and blend the soup. When serving, add some soya cream for good flavor.

Pumpkin and Lentil Soup

This is a soup rich in carotene and a good antioxidant, with magnesium and iron good to strengthen the body. It also contains good proteins.

Ingredients for 4 persons:

120g of green brown or green lentils
400g of pumpkin
1 tablespoon of cold pressed virgin olive oil
2 branches of cilantro
1 pinch of cumin powder
1 small onion
500 ml of vegetable broth

1 pinch of vegetable salt
4 tablespoon of soya cream

Wash the lentils, peel the pumpkin, and cut it up into small cubes. Peel the onion and cook it rapidly to give it color in the olive oil in a pan and then add the cumin.

Add the pumpkin and the lentils, mix well and pour in the vegetable broth and then bring to boil. Reduce the fire and let it cook covered for 15-20 minutes until the lentils are tender. Put all the ingredients in a blender and mix well. Add the vegetable salt, a little black pepper if you wish. In each serving plate add one tablespoon of soya cream and chopped cilantro on top.

Leeks and Parsnip Soup

This is a really an excellent detox soup especially with the leeks and parsnip, rich in fibers magnesium, and potassium to activate the colon.

Ingredients for 4 persons:

3 parsnips
4 leeks
1 onion
1 head of garlic
1 small handful of parsley
1 tablespoon of cold pressed virgin olive oil
1 liter of vegetable broth
1 pinch of vegetable salt and pepper

Peel and slice the onion. Peel the parsnip and cut it in small pieces. Wash the parsley and chop it up. Wash up the leeks and chop them finely. Into a pot pour in the olive oil, warm it up and add the onion, garlic and the leeks and cook them for 5 minutes with low heat. Then add the parsnips, cover with the vegetable broth and bring to broil. Then reduce the fire and cook the ingredients for 15 minutes.

Put all the ingredients in the blender and mix well. Add the salt and pepper. Serve the soup hot with some chopped parsley in each bowl.

Four Important Cereals for Intestinal Health

Oats

I have always advocated the use of oats can be one of the best medicinal foods for gastrointestinal problems. Oats, and particularly oat cereals, were recently acknowledged and classified in a list of the "Ten Most Healthiest Foods." One of the most interesting qualities of oats is the presence of phytosterols that help to control the level of cholesterol absorption of food at the intestinal level. A characteristic of oats is they also surround the fats to eliminate them, without being absorbed.

Oats play an important role in the diet of children, patients, and even in the diet of healthy people. Indeed, the oat is an extraordinary cereal that contains a variety of substances beneficial for health.

First of all oats, as opposed to wheat and other cereals, after processing still retain the bran and germ containing the highest concentration of nutrients. Oats also contain important soluble fibers useful in combating and preventing constipation.

Oats used in the form of flakes contain more proteins than any other cereal (13.8% mg). In comparison to other cereals, the lipid content is high, up to 7.9%, whereas it varies between 0.6% and 3.9% in other cereals. Proportionally it is excellent as 80% of the fatty acids contained are unsaturated, which makes this food good for the heart. Oat flakes for example, contain 365 calories per 100g and high levels of potassium and magnesium that maintain the acid alkaline balance. Another advantage of oats can be found in their low sodium content (8mg/100g). They are equally rich in:

Magnesium – 129 mg / 100g
Calcium – 80 mg / 100g
Especially in Phosphorus – 342 mg / 100g

The composition of oats shows that it is an appropriate food for the nervous system because of the high level of phosphorus and magnesium. Besides these qualities, oats, thanks to the presence of phytosterols control the intestinal level of absorption of the cholesterol content in food. They are able to lower total cholesterol, but above all they exert action on the bad cholesterol (LDL) maintaining the balance of the good one (HDL).

> ## *Oats Make Iron Men*
> ## *Traditional German Proverb*

Oats also contain a very special fiber called betaglucan, which also acts on cholesterol and dietary fats. It forms a sort of jam that that goes through the intestine, without being absorbed, enclosing these fats and eliminating them. Oats also contain antioxidant compounds capable of neutralizing free radicals. One of these compounds, tocopherols, is abundant in oats. These oat nutrients are very effective in preventing cardio-vascular disease and certain types of cancer, above all against colon and intestinal cancer. Tocopherols protect against oxidation process, which makes cholesterol rancid resulting in oxidized cholesterol deposits on our arterial walls. Tocopherols contained in oats are 50% more efficient that vitamin E alone.

Apart from these important factors, oats are an excellent and high energy source food. Oat flakes, for example, contain 365 calories per 100g. For this reason oats are used instead of wheat in the diet of race horses. You never see a race horse fed with wheat since it will create too much acidity, reducing its muscle capacity during racing. We consume too much wheat: spaghetti, pizza, wheat bread, and pastries, which increase our acidity level, obliging the body to use its mineral reserves from other tissues.

Oats is the perfect food for the treatment of gastrointestinal disorders, when people suffer from intestinal colitis, from gas, bloating, or any inflammatory condition. I usually prescribe this to my patients suffering from intestinal disorders that need to detoxify or just to keep healthy. Oats is also the perfect evening meal for elderly people to have a light and nutritional meal.

This food is suitable for people of all ages, even for babies with intestinal problems. A bottle with porridge will relive any disorder. It is the perfect evening meal for elderly people.

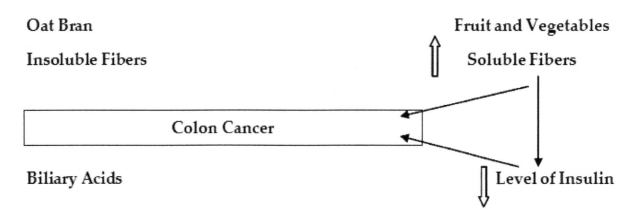

Nature always supplies us with effective and repairing foods, not to mention medicinal foods, which do not present the same risk as medicinal drugs. I believe it is now up to us to rediscover what God has given us in terms of food to keep us healthy.

Currently there are specific and justifiable theories about colon cancer attributed to the presence of an excess of biliary acids. These play a role in the digestion of fats but on the other hand, in the intestine they turn into secondary and very harmful biliary acids, due to bacterial action. According to this theory, they may attack cells and this may originate a cancer. On one other hand, exposure to an elevated level of insulin in the blood can also promote cancer development. Oat and fibers seem to be the answer to maintain moderate levels of insulin and therefore may also prevent cancer development.

Whole Rice

Rice might be the most widely used food on the planet. It is the staple diet of most Oriental and European populations, and forms the base of many traditional dishes. Rice has an exceptional dietary value; it lends itself to different kinds of preparation being easy to prepare. It is especially recommended for people with a fragile digestive tract. There are many varieties of rice, from basmati to wild rice, scented rice from Thailand to Italian risotto. But the most nutritional one is whole grain rice that contains a large quantity of minerals, vitamins, enzymes, rice bran fibers, and complex glucose. Overall, whole grain rice offers more nutrition, vitamins, minerals enzymes, fibers, and complex glucose.

Its richness in fibers stimulates the intestinal peristalsis facilitating elimination. The exterior layer (bran) contains a substance called oryzenin, which limits the organism's production of cholesterol. Whole rice along with a diet free of fats is one of the best ways to lower cholesterol and keep away from Statins, a pharmaceutical anti-cholesterol drug that may damage the liver and may even lead to the development of cancer.

A serving of 150g of whole rice contains about 2g of insoluble fibers, which are the most essential for the organism. The fibers contained in whole rice reduce the risk of colon cancer. According to some scientists, if we were to increase the daily consumption of these fibers by 40g, the risk of intestinal cancer would diminish by 31%.

It is easy to digest rice, which is why it is recommended both for patients, convalescents, and healthy people. It has great power of absorption that reduces the risk of intestinal putrefaction. It is always the food recommended in cases of enteritis.

Diets based on whole rice bran help to lower arterial pressure and help to strengthen heart function, and therefore suggested in cardiac insufficiencies. Whole rice favors the elimination of salt and toxins that adhere to the tissues and cause fluid retention.

For patients who need to lose weight and detoxify, I recommend a diet of whole grain rice over a four-day period. You eat rice at breakfast, lunch, and dinner. At breakfast you can flavor your rice with some honey to look more like breakfast. At lunch and dinner you combine the whole rice with few slices of tomatoes. In between, of course, you can drink some vegetable juice cocktails as well as herbal teas. Drink 2 liters of water a day, only water or infusions and 1 glass of fresh fruit juice a day.

I suggested this diet to the U.S. Ambassador, Elizabeth Frawley Bagley who complained about gaining weight after protocol dinners, and it really worked well. The ambassador became my patient during a four-year period. Ambassador Bagley often invited me and my wife to dinner or for meetings at the U.S. Embassy. Twice she invited the world famous spiritualist, Deepak Chopra, for a private lecture, and it gave me opportunity to meet him and for us to have discussions together.

Whole rice is easily altered at room temperature. It must be kept in a hermetically sealed container or in the refrigerator where it will maintain its freshness for an entire year.

Whole grain rice offers two times more vitamin B2 and three times more niacin than regular rice. While I was in Los Angeles, Dr. Bernard Jensen developed a rice bran syrup to prescribe to people with nerve disorders and it was quite efficient. It contained large quantities of B complex and was high in proteins. I personally experimented with this rice bran syrup per Dr. Jensen's prescription, and I remember how it really energized my nerves, but also felt relaxing. I believe that this product is still available online from, "Dr. Bernard Jensen Products."

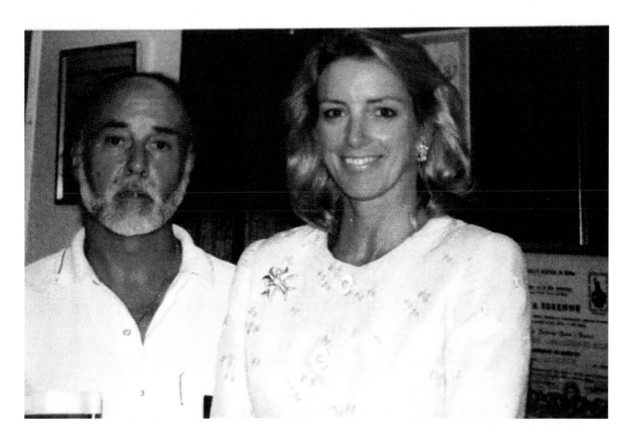

Professor Serge Jurasunas and U.S. Ambassador Elizabeth Frawley Bagley

Bulgur or Boulgour

In spite of these commercially adopted names, it is actually prepared from wheat germ. Its composition is also similar to whole wheat grain. These foods are traditionally prepared in the Middle East where the wheat grain is precooked, dried, husked and ground finely or coarsely.

Bulgur is a cereal food that keeps the people of the Middle East very healthy, such as in Turkey, Lebanon, and Tunisia. I often travel to Middle East, especially to Turkey, and made observations about their food habits, noting how strong and healthy these people are. It contains important quantities of minerals that help our body to be healthier and stronger: iron, phosphorus, zinc, magnesium, and selenium, to strengthen the immune system, improve nerve function, muscle, and bone. If you regularly eat bulgur three times per week, rotated with other cereals, you can supply your body with a well-digested food rich in nutrients, and you will be healthier with more energy.

Being a precooked food, this cereal is easily cooked and prepared. It is sufficient to immerse it in boiling water and let it stand for 15 minutes, or simply steam it.

It is rich in various essential nutrients, containing 12% proteins, 75 % carbohydrates, and 2% of fats, with 368 calories per 100g.

It is, therefore, transformed into an easily assimilated food and is well tolerated from a digestive point of view. It contains almost the entire germ, a large quantity of B complex vitamins, and an abundance of protein. It is also rich in fiber, which prevents constipation and feeds the friendly bacteria.

Bulgur contains a complex substance known as folic acid, which prevents certain chemical substances absorbed with food from transforming into nitrosamines, which are highly carcinogenic substances. It has been scientifically proven that nitrosamines are a predominant factor in the genesis of cancer, particularly colon and breast cancer. Today, because of industrial foods, it is not always easy to avoid foods that can lead to the formation of nitrosamines in the intestine. But the frequent consumption of this cereal can really reduce the harmful effects of nitrosamines.

Bulgur being high in cellulose protects the heart and prevents bad cholesterol absorption as well as many other digestive and intestinal disturbances, because of its high content of insoluble fibers, which do not decompose but remain in the intestine much longer than other food. They absorb large quantities of water, important to build up a proper texture of feces, which allows for faster elimination. Therefore it also fights against constipation and hemorrhoids, which today has become a major problem in middle age women.

Comparative studies of individuals suffering from intestinal polyps have shown that the polyps were reduced in volume or disappeared completely in the group that was consuming cereals containing 22g of insoluble fibers.

Barley

Barley was possibly one of the first cereals cultivated by man and was introduced to Europe before wheat. It is cultivated widely from the Nordic countries to remote deserts. The national Tibetan dish is "Tsampa," which is based on toasted barley flour also used by the Moroccan

Berbers in typical dishes. It is an easily adaptable cereal, resistant to drought and extreme climates, and also grows in poor soils.

Barley is one of the healthiest foods, containing valuable nutrients, a variety of minerals and antioxidants such as manganese, selenium, copper, calcium, zinc, chromium, phosphorus, magnesium, niacin, and vitamin B1, being high in fiber. These antioxidants combat and prevent oxidation from attack by free radicals, while simultaneously promoting liver function and limiting excess cholesterol production in the body. Barley is also rich in amino acids. First we have a good antioxidant with selenium and zinc that may prevent against prostate cancer and breast cancer, which always harbors a zinc deficiency. Same as with the other cereals mentioned, potassium and magnesium are important for the nervous system, but also to keep the colon healthy.

According to the FDA, barley's soluble fiber reduces the risk of coronary heart disease. It also contains antioxidants and prevents the blood from coagulating. Barley also keeps the colon healthy having very valuable fibers which improve digestion and manage to absorb the possible carcinogenic substances in the intestine, reducing the risk of colon cancer by their elimination.

Soluble fibers capture large quantities of water in the intestine, accelerating the digestive processes and combating constipation Barley is one gentle middle laxative that fights constipation and increases the digestive process. We also can use it in case of diarrhea because barley can adapt either against constipation or combat diarrhea, which makes it a unique food.

The following laxative recipe is one of the secrets that Dr. Jensen taught me when I was at Hidden Valley Health Ranch. Dr. Jensen never prescribed laxatives to patients but only healthy food combinations of vegetables and fruits, juices etc., with natural fibers. Colonic therapy was used, and sometimes to help, Dr. Jensen prescribed a medium strength laxative made from herbs, but definitely this was not the general rule.

> **Laxative Recipe**
> **Gentle and Natural**
>
> *Place two handfuls of whole barley in a liter of lukewarm water (once husks have been removed) for twenty four hours. Consume one cup during fasting and repeat throughout the day if necessary. When ready to eat, strain and mix with a bit of honey and lemon juice, to your taste and liking.*

Besides its high content in minerals, barley is rich in vitamin B3 and B12 that makes it perfect for the nervous system. In historic Rome the gladiators were fed barley in their diet and farmers knew that it is one of the best cereals to stimulate milk production in cows.

Barley is consumed without the exterior husk, which is not edible, and is therefore considered whole barley. Another kind can also be found is called "pearl barley," the grain of which undergoes a process of polishing. It is excellent for enriching soups and broths. Roasted barley may be used as a coffee substitute.

> *Whole barley nutritionally contains 348 calories per 100g. 10% water, 9.7% proteins and 75 % carbohydrates.*

Detoxification Crisis

All the great pioneers in Naturopathy such as Drs. Tilden, Lust, Ehret, Platen, Jensen, and others have spoken about the mechanism of detoxification crisis in their works. What does it mean? This is a process where during a detox treatment and diet, the body starts to accumulate and throw out toxins and poisons through the emunctory organs, often causing some reactions. However, this crisis leads to cleaning up the body that further leads to curing itself.

I personally experimented with this reaction when Dr. Jensen first put me on detoxification and I had a severe skin rash and fever lasting several days, and afterward, I was feeling much better. Fever is good since it helps to burn up toxins and kill bacteria.

In his book of over a thousand pages called *The Golden Book of Health*, published in Germany in 1930, unobtainable today, Professor Platen wrote as follows: "Chronic illness alone could be cured if the germs were thrown out from the interior towards the exterior of the body." He could not have been clearer about how we should start to treat the body.

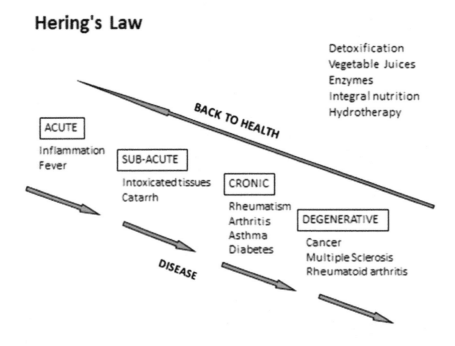

The Law of Hering

The human body is not an inert machine, which medical doctors have been proclaiming. The body possesses a real intelligence to engage defense mechanisms, auto-regulation, and activate its own process of healing. Fasting is one example of when not busy digesting food, the body activates an auto-regulation mechanism that balances the disturbed mechanisms. That is why it needs assistance. Hippocrates said, "It is not the doctor who heals but nature, the doctor uses nature and reaps the benefits.. Before Platen, already in the nineteenth century, Dr. Constantin Hering (Jan 1, 1800- July 23,1880) became famous for discovering that cures start on the inside, pushing the harmful elements outwards. This is how the body should be treated during disease.

All the toxins must be removed and eliminated from inside to the outside, that meaning from intoxicated cells and cell tissues through the blood circulation to be expulsed via the emunctory organs, leading to a better health status condition soon after.

Induction of Apoptosis

The healing process starts after the body is no longer busy repairing itself or self-destructing damaged cells from excessive oxidative stress after the body detoxifies through the active functions of the liver, kidney and colon to expulse and excrete waste products. Healing process means that now the body is changing the old bad tissues for new ones. This means that the body is accelerating protein biosynthesis instead of busily repairing damaged cells with repair enzymes. This is what happens when we are under chronic stress or constantly poisoning our body with industrial foods or taking medications. The cell's mechanisms are keeping active to repair damage or activate the apoptosis mechanism through the P53 tumor suppressor gene, in order to self-destruct damaged or abnormal cells. After you detoxify your body, you start eating better food and do not forget to have enough rest and sleep, reduce stress load. Then you start to increase the energy force or "vital" force and your body can activate its mechanism of regulation. This also allows our bodies to start synthetizing proteins and make new tissues, by producing new healthy cells for a healthy body. Mitochondria are also a crucial key in the production of healthy cells. Excessive free radical activity, toxic drugs, pollution, antibiotics are all damaging to the mitochondria respiratory chain which results decreasing ATP production and cellular dysfunction. We therefore have to keep in mind that the healing process means that we have to change something that permits us not only to clean up our bodies but afterwards this implicates a biological rejuvenative cellular process.

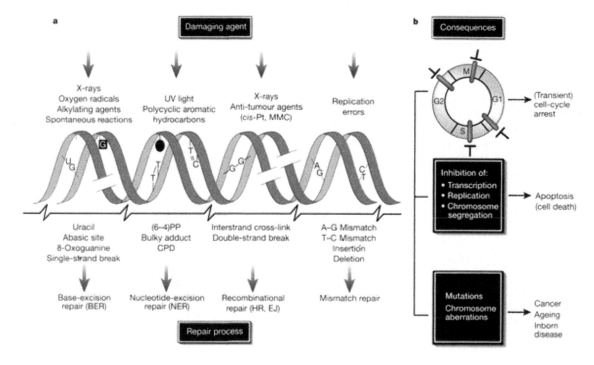

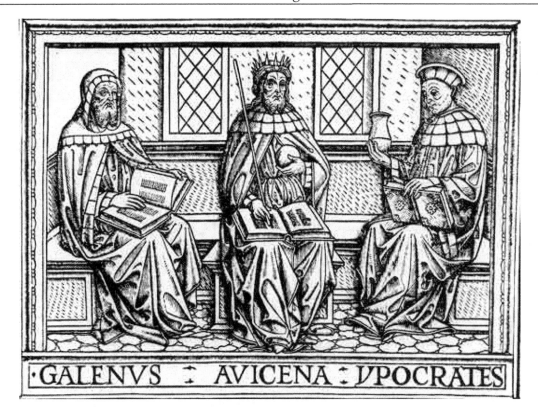

·GALENVS ⁑ AVICENA ⁙ VPOCRATES

The Naturopathic System

The Naturopathic system is based on the theory of "vitalism" or "vital force", as proclaimed by Hippocrates. In the Eastern traditions it is essentially the same thing as "QI" from Oriental medicine that I refer to in this book. The vital force in Naturopathy is based upon inherent capacity of the organism to live, grow, develop, and heal. Therefore, according to its energy capacity, the body excretes those toxins to allow better functioning of our organs. Our body can oppose disease with resistance and/or increased energy level in order to help the detoxification process, same as it can balance itself against hypertension, and inflammation. The body can then cure itself through its system of auto-regulation.

Only in this way, can it be called the Healing Arts. Indeed, practicing true Naturopathy is a Healing Art that requires intuition and knowledge.

Medicine cannot be only about tests and statistics using only drugs to choke off the symptoms. Healing cannot be achieved by the use only of drugs since this intervention doesn't produce a change in the body since it blocks all the regulatory mechanisms and may lead the body to move towards chronic and degenerative disease. Fifty years ago we were mostly dealing with 80% of acute disease and 20% of chronic/degenerative disease, today we are dealing mostly with chronic and degenerative disease no matter the age or sex.

Children can suddenly be affected by cancer, leukemia, autism, diabetes, and even now, with mitochondrial disease. A newborn child is literally bombarded with vaccines and antibiotics. Today many voices point to vaccination as one cause of the increasing rate of autism, not speaking of other diseases and sudden death of babies, but never mind, we just keep on vaccinating. Lately in France, three children died after being vaccinated against so-called "baby colitis," which according to pediatric doctors, is simple to resolve, but the vaccine will continue to be used, only with the mere mention that it may be dangerous, so it was up to the parents to decide. After all this, we are still criticized that our Naturopathic treatments may be dangerous, which makes no sense!

I remember around 1964, while still living in Los Angeles, they opened the first cancer hospital for children in Boston and applauded it. How can this be true? Everyone seemed very proud of such hospital, yet twenty years before, cancer in children was practically unknown. In 1900, cancer of adults was in the 10th position while now it arrives on the first position among other diseases.

Let us return to the different degrees of inflammation and intoxication. During a detoxification treatment, subject to the degree of intoxication and vital reaction, the body excretes toxins and wastes, more or less with difficulty. This type of reaction, depending on the quantity of toxins on their way out, may cause reactions and symptoms according to the power or weakness of the body as the organism excretes these toxin causing substances.

But people affected by degenerative disease such as cancer or multiple sclerosis, reach such an inert state, that their bodies are unable to properly react to heal themselves. In these cases it would be more important to help and revitalize such weak bodies, which are usually bombarded with highly toxic treatments, often antibiotics which results in a weakened capacity for the body to react to disease, as well as decreasing immune response. In the case of cancer patients with poor vitality and a bad nervous system, this allows cancer cells to spread faster and to metastasize to other organs and this is true for breast cancer patients but other types of cancer as I often observed myself.

Usually stage III, and even IV, cancer patients have a body that reacts poorly to the mechanism of auto-regulation depending also on the toxic effects of chemotherapy unless you help out with procedures that protect organs such as the liver, blood components, detoxification, increase bowel function and of course to stimulate the immune function. Based on my wide clinical experience this is the best way to approach the disease. While undergoing chemotherapy, if the apoptotic channel is not activated, often cancer cells may be destroyed through necrosis but in turn it increases inflammation which stimulates tumor growth and/or metastasis invasion. The observation through LBA of cancer patients under chemotherapy has often shown necrotic tissue in blood circulation, proof that cancer cells been destroyed by necrosis and not apoptosis, which in turn the body cannot eliminate and intoxicates the blood since the kidneys cannot eliminate dead tissue which in turn may even block their function. So again, her detoxification is important including the intake of proteolytic enzymes to help the breakdown of necrotic tissue. Most importantly you need to revitalize your patient before doing a regular anti-cancer treatment and/or returning to chemotherapy.

The other day I had a middle aged woman with a story of breast cancer recurrence, and after three chemotherapy sessions, she could hardly get up of her bed and come to my clinic. This is a very weak constitution and low vitality. I gave her a treatment to increase her energy level taking 60ml of chlorella growth factor per day mixed with carrot, red beet and apple juice (divided into three servings). After three days, she was already much better. This is one thing we need to understand and show that each patient is an individual and reacts differently according to his or her state of vitality.

Let us see how an intoxicated organism reacts to detoxification.

A – The intestines begin to function two or three to times a day, with dark feces and the expulsion of gas.
B – The skin erupts, sometimes with boils.
C – Body temperature can increase in the form of fever.
D – Vertigo appears when there are too many toxins circulating in the blood.
E – The urine becomes darker.

F – Headaches can manifest.

Generally, these symptoms manifest according to the condition of the emunctory organs, and their ability to eliminate.

For example:

- If the colon works well there will be hardly any other symptoms.
- If the colon is momentarily blocked, the organism will find a diversion through the skin and that is how eruptions appear.
- If the toxins are rapidly concentrated in the blood, then vertigo and headaches appear.
- A body that reacts well will support and facilitate the elimination of toxins, by burning them up through the mechanism of high temperature.

The body then excretes toxins and wastes with (more or less) difficulty and this type of reaction, from this quantity of toxins on their way outwards, may cause reactions and symptoms according to the power or weakness of a person's body.

In some cases, detoxification occurs normally without symptoms, proof that the organism is resistant and is not overly intoxicated. However, detoxification should necessarily follow a program of body revitalization, so it can regain its normal functioning to stabilize health status. Detoxification can also weaken the body, but revitalization may help to renew good, healthy cells. As a suggestion, based on my own wide experience, both Chlorella Growth Factor (C.G.F.) and Enzyme Yeast Cells preparation contain all the nutrients that the body needs including nucleotides, nucleic acid, RNA, sequences of mitochondria, coenzyme A, and glutathione. These are all in natural form and are highly indicated to revitalize the body.

Regeneration means to synthesize new proteins but only good proteins, not mentioning the restoration and activation of mitochondria and increasing ATP energy. We are currently living in a society that generates permanent stress. Fortunately, the body is protected by endogenous antioxidant enzymes, but it can fail with an excess of stress, especially after reaching a certain age. The same holds for our enzyme repair mechanism, which becomes less efficient with age. This is why these people are under cancer risk, especially when the apoptosis mechanism is decreasing. Here is an example from one of my patients.

Here is an example from one of my patients: A fifty-year-old woman, who had taken a molecular markers test for purposes of cancer prevention, was always under heavy stress. The test which includes the P53 tumor suppressor gene that activates apoptosis had shown in her case a high activity, meaning that damaged/abnormal cells from oxidative stress conditions are destroyed, which demonstrates that the apoptotic pathway is functioning. It can be seen as an "apoptosis defense mechanism against bad cells." However if it is not functioning, damaged stressed/transformed cells accumulate, and mutate, becoming cancer cells. It also shows there is a future risk of tumor development if the patient continues with oxidative stress, especially if the immune defense fails. See www.sergejurasunas.com: "How to Treat Cancer by Targeting P53, BCL2, Surviving and P21, Prevention, Diagnostics, Targeting Therapies – 2nd International Conference on Complementary Oncology – 15th-17th June 2012 – Munich, Germany."

About ten years ago I developed a breast cancer iris profile based on my years of experience observing hundreds of cases of breast cancer patients and women with breast cancer family risk. It gave me an opportunity to list the various iris signs associated with breast cancer profile. Later on I have been able to double check my breast cancer profile, tumor activity or precancerous condition with the association of P53 tumor suppressor gene, inactivated or mutated and other apoptotic players: In other words, after observing a patient's iris with cancer profile or risk, we can now take a further step by actually proving what we have observed by performing Molecular Markers Testing. I have collected many more iris case studies with results from Molecular Marker Testing (See www.sergejurasunas.com – "Breast Cancer Diagnostics and Prevention.").

This is how diseases can develop if our body is poorly protected from bad dietary lifestyle, chronic stress, pollution and excessive drug intake. This may damage many cells that need to be repaired or if not, self-destructed through apoptosis. Cancer cells fail to die because the apoptosis channel is not functioning and therefore unchecked cells continue to divide. The P53 suppressor gene may be inhibited or mutated from exogenous factors such as pesticides, tobacco, social stress, or endogenous bacteria, while the anti-apoptotic oncogene Bcl2 is over-expressed and increases survival of bad cells. For instance, the Nuclear Factor Kappa B (NF-KB), an inflammatory mediator, is mostly associated with tumor growth, because when activated by excessive free radical activity, it increases the expression of BcL2, that in turn increases resistance of cancer cells from their destruction by apoptosis. The NF-KB factor when activated also inhibits the immune cell defense and stimulates angiogenesis. Therefore this greatly contributes to the cancer initiative, progression, and resistance against their destruction through apoptotic channel which includes chemotherapy regimens.

But this is not good for a body that is constantly activating the DNA repair mechanism. If under chronic stress the DNA repair mechanism fails, cells may transform into cancer cells or they adapt themselves to oxidative damage and continue to divide, however they age prematurely. Old cells have less repair mechanism potentiality being deficient in nucleic acid, which also associates with aging. Because of failure in the apoptosis pathway, these damaged cells keep dividing, but each time with more damage, fewer mitochondria, each time being less efficient. This is what we usually see in old people with much less physical capacity, less immune capacity, and very bad bowel structure.

The true medicine should be based on exploring the various self-defense mechanisms of the body, the auto-regulation system, the healing power of the body, the body's own detoxification system, the mitochondria the power house of the cells and intervene with more precaution ,less toxic drugs and to help the body to recover. This is what Naturopathic medicine teaches, but in our modern world, a new definition as such of Integrative Medicine could be more appropriate.

Curiously enough, medical doctors and especially biologists do not seem to connect what they learn to associate with a better way of living and health status. This is why medical doctors are unable to help us if we are ill, since they themselves often eat the wrong food, drink and smoke, and die of cancer themselves, the same as their own patients. Their deep seated paradigm doesn't permit them to open their minds into other directions and this is real tragic, since often we put our life into their hands. How many times patients, biologists, nurses, chemists came to me for consultation, showing how poor their own knowledge really was about nutrition, about health, or what should be done. Recently a middle age women biologist who had been smoking daily three packs of cigarettes came to me with an advanced lung cancer. What can we say? She should know better about the consequences of such smoking, being a biologist?

The association of oxidative stress with pathologies and the aging process is a relatively new science. Today it is widely recognized how free radicals may damage cells and accumulate mutations that can lead to cancer or aging. Our body is built with an antioxidant protective mechanism within each single cell, however the system can often fail to protect.

More recently some researchers from the University of Wisconsin submitted a group of rats to a hyper caloric diet from regular supermarket food and demonstrated that cells became older quicker when they have to work incessantly to protect against free radical damage and toxins, and perform genetic repair. If we live with permanent stress many cells are damaged and usually they are self-destroyed through apoptosis as previously explained, but this is not good for a body that is constantly activating cellular repair or immune defense because it overtaxes the induction of repair enzymes and overstimulates the immune system. Both systems may fail and the cells may become prematurely aged unless they become cancerous cells.

The same type of experiment with a hypo caloric diet showed that even old rats were stronger and vigorous like young rats and lived longer. This is because cells from rats fed with hypo caloric diet produce much less free radicals and do not waste time in repairing process and concentrate on the biosynthesis of making new proteins and other cellular components. Today it has been shown that the telomeres decrease their length under oxidative stress increasing cellular aging. Lifespan extension can be also increased by activation of autophagy, from the Greek Self eating. One characteristic of aging is the accumulation of damages in the cells which through autophagy should be break down and be digested into vacuoles; older structures need to be broken down for self-renewal allowing for new ones to be built.

In old rats, caloric restriction, fasting every other day or for one week restored levels of autophagy. Today it seems that mini fasting (14 to 16 hours without food) and a detox diet may decrease the production of IGF 1 (Aging factor) and CRP (C Reactive or inflammatory protein). So undergoing a diet and detox treatment by decreasing the quantity of food (low calorie) for some time, and by resting with a 14-hour interval between diner and breakfast, increases autophagy to keep the body younger. It also decreases the production of free radicals, one important factor of aging. One other important discovery is about what we call genomic food that protects cells from aging and cancer.

In 2012 we saw the experience of professor Gilles-Eric Seralmi's research group that fed groups of rats GMO corn and pesticides compared to a control group. After the thirteenth month, the GMO fed rats started to develop large tumors. Definitively we are playing with fire when it comes to man-made evils.

Our body needs natural non-processed food to feed its 60 trillion cells and activate all the mechanisms of our body. We know that nutrients such as minerals, vitamins, enzymes, proteins are necessary for making new tissues, bones, hair, and blood.

You don't make new tissues in your body out of pharmaceutical drugs but through proper nutrition that we know is also important to boost our immune defense, support liver detoxification and activate a number of biological mechanisms.

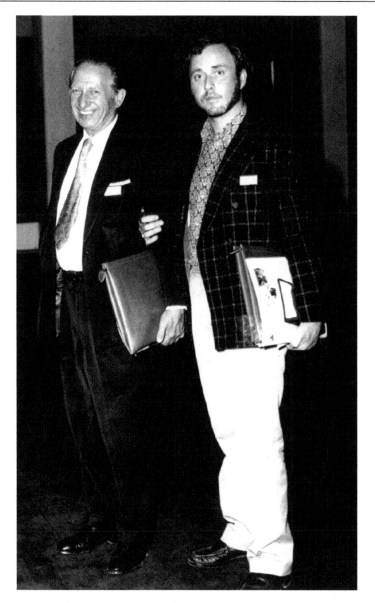

Dr. Bernard Jensen was one of the greatest pioneers in nutrition and detoxification in the twentieth century. He also contributed to the development of Iridology on a worldwide basis. Our photo was taken at the 1st World Congress of L'Altra Medicina – San Remo, Italy – 1972

As Dr. Bernard Jensen used to say, "Iridology is a science associated with nutrition and nutrition is a science associated with Iridology." Hence, through Iridology one can determine a person's eating habits by the observation of the iris. But it is even more probable that Iridology is related to biology and embryology. In order to understand and treat the human body we must first have an appreciation of life and its biological tenets. Maybe someday with the review of old methods and facing the disaster of medicine, we will get to the point of no longer treating symptoms but actually treat the cause of the disease.

The paradigm of cancer back in 1866, was based on the fact that a tumor was caused solely by a mutation of the nuclear DNA cells, where in the beginning medical science implicated a virus to be the cause of this mutation. Today many new lines of research implicated mitochondrial DNA mutation as one other probable causes of cancer. A map with the mitochondrial regions in various segments of the MT DNA (Mitochondrial DNA), harbor a common mutation associated with different cancers had been developed (1). Furthermore we know today that a tumor responds to environmental tissues, that it is not isolated from the body. Inflammation is one new avenue, or to be more correct, an old theory subject today to serious consideration by modern science. This is an enormous step in the way of explaining disease and now we really have a new paradigm in the way we approach disease and cancer. We can try to reduce the madness of excess pill prescriptions that in turn damage more than curing our body, not to say often makes it worse.

That makes an overwhelming difference when it comes to treating cancer since we understand that now the disease should be approached from several directions to better control or attack the growth of the tumor by destroying cancer cells, not only from chemotherapy alone. Chemotherapy alone cannot cure cancer since it also damages healthy cells including mitochondria, which are fewer in cancer cells, may disorganize the homeostasis balance and often lead to death. A complementary approach including an anti-cancer diet and dietary agents to boost the immune system, protect healthy cells including the liver, that stimulates apoptosis may be seen as a better way to increase the percentage of remission and to reduce risk of recurrence. How many cancer patients are coming into my clinic with cancer recurrence after a period from two months to fourteen years after undergoing surgery, chemotherapy, or radiation? We cannot say that conventional medicine is doing everything possible to cure your cancer or to prevent recurrence despite the advancements and technology utilized. I strongly believe that healthy food, fresh organic vegetables juice and intake of anti-cancer dietary agents are now a breakthrough approach in treating cancer with better care.

(1)"Dynamic Mitochondrial Network in Cancer" – blogs-scientificamerican.com/dynamic mitochondria

Healing Process

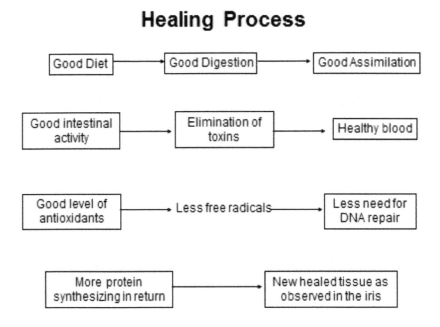

Today we have enough proof about the therapeutic value of dietary agents, vegetables, spices, and foods that can be used in different ways together with detoxification, fasting, and dietary supplementation to increase the healing process in the body, even if you need some emergency medicine with which to start. This is the same way you may treat bad health status through diet, detoxification, and better nutrition by stimulating all the different mechanisms of immune defense, auto-regulation in the body, and by decreasing inflammatory cytokines, to achieve healing process.

What is important is to be able to perform a follow-up check in regard to real patient improvement after completing a detox and revitalization treatment. We can use different methods such the Vega apparatus, LBA, or MBT. Iridology is also a good way to make a confirmation of how bodies start to heal themselves through the observation of what we call healing signs in the iris, written about by Dr. Bernard Jensen in his books and presented during conferences. According to Dr. Bernard Jensen, perceptible changes in the iris appear as white lines or fibers which fill inside of lacunas showing that new tissues are forming in the body after detoxification and a period when the body revitalizes itself through a nutritional program. It is a real healing. Today some iridologists claim that they never see healing signs appear, but over the years I found out that many iridologists are unable to recognize these new signs, so really this is a question of experience and expertise.

I remember taking a group of Canadians to Hidden Valley Health Ranch and one important man, who under my contact and guidance changed his way of life and dietary habits, which were very bad in French Canada (he was overweight by forty pounds) and started drinking large quantities of carrot and other vegetable juices. So, when Dr. Jensen made his iris observation, he told him, "I see some good healing signs coming. You are improving and probably you drink a lot of carrot juice." One may understand how the patient was impressed and me too. So this is up to each practitioner to define observable healing signs in the iris or changes in the color from darker to brighter. But as I mentioned, today the LBA observation is also important since it shows how your blood is detoxified and how it improves after detoxification with better nutrition. We make new tissue, new healthy cells after the body is detoxified and with the proper nutrition and the use of some dietary compounds, the same as I have done and observed for nearly fifty years. A good way to learn about nutrition and active dietary compounds is from reading the *Handbook of Nutraceutical and Functional Foods*, edited by Robert E.C. William (CRS series in Modern Nutrition)

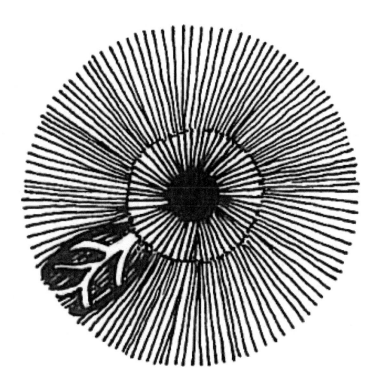

Healing lines

Over long periods of time we can even better observe patients and how they live a healthier lifestyle, being younger and feeling stronger than many middle-aged persons. One of my patients, an eighty-three- year-old woman I treated for over thirty years, surprises everyone in her yoga class. She performs movements more easily than much younger participants. She is still in very limber condition. She doesn't get flu during winter and she is not bombarded with pharmaceutical drugs or with vaccines against flu or other infections like most elderly people who constantly get sick and hospitalized. She is on an almost 100% natural food diet, dietetic supplementation, takes enzyme yeast cells, fermented chlorella, and NADH, which makes a dramatic difference, where her brain is still very agile.

And she has no Alzheimer's whatsoever, while conventional medicine is still in the midst of a search for miraculous blockbuster drug against cancer or Alzheimer's. Elderly people with cognitive disorder and other complaints and diseases have become a big market, where healthy aged persons become an intruder in this diabolical system.

After a detoxification crisis during which time you have to use only natural foods, the body will now react differently. You feel better, stronger and less tired with a better mental disposition and above all your body may reject bad and heavy meals. You really feel repulsion for industrially processed foods and over-cooked food. Your body is now clean, your taste buds have changed, and your body starts to reject bad food in favor of healthy food. It has a real intelligence and is able to fight off disease, if you choose to utilize this intelligent power of nature and are able to fight the disease by using its own system of auto-regulation, no matter what doctors think. Remember that the intestinal neurons communicate throughout the enteric nervous system with the brain and as soon as you eat, it sends a message to the brain indicating what food you have eaten. Your body can adapt itself to bad food and you feel nothing, but you still intoxicate yourself.

Colon cancer is not developed overnight but through a process that takes many years, that includes transformation, initiation, and tumor growth, but you feel nothing. You may have some gases in excess but who worries about this! Maybe your doctor will prescribe you some drugs or enzymes for relief but nothing else. Lately I had the case of a fifty-two-year old woman with the diagnosis of a colon rectal cancer, metastases to liver, lung in terminal phase only three months after being diagnosed. When she started bleeding her doctor told her that it is nothing, probably hemorrhoidal, no need to worry, and that occurred over a couple of months. She was raised on common food like most people and nobody was really thinking about some consequences that may arise from bad diet. I hadn't seen her yet, she had been hospitalized, but her daughter came to see me asking some help. I readily asked her to let me observe her iris, and what do you know I saw? A bad sigmoid colon and a very small lacuna on the rectum area so the iris speaks for itself and there was a risk for the daughter as well, unless she changed her diet.

On the other hand if you abuse your body with bad food, poisoned food the digestive system sends a message to the brain and it will activate some mechanisms, for instance like vomiting. If you keep taking pills it becomes evident that your body gets worse and more intoxicated, if you do not change your dietary style and later on, it may turn to disease.

By eating industrial food, and bombarding your body with an excess of toxic pills, it becomes evident that you may intoxicate your body including the cellular function, the mitochondria, but also you opened the road to diseases. One of the consequences of wrong food and pollution is to impair the immune system, where immune cells become much less effective in activating their toxic granules that kill cancer cells. In a normal healthy person having a ratio under 100:1, Natural Killer Cell activity ranges between 60-75% while in a cancer patient it drops down between 0 to 30%. It means that first you can be subject to infections, colds, flus, and viral disease if not, a cancer. Today, so many people, especially older people are dependent on pills, which surely are unhealthy creating an artificial state of life, with poorer overall quality. The other day I had a seventy-three-year-old woman come in for consultation. She had chronic urine infections, one after another treated with antibiotics, that she needed to carry with her while traveling, and had taken drugs to control her cholesterol and high blood pressure. Are we happy with that?

Now if you detox your body, especially the liver, colon, and kidney, then clean up the blood, you may be able to expulse not only toxic wastes, but drugs that accumulate in the blood and tissues, because the liver has not been able to eliminate them in the first place. When you use natural foods, the message sent to brain is now different and you don't feel like eating again like before. Contrary to the doctors thinking, your body has a real intelligence governed by biological laws and is able to fight off disease and restore health, if you use the power of nature and healing laws.

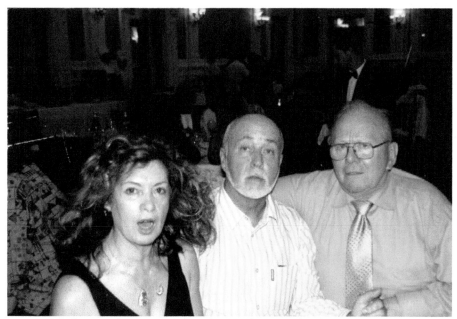

Serge Jurasunas with his wife Lucie on right, Bob Bradford Ph.D. the pioneer of Live Blood Analysis and HLB test. One of the founders of Capital University of Integrative Medicine - USA

My wife, Lucie, is a very alert and busy woman, looking like a young woman. She knows how to listen to her body and what kind of food is best to keep herself healthy. She never takes drugs, but good vitamins and supplements, and during medical check-ups, medical doctors are astonished and keep asking, "Why don't you take any pharmaceutical drugs?" To them, this seems impossible, but doctors do not ask what she is doing, how is her diet, or does she take supplementation.

Special Diet for Gastrointestinal Problems

Constipation

Recommended Foods:

Water (2 liters per day) – seasonal fruits – dried fruits (especially prunes) –papaya - carrots – pumpkin – leeks – spinach – asparagus – corn – barley – oats – algae - bulgur wheat – millet – oat and wheat bran – kefir – yogurt –fiber – virgin oil – whole foods – lacto-fermented vegetables – peppermint tea (1 cup after meals).

Foods Not Recommended:

Processed foods – white flour – white rice – white sugar –fried foods – stews – spicy food – saturated fats – etc.

Recommended Supplementation:

Probiotics – Enzyme Yeast Cell Preparation – Chlorella –Liquid chlorophyll – SOD enzyme – Glutathione – Papaya enzymes – Magnesium – Ground linseed (20g per day) or capsules – Flax seed oil capsules.

Observations:

Drink a glass of hot water with 1 tablespoon of cider vinegar and 1 tablespoon of honey two times a day, before meals and at bedtime. When constipation is connected with hepatic disorder you can take some artichoke extract, milk thistle, dandelion root in supplementation, try the extract of fresh herbs from Dr. Vogel for the liver called Arabioforce, since it has much more power than dried herbs.

In these cases it is beneficial to take a daily walk or to do some abdominal crunches. Abdominal massages are also recommended. Avoid sitting or standing for too long in the same position as it makes digestion and circulation more difficult.

Drink to Combat Constipation:

    1 glass of carrot juice
    1 tablespoon enzyme yeast cells
    1 tablespoon liquid chlorophyll or grass juice
    1 tablespoon of black molasses

Kefir Drink:

    1 glass kefir
    1 tablespoon oat bran
    1 tablespoon raisins, previously soaked 1 tablespoon crushed nuts
    1 tablespoon honey
    1 teaspoon linseed
    1/2 juiced lemon
    Mix all the ingredients in an electric blender or with a hand blender.

<u>**Energy Drink to Combat Constipation:**</u>
 1 carrot
 1 large apple
 1 kiwi
 2 oranges
 100g fresh pineapple
 1 teaspoon linseed
 1 teaspoon sesame seeds
 2 teaspoons lemon juice

Juice the fruit and the carrot. Then, place in a blender and mix with the remaining ingredients and blend for about 2 minutes.

Rules of Hygiene for Combating Constipation

A - Avoid heavy meals for dinner.

B - At breakfast, eliminate croissants, industrially made cakes and white bread.

C - For breakfast eat: cooked apples, whole cereals, seasonal fruit or dried fruit soaked overnight.

D - Eat muesli cereals to which one can add soaked dried fruit, 1 or 2 tablespoons of bran, 1 teaspoon of ground linseed.

E - Frequently eat meals based on oat flakes or barley, which are rich in fibers, which absorb water.

F - Avoid all fried foods, charcuterie, pastry, and red meat.

G - Introduce fresh vegetable juice to the daily diet.

H - Get used to drinking water between meals.

I - Perform abdominal crunches or walk a bit every day. This is excellent for activating the intestinal muscles.

J - Take a few minutes to relax, especially at night before bed.

K - Listen to some background music at the same time (sound of waves, running water, sounds of the forest). Do not forget that the brain communicates with the intestine.

L - Once a week detoxify by eating only whole cereals, whole rice with cooked apples, or just fruit.

M - Drink at least 2 liters of water a day, natural still water, herbal teas, teas, fruit or vegetable juices.

N - After the evening meal, move, do not sit. Do some housework, gardening, walk an animal, or time permitting, go for a walk.

O - Do some intestinal massages.

Diverticulitis

Recommended Foods:

Whole cereals – vegetables rich in fiber – oat bran – wheat bran - spelt – oats – carrot and oat soup – whole oatmeal porridge – pearl barley soup.

Non Recommended Foods:

White sugar - white flour – industrially made food – charcuterie – pickled foods.

Recommended Supplements:

Bran supplements – wheat and oat fibers – kefir – probiotics – pectin – liquid chlorophyll – Enzyme Yeast Cell Preparation – Chlorella – pollen.

Observations:

Diverticula are small sac-like cavities or sacs formed in the intestinal walls that often contain toxic material, bacteria not removed alone with other wastes. With time chronic diverticula can become infected and responsible for further disease. It is thought that forty percent or more of people, who suffer from diverticula, demonstrate weaker intestinal membranes, wrong food, and bad elimination. These small bowel pockets, as named by Dr. Jensen, should be treated with better food diet, especially avoiding some vegetables that can irritate, like French beans, but other natural foods rich in calcium, potassium, magnesium, and fiber are recommended. It is not easy to combat this problem only through detoxification and diet, although detoxification of the colon is the first steep, some abdominal exercises with a slanting board seems very important, even necessary in order to remove the bowel pockets.

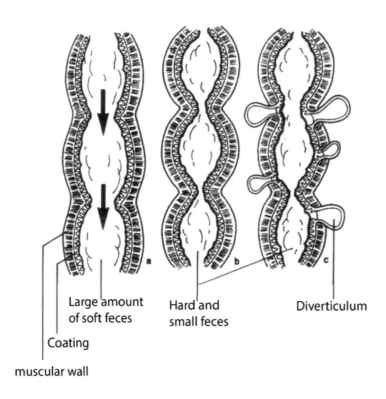

Large amount of soft feces

Coating

muscular wall

Hard and small feces

Diverticulum

Flatulence and Intestinal Gas

Recommended Foods:

Carrot juice – vegetable purees and mashes – whole cereals – cooked apples and pears – pineapple – kefir – soy yogurt

In these cases the diet must be basic to respect the laws of food combinations

1) Consume proteins with vegetables and greens
2) Carbohydrates must be eaten with vegetables and greens
3) Fruits and sweet foods must never be consumed during meals but in the interval, or else eaten as a meal.
4) Do not mix proteins and carbohydrates at the same meal.

Example: meat and potatoes (wrong)
> Proteins + vegetables
> Proteins + fruits
> Carbohydrates + fruits
> Carbohydrates + vegetables

Foods to Avoid:

White bread - cabbage - milk - white chocolate - pork meat - fat - matured cheese.

Recommended Supplementation:

Probiotics - pollen - cider vinegar - lacto-fermented foods - charcoal - enzyme yeast cells.

Observations:

If you have an attack of flatulence, undertake a two-day diet eating only whole barley cream or whole grain rice with grated or cooked apples. You can mix in some steamed carrots with your cereals.

If necessary, some enemas may be beneficial, especially with clay mixed in with an infusion of chamomile. It will absorb and eliminate gas.

Application of an Abdominal Wrap

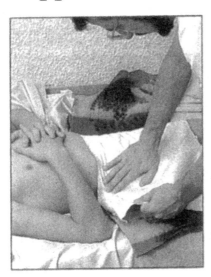 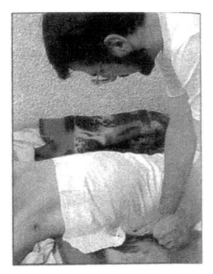

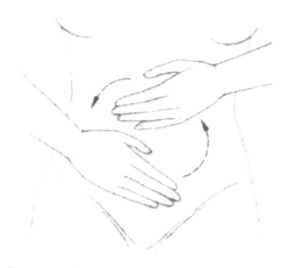

Apply a hot and humid cloth soaked in cider vinegar on the abdomen. Wet a cloth in hot water, wring out and spray with cider vinegar. Apply around the abdomen and cover with a blanket for 15 minutes. A very old method may be used which gives wonderful results. Try abdominal message with some warm olive oil (use a double boiler or slow warmer), which may help the intestinal function in case of constipation. About 30 or 40 rotations, following the mechanism of a clock on the abdomen, along with some gentle pressure with the hands, so as to penetrate the olive oil into the tissue.

Diarrhea

Recommended Foods:
Whole rice – rice noodles-whole pastas – bananas – buckwheat – rice flakes – whole rice cream – bulgur wheat – eggplant – zucchini – apples (grated or pureed) – rice broth – pearl barley broth – soy yogurt.

Non Recommended Foods:
Avoid dairy products and products rich in fiber.

Recommended Supplements:
Probiotics – pollen – vegetable charcoal – clay – Echinacea

Observations:
During a diarrhea crisis, eat only whole bran rice alternated with oatmeal, banana and apples that you eat either raw or cooked. Blueberry juice is recommended in case of diarrhea to drink between meals. Drink a lot of water between meals and if the discharges are very strong, drink fruit juices or you may drink a mineral formula such as the one's used by runners to re-mineralize their bodies.

In cases of diarrhea, the World Health Organization recommends:

Dissolve 8 tablespoons of raw sugar, 1 teaspoon of brown sea salt in 1 liter of water. Drink throughout the day in order to avoid the loss of fluids and the danger of dehydration.

Hemorrhoids and Anal Fissures

Recommended Foods:
All food rich in fibers - whole cereals - carrots puree - pumpkin - cooked apples - vegetables juice - blackberries - blueberries - psyllium - cherries - apple juice.

Non Recommended Foods:
Pasta - coffee - white wheat bread - chili and spicy food - fried food - red meat.

Recommended Supplements:

Liquid chlorophyll - wheat germ oil - garlic - horse chestnut extract - witch-hazel (*hamamelis*) extract.

Observations:
In case of crisis, follow the colitis diet and refer to the chapter on vegetable juices. A sitz bath with lukewarm chamomile water, one handful of clay and 1 cup of cider vinegar (make a cup of

chamomile tea). A sitz bath is excellent relief from hemorrhoid crisis and could be done before retiring.

Sitz Bath

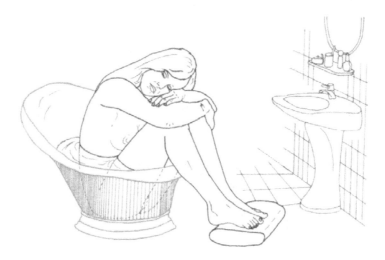

Inflammation and Irritation of the Colon

Recommended Foods:
See chapter on vegetable juices
Oats – barley – bulgur – millet – sesame puree (Tahini) – pureed vegetables – nonacid fruit, cooked, plain, or juiced – soy milk – almond milk

Non Recommended Foods:
Soft drinks – all wheat based foods – reduce coffee or best substitute with cereal- or chicory-based coffee. Avoid beans that irritate the colon.

Recommended Supplements:
Enzyme Yeast Cell Preparation – Chlorella – Liquid chlorophyll – Papaya enzymes – Oat bran (25g per day) – Ground linseed (20g per day) – Psyllium – Peppermint tea (1 cup after meals)

Observations:
Often in these cases, everyone reacts differently to the different foods. There are no absolute rules. Everyone should discover which foods are not suitable. I suggest the diet for colitis.

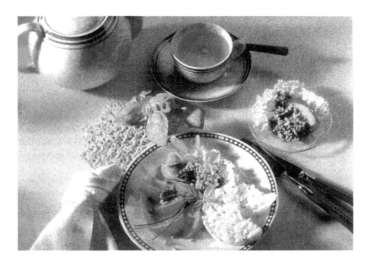

Gas – Intestinal Inflammation or Colon Irritation

In a blender puree or liquefy 200g of fresh pineapple, 1 ripe banana, then add 1 glass of sesame milk, 1 teaspoon of honey and a little water to dilute it.

You can make sesame milk with some sesame cream that you can buy in health food store (called Tahini). Just blend one tablespoon of this sesame cream with one cup of water to obtain sesame milk.

Or you may put in a blender 1 cup of sesame seeds mixed with water and blend to obtain your sesame milk. Use the quantity of water according to the concentration you want to obtain.

If these disorders are accompanied by pain, drink 2 to 4 papaya enzyme tablets at the same time.

Colon Cancer

Recommended Foods:
Beetroot - carrot and fruit juices – oats – bulgur – buckwheat – kefir – foods rich in fibers – Vegetables: beetroot – broccoli - asparagus – eggplant – mushroom – onion – yellow pepper – zucchini – abundant seasonal fruit – papaya – graviola (soursop fruit) - whole cereals and flakes – consume many soy based foods: milk, different drinks, yogurts, tofu, etc.

Non Recommended Foods:
Processed foods – white flour – white rice – white sugar – table salt - fried foods – stews – spicy food – saturated fats – etc.

Eat frugally, light meals and avoid the mixture of various foods at the same meal. Avoid canned foods, pork and smoked meats, processed foods.

Recommended Supplementation:
Enzyme yeast cells preparation, Chlorella extract, Probiotics, Flax seed oil, Nucleic acid, Ganoderma, and Maitake mushrooms, Pau d'Arco, Chlorella Growth Factors, Probiotics, liquid chlorophyll – oat and wheat bran – flax seed – flax seed oil. Both supplements, Enzyme yeast cells preparation and chlorella are important for the detoxification process of the entire body, but especially the colon. They revitalize the entire body, especially to activate cellular respiration in damaged mitochondria, and increase ATP energy.

Chlorella – Best to use the Sun-Chlorella or fermented chlorella which I use in my clinic, specially developed for my patients.

Enzyme Yeast Cells: The Bedrock of My Treatment

The success in treating patients without harm while detoxifying relies on years of experience in the healing arts, particularly in the choice of remedies that we utilize. Today in the jungle of vitamins and dietary supplements one may have difficulty to make choice and may be influenced by publicity.

More than four decades ago, when we first started treating and detoxifying patients, we moved forward depending on intuition, and protocols based on old methods. At the same time, we began to develop and manufacture our own remedies to make sure we had the best available, to obtain a successful cure for our patients. Dr. Jensen was an excellent example. When I first met him, he started developing his own branded products, such red beet tablets, hemaglow, alfalfa tablets, liquid chlorophyll, whey, and bone marrow capsules. When I open my first consulting office in Montreal, Canada, I worked with Dr. Jensen's products while at the same time I discovered the fresh herbal extracts from Dr. A. Vogel and the famous Rasayana cure for total detoxification, absolutely unique, but I believe it was taken off the market today because of restrictive European import laws (Available in Canada and possibly in the USA) for medical herbs.

Later on I moved back to Europe, tentatively, to learn more about German biological medicine. My interest was to search for new remedies that could heal the body, treat cancer, and maybe detoxify the body. While traveling I was fortunate enough to meet Otto Warburg's co-workers, especially Dr. S. Wolz, the scientific co-worker of Nobel Laureate Professor Feodor Lynen, who worked on isolating Coenzyme A from yeast. For this research he received the Nobel Prize in medicine in 1964. Dr. Wolz is an engineer specializing in biotechnology and fermentation processes. For many years he collaborated with the great cancer pioneer Paul Seeger, who was working on the theory of cellular respiration and mitochondrial function in regards to cancer, which, of course, was completely unknown and new to me.

Dr. Wolz developed something new to fulfill the need of Dr. Seeger that could reactivate the cellular respiration in cancer, but also to detoxify the body and protect it again environmental toxins. He developed the famous enzyme yeast cell formulation, which contained the same substances available in human cells which I am now going to discuss. Since its inception, these enzyme yeast cells have been my most important biological intervention over the past forty-five years. I take this opportunity to explain that enzyme yeast cells preparation is a live product, not dried yeast, to the contrary not stimulating Candida growth as many Naturopaths believe. This is totally false. Live enzyme yeast cells kill growing Candida in the blood as one can see while performing a LBA before and after, in a period of few days.

What is enzyme yeast cells preparation?

This is a dietary product that essentially contains only enzyme yeast cells, using saccharomyces cereviscae made from a process of fermentation in presence of oxygen, which stimulates the mitochondria's cells during the process of growth. The product is provided in a natural concentrate, offering all the nutrients required by our body. What is also important to remember is that the nutrients contained in the young yeast cells are almost identical replications of the biological substances with naturally occur in cells of the healthy human body.

Within the enzyme yeast cell preparation we have a balanced combination of vitamins, minerals, enzymes, antioxidants, nucleic acid, and biocatalyzers; perfect for restoring a sick body and/or detoxification.

- 17 vitamins, 14 minerals, 16 amino acids, nucleic acids, redox enzymes, and biocatalyzers.

- Proteins – 46/50 for every 100g of dried yeast

- Practically all amino acids and particularly essential amino acids and methionine, cysteine important for detoxification.

- Vitamins A, C, E, K, beta-Carotene, and growth factors such inositol, biotin important in cell division and differentiation.

- Minerals and trace elements include iodine, Phosphoric acid, copper, magnesium, potassium, molybdenum, iron, selenium, and zinc. The last two selenium and zinc are important to improve the immune resistance, acting as antioxidants.

10g of yeast covers our daily need for vitamins B1, B2, B5, and B12 which is substantial since with pollution and stress, our need for B Vitamins increases. B complex vitamins are used for all cellular energy production and repair. Deficiency of B complex may decrease immune function. The combination of magnesium, and vitamins A, B2, B5, and B6, along with iodine found in enzyme yeast cells is central for activating the Krebs cells and cellular respiration.

What is important is that enzyme yeast cells contain Coenzyme A, cytochrome, a high level of coenzyme Q10, and other small molecules critical for increasing cellular respiration, but also to reactivate any blockage in the respiratory chain. Our entire life on this planet is based upon cellular respiration necessary for survival and recovery of health.

Glutathione is a very important component of the enzyme yeast cells worthwhile addressing. First glutathione is found in high concentration in the enzyme yeast cells, about 10mg/100 ml of the preparation. Glutathione is one important substance that works as a powerful antioxidant and a strong detoxificant necessary for activating the liver's detoxification process. The liver contains a high level of glutathione (10 monomolar) which indicates how important glutathione is for both detoxification and for our liver to protect itself against pollutants (or to protect cells against the adverse effects of chemotherapy and to detoxify mutagenic chemicals). Enzyme yeast cells also contain cysteine, sulphur, and methionine to increase the liver's detoxification system. However, glutathione also plays an important role in the redox system. The bioelectrical potential of the human cells show a redox between 175mv and 282 mv, while glutathione is about 220 mv. Therefore it increases the redox and energy level and raises membrane potential which may fall by 1/10, as a result of the effects of environmental pollutants.

Enzyme yeast cells are a strong detoxificant, first against environmental poisons, which on 17th October, 2013 the WHO officially recognized as a direct cause of cancer, rather than just only a risk, which is a major step in our own fight. This underscores the need to detoxify the whole body from excess toxins and mucosity circulating in the blood which negatively affects and decreases the oxygen level, slowing down blood circulation.

Enzymes and other protective substances contained in enzyme yeast cells adhere to cellular receptors where the toxic substances become fixed, preventing membrane damage. These enzymatic protective substances react with those toxic substances which are transformed fermentatively by hydrolytic cleavage (hydrolysis), oxidation, and splitting-off side chains and toxins, thus rendered harmless by complying with such active substances such as glutathione, coenzyme A, glucuronic acid, and cysteine.

The inactive compounds produced during the transformation are readily excreted by the urine through the kidney. Chemical toxins from the environment such as xenobiotics if not eliminated, accumulate in the body, being responsible for organic disorders and diseases. Xenoestrogens such as PCB's and Phthalates have estrogenic effects on living organisms, having been implicated in a variety of medical problems and may even cause breast cancer.

What is important at this point is to focus the high biological value of enzyme yeast cells to basically act as a true cellular regenerator. They really contain all the ingredients in a natural form to activate the Krebs cycle and increase the ATP energy, which is substantial for most

272

body's function, including detoxification, apoptosis, and the replacement of dead cells by new cells. Indeed the combination of magnesium, iodine, vitamins B1, B2, B5, B6, and B12 not only increase cellular respiration but is potentially helpful in depression, anxiety, nervousness, and even Parkinson's disease. This is really the perfect substance required by the mitochondria to protect the body from diseases especially cancer.

However, we would like to focus on the extraordinary preventive and therapeutic action of enzyme yeast cells preparation as one of my main targeting treatments for detoxification, which enters into most of the treatments for gastrointestinal dysfunction, or disease in this book. I have been using Enzyme Yeast Cells for now for over four decades on over 80,000 patients with all kinds and grades of disease, to detoxify and to treat cancer as a complementary treatment. Now, if we are talking about the intestine to maintain good function, to treat intestinal dysfunction, or on the level of regenerating a sick or old colon, once again Enzyme Yeast Cells preparation is the most perfect natural compound for this purpose.

Enzyme Yeast Cells contain in high quantity potassium, magnesium, calcium, manganese, and nucleic acid, important for the brain and maintaining good muscle and tissue in the intestine. Enzyme yeast cells keep a colon healthy especially for older persons with poor intestinal structure.

Some of my patients, now at eighty-five years of age, are taking Enzyme Yeast Cells preparation for now thirty years and shown very good physical and mental activity as explained before. They don't need pharmaceutical drugs for blood pressure, cholesterol, bad memory, nerve disorder, pains, aspirin, etc. They just are healthy, and this is great! Nonetheless, in my opinion, Enzyme Yeast Cells is the most highly recommended rejuvenating compound that increases the body's overall detoxification as a whole, including the colon, liver, kidney, and blood.

The best example to verify how enzyme yeast cells modify the blood status is to perform a live blood microscopy cell's analysis before and after. The result is visible in a matter of thirty days, when the patient comes back for consultation, but actually you can observe result earlier in a matter of 8-10 days. Patients feel better and stronger since Enzyme Yeast cells preparation boosts the immune system, increases energy level, and strengthens the nervous system. I'm not ashamed to say that I personally take enzyme yeast cells every day, that this maintains my youth and strength. I have participated in various triathlon competitions, undergoing considerable physical training, running, and swimming, which I still do today. No doubt that Enzyme Yeast cells preparation has given me more strength during training. In fact, there is one special formula for athletes which has been used by the German Olympic team. In our busy life, it is important to support our body to preserve it from pollution, oxidative stress and societal pressure, compensate denatured food in the diet, and sometimes to detoxify ourselves.

I am always shocked when I hear about a colleague who died from cancer. How can it be if we ourselves are supposed to be the ones giving an example with prevention, especially if we understand how to treat our cancer patients? How it is possible if we know what to do!

About four years ago, a woman PhD. graduate, wrote a very good article in *The Townsend Letter Magazine* about the Oncogenic Effects of Rice Bran Arabinoxylan Compound (RBAC). Personally, I use this compound widely with my cancer patients. More recently I heard she died from breast cancer which, to me, was incomprehensible, demonstrating perhaps a lack of experience as well as her incapacity to treat herself in the best manner, essentially failing to use her own best judgment regarding
what should have been done and\or to contact some experienced integrative cancer doctors. According to my experience there is a better way regarding the follow up of cancer, although

prevention is also important. If we perform molecular markers testing which provides information, permitting us to tailor a treatment adapted to the result of the test. But of course we need to be open to new theories and believe ourselves how cancer can be targeted. Many Naturopaths are practicing a profession but this doesn't mean they believe in what they do. I have many examples. I do believe that taking enzyme yeast cell (Zell oxygen) or even some chlorella extract on daily basis improves our health status. This is also a way to keep away from disease with of course a good food intake.

My new document about integrative cancer, "New Theories, New Treatment," is on the leading edge of progress with new discoveries in molecular medicine, but also includes new Naturopathic approaches (please contact: sergejurasunas@hotmail.com)

One great advantage with Enzyme Yeast Cells is that first it is a natural product, not manufactured tablets, since it contains young yeast cells similar to human cells. Second, you do not need to feed your patients with a large quantities of tablets as I often see in books where doctors giving up to 70-100 tablets of vitamins, minerals, and enzymes daily. It is not possible for the stomach to digest such quantity and probably most of the nutrient value is lost. On the contrary, the enzyme yeast cells, orally administered, pass via the thoracic duct into the right side of the heart and immediately into the blood stream where all the broken young yeast cells release billions of enzymes for immediate healing.

Biological and Therapeutic Intervention of Enzyme Yeast Cells

Glutathione, cysteine, methionine, sulphur, glucuronic acid	Increase detoxification, increase redox, antioxidants, protect from pollutants
Vitamins A, C, E, K, beta-Carotene, inositol, biotin	Cell division, antioxidants , cellular differentiation
Selenium, zinc	Crucial to activate metallic antioxidant enzymes, prevention of cancer
Glutamine, magnesium, potassium	Repair leaky gut (damaged intestinal membrane
Magnesium, Vit. B2, B3, B5, B6, B12, iodine, iron	To activate the Krebs cycle, increase cellular energy production
Coenzyme A, cytochrome, coenzyme Q10	Increase cellular respiration and boost ATP production in mitochondria
Coenzyme Q10	Strong antioxidants, support heart against chemotherapy adverse effects.
Nucleic acids, adenine nucleotides, ribonucleic acid	Anti-aging – rejuvenation – necessary for cells response and replace old cells by new cell's – to synthesis de Novo from exogenous nucleotides by the liver
S.O.D., glutathione, catalase, selenium, beta-Carotene	Powerful combination of antioxidants
May target pro-apoptotic and anti-apoptotic genes	

Mitochondria	To regenerate the whole respiratory
Enzyme yeast cells contain billion of active mitochondria that release the enzymes of the respiratory chain.	chain of mitochondria blocked such in case of fibromyalgia, chronic fatigue, P.D., cancer, and aging.

Therefore, I can only suggest to doctors and the ones called Naturopaths to include Enzyme Yeast Cells Preparation in their panoply of Naturopathic treatments, especially for detoxification. You can get more information about Enzyme Yeast Cells and my work into this particular field by reading:

"The Therapy of Enzyme Yeast Cells in Cancer Disease, C.F.S. and Aging Process"

"The Clinical Evidence of Cellular Respiration to Target Cancer" – *Townsend Letter* – **Aug/Sept 2012**

"Mitochondria and Cancer" – *Townsend Letter* – **Aug/Sept 2006"**

Available on the Internet: www.sergejurasunas.com

Enemas and Hydrotherapy of the Colon

Enemas and purges have existed for hundreds, or even thousands, of years. They are mentioned in Ayurvedic medicine, in Tibetan medicine, as well as by Hippocrates, while the Bible makes mention of purifying the body with the use of an enema.

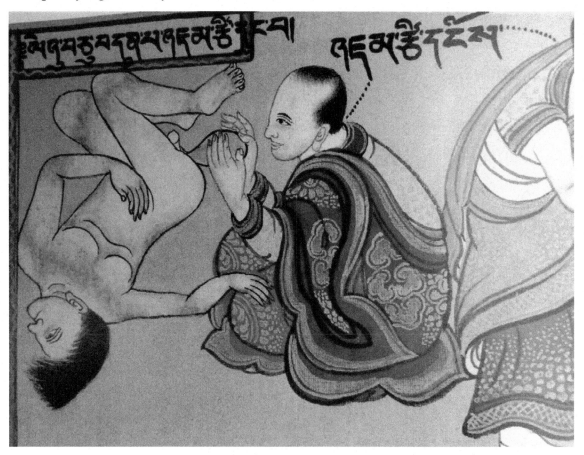

Internal Wash

Image from Tibetan medical practice of the eighteenth century (Art of Healing in Tibet). A Tibetan doctor purges the patient in spring and autumn, to purify the body.

This technique is most important in order to detoxify the colon and clean up the whole body. In the past people were used to purging themselves, especially in spring and autumn, as a way to get rid of the accumulated toxins that weaken the body. Those people were healthier and not subject so much to flu and infections as we experience today.

At the beginning of my career, I was greatly inspired by Dr. Bernard Jensen in regard to detoxification and colon irrigation protocols that he widely used. At the time, Hidden Valley Ranch was the World Mecca of Naturopathy. Later on I studied the work of Max Gerson, whose book, *A Cancer Therapy – The Result of 50 Cases*, emphasized internal cleansing. This book is still available today. Through it, I discovered the properties of coffee-based enemas, which he used with cancer patients.

In fact, just before meeting Dr. Jensen, around 1962, I met in Los Angeles a very cultured, highly spiritual lady recently coming from India where she had learned from great Indian Naturopathic doctors, after herself recovering from an incurable cancer. She then told me about enema therapy and its purpose, and that she was taking them regularly besides a very strict diet including daily intake of carrots and other vegetable juices. That was the first time I heard about carrot juice, about detoxification of the colon, and it also made sense to me. Later on this lady introduced me to Dr. Bernard Jensen. I then started taking my first enema and it had really shown me firsthand how we can detoxify ourselves.

Later on, coming back to Europe, I studied the work of great German pioneers, such as Abbot Kneipp, Louis Khune, and Vincent Priessnitz, especially their detoxification systems that were used as their special medicine called Hydrotherapy. This was practiced in some Sanatoriums and very large health establishments such the one founded by Louis Khune in 1883 that could treat 1000 patients per day, or water Spas such as Sebastian Kneipp's Bad Wörishofen.

Fasting is also one technique which was used by the German pioneers to help the body to detoxify and rest the digestive system for a few days. It was also used by some Soviet doctors who performed experimentation, and became widely developed in the USSR's territory under government order. In the USA, Herbert Shelton was a real pioneer of fasting, unfortunately he was arrested several times and even sent to a labor camp because he was teaching fasting, while years later he was accused and sent to court because he conducted fasting with hundreds of patients.

Today in Germany several public hospitals have a large space for patients willing to fast. One example is La Charité Hospital in Berlin, the largest public hospital in Europe. Fasting initially for 3 or 4 days is beneficial to patients doing this detoxification program, especially for patients who are affected by chronic and degenerative disease, which mostly were always subject to chronic constipation.

Furthermore, a subsequent 10-12 day fasting period is beneficial for patients that have suffered many years from rheumatoid arthritis, obesity, high cholesterol, high blood pressure, or nervous disorders. They also need to be closely followed with medical care. Generally, people who are affected from chronic and degenerative diseases are almost always subject to constipation.

Colonoscopy can be useful in a way to observe the presence of compacted feces accumulated in various segments of the colon, while few people seem to even understand about this consequence. What can be done to expulse the compact feces that stick on the wall of the colon? Here we have one solution using a coffee enema, which is an excellent stimulant that acts on the peristalsis. It also acts indirectly on the liver by detoxification of the colon, removing toxins and other poisons that damage liver function. Coffee enemas can cause deep elimination of dark, nauseating feces. By stimulating and detoxifying the hepatic enzyme system, coffee enemas alleviate or help to eliminate various health problems.

A liver free from amine and toxic ammonia prevents their infiltration into the body. This also stimulates hepatic detoxification and the enzyme system, relieving the body from various symptoms including headaches, migraines, pains, and ballooned colon.

Some recent experiments carried out on animals have demonstrated that coffee enemas stimulate the liver's production of glutathione S-transferase-enzyme, increasing detoxification of the small intestine by 700%. Overall it relieves the body from toxins, increasing the immune cell's activity, patients feel a sensation of well-being and in normal cases, it relieves the body from various symptoms such headaches, migraine, pains especially of the legs, back, and discomfort from a ballooned colon.

A clay enema is also interesting as it allows for a significant absorption of toxins, without irritating the intestine, unlike the coffee enema, which is not advisable in cases of colitis and colon inflammation. In these cases a clay enema should be used along with an infusion of chamomile or mallow.

Over forty years ago I was in Paris and met an interesting man known as Mr. Xanty, who originally came from Bulgaria. His real name was Joseph Josifoff and he changed it because Jews were persecuted and sent to death camps during the French occupation by the Germans. Mr. Xanty was running an Institute also called Xanty. It mainly was based on the detoxification of the colon through a special formula he developed to use in special enema while making a reflexology process on the colon. His formula was made from a variety of herbs, potassium, mineral salts and other ingredients that he kept a secret. He called his treatment a rectal shower done in various rooms in the Institute while other rooms were equipped with tub baths for taking a bath with a formula of herbs after the rectal shower. I was working at the French School of Naturopathy, where lectures were organized during the week, and in fact Dr. Bernard Jensen came over to lecture. Mr. Xanty who assisted was a nice man, impressed by my personality and what I was using. I told him about the colonic treatment used at Hidden Valley Health Ranch. One week he invited me to try out his rectal shower. In fact, at that time I was suffering from some severe skin eruptions from stress after returning to Europe, not being well established in my profession but lucky to teach some iridology and naturopathy classes at the French School of Naturopathy. I accepted the offer to take the cure every morning before eating any food over 8 days. The result was absolutely unique the way these treatments cleaned up and eliminated enormous quantities of toxic wastes. In meantime it permitted me to learn more about Mr. Xanty and the reason why he developed this colon cleansing regimen, of course based on disease that medicine cannot cure.

After that one week, I decided to continue about three times per week, and soon the skin eruptions totally disappeared and I felt much better and slept in such way that even a thunderbolt could not wake me. Later on, after moving to Portugal, I started to use his rectal shower in my clinic for the benefit of my patients.

This clearly proves that auto-intoxication which slowly comes about, ends up poisoning the organism. In some people, this enema can cause painful spasm or colic, during the elimination of matter. Indeed, people eat food that irritates the intestinal mucosa and moreover, the dried up feces, encrusted on the intestinal walls become difficult to release, causing spasms. But the well-being, which is restored after these pains, due in some cases to the elimination of such a large quantity of matter, which in retrospect can make the pain seem trivial. You can attenuate these cases by dieting for two days prior to the treatment, eating no meat, no spices, or fried foods, but only vegetables, fruits, drink vegetable juices along with natural aloe/papaya mixture to promote detoxification and to protect the intestinal mucosa. A mucosa irritated by unsuitable foods can be a major source of the pain caused by elimination. After a few days of diet, this situation will be resolved.

A retention enema is also used with another purpose against intestinal inflammation to protect or restore the mucous membrane. Dr. Kousmine suggested adding in 2 tablespoons of virgin, cold pressed sunflower oil in some water. Otherwise, add it to the enema mixture to be administered, which can be better absorbed by the colon mucosa rather than being expelled, as with regular enemas. The substances retained are absorbed through the intestine and enter the organism through the blood stream. For example, in cases of inflammation or of intestinal ulcerous colitis, a drink made from a combination of Linseed, Aloe Vera, and Carrot Juice is used to take away the inflammation of the mucosa.

In fact, Dr. Kousmine's method relied on four columns, the same as a chair with four feet. Remove one and the chair topples. Food and nutrition is the first, clean bowel and the regeneration of the intestinal mucous is the second, the acid/alkaline balance is the third, and vitamin and trace element supplementation is the fourth.

We can not only rely solely upon medical doctors and permit ourselves to remain ignorant. What about our children and their health and future? They will end up the same as we are or even worse, since diseases are the result of incorrect life style choices, and not taking the opportunity to learn and to educate ourselves. This should most definitely be corrected and implemented at our earliest opportunity.

Colema

Today, there is a modern method of detoxification which uses a sophisticated apparatus called the "colon hydrotherapy system," which is a modernized system compared to the original colonic, or colema board system developed by Victor E. Iron, who introduced it to Dr. Jensen, who in turn recommended the colema system to his patients.

Colon cleansing at home is a very good way to keep the colon and the body clean and feel healthier especially keep the mental alert since toxins can circulate up to the brain. If utilized in a clinic, colon hydrotherapy requires well-trained technicians to assist the patient, because it can occasionally be painful, especially if one has a very intoxicated colon with dry feces retention stuck on the wall. You can take a colema at home by buying the colema board, which is also efficient to detoxify, but again you need to follow the instructions carefully.

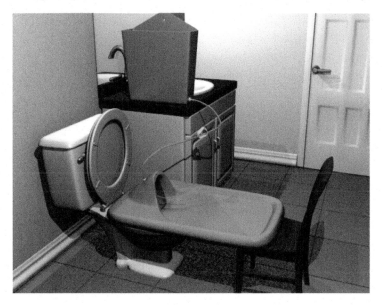

Modern Colema Board System (www.colema.com)

In today's Europe, colon hydrotherapy is taught at Naturopathic colleges and in schools of Integrative Medicine, especially in the U.S. and Germany.

I have a couple of friends managing a clinic in England. Barbara is an eighty-four-year-old woman who continues her activity in the clinic as an acupuncturist with incredible energy. Every morning before breakfast she does a colon cleansing with one of these personal machines.

It is undeniable that an inefficient elimination of toxins disturbs the organism especially at an advanced age, which demonstrates, in Barbara's case, how colon hydrotherapy keeps her very active.

Colon Hydrotherapy

Colon hydrotherapy is different compared to an enema. The latter only detoxifies the lower part of the colon, while a colon irrigation or hydrotherapy detoxifies the entire colon. It is actually a thorough cleansing with a special apparatus that uses large amounts of water that allows it to suck out the matter intoxicating the descending colon as well as the transverse or ascending colon. The patient can even see old or toxic fecal matter exit through a lighted glass tube. Again, it can be occasionally painful during a few minutes, especially when dried feces have accumulated on the wall of the colon and are difficult to break up. An excess of hard feces can also block up the colon until a large quantity of injected water can dissolve it in combination with an abdominal manage to relax the muscles. It is always best to eat a light meal and drink vegetable juice a couple of days before doing colon hydrotherapy and to take some dietetic supplementation to increase detox, but cleansing of the colon is one of the best ways to help your body against disease and improve your health status.

Everyone can benefit by undergoing colon hydrotherapy or using a colema board. In Europe, for instance, in Germany and England, there are colon institutes which treat the patients through diet and colon cleansing. Dr. Erich Rauch, who distinguished himself for his research on the colon, is famous among them. In fact, today there are institutes and schools of colon Hydrotherapy all over the U.S. and Canada, since these days more and more people are looking to detoxify themselves.

Recently one of my patients came back I haven't seen for quite a few years. She was twenty-three years old when she first came in to see me and now she is forty-three. In the beginning her colon was functioning every six days and I could easily give you the list of her symptoms. What a quantity of feces she had accumulated in her colon! She first started taking enemas to clean up her colon, but some years afterwards, she agreed to take colon hydrotherapy treatments in our clinic.

This system often makes certain symptoms disappear immediately.

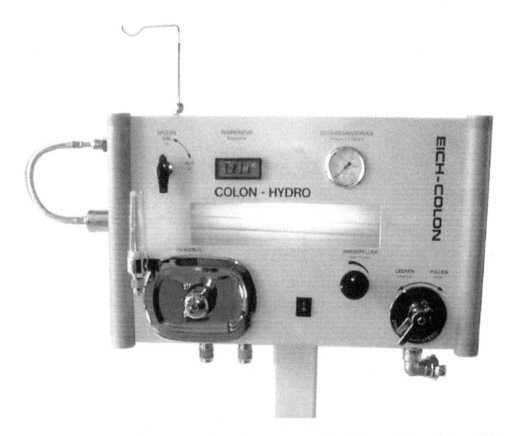

Professional Colon Hydrotherapy Machine Used in Clinics

Colon hydrotherapy is undergoing a deep cleansing of the entire colon and helps to restore normal intestinal functions. It permits the elimination of accumulated dried feces that sticks to the wall of the colon, which includes dead skin, non-digested food, toxins and bacteria. It prevents auto-intoxication, relieves the body from symptoms of illness, restores bowel function and overall improves one's health condition.

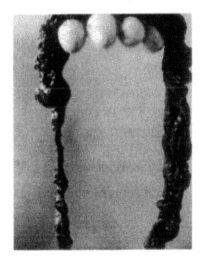
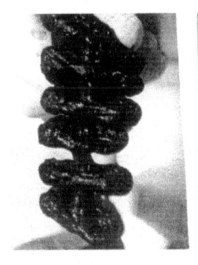
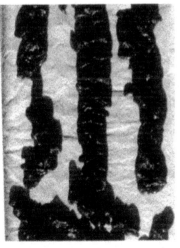

Elimination of Feces after Colon Hydrotherapy

<u>Benefits of Colon Hydrotherapy:</u>

- Improves the general state of the organism
- Relaxes
- Tones
- Reduces the abdominal volume and waistline
- Eliminates parasites
- Reduces and eliminates local inflammation
- The skin becomes lighter and brighter
- Improves blood circulation
- Diminishes or eliminates joint and muscle pains
- Improve the immune cells function
- Balance the nervous system
- Indirectly improves the hepatic functions
- Thoroughly eliminates toxins

In summary, the beneficial effects on all the functions of the organism can be seen.

How Do You Take an Enema?

In order to take an enema, one needs to buy a small plastic kit in a drug store. Normally it has the capacity of 2 liters, but generally we only use one liter of liquid for this type of enema.

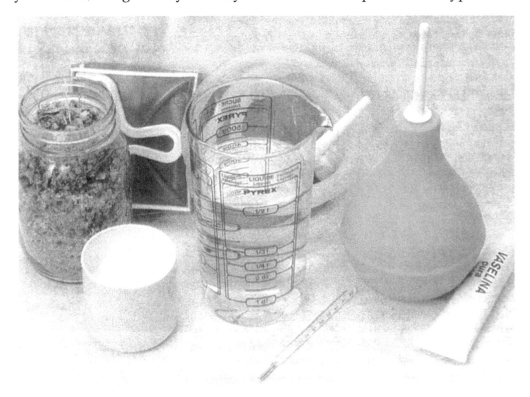

Equipment Used to Take Enemas

Hang the container on the wall in the bathroom. These containers have a flexible rubber tube to which an anal cannula is attached. A small clamp controls the liquid flow. The liquid must be at body temperature, never exceed 98.6° or 100° maximum, to avoid any spasms.

Procedure:

- Lie on your back on a carpet on the floor, turn onto your left side with your legs drawn up to your body.

- Introduce the cannula dipped in glycerin, sesame oil, or a greasy cream (Vaseline) for gentle insertion. Allow the liquid of the enema to enter, relax with a slow rhythmic breath. If you feel any spasm, stop the inward flow of liquid for a moment and then continue. Should there be need to interrupt the enema, take it out and start later as the colon will be more relaxed. It is not wise to take a colonic and under stress. First relax, take a few deep breaths, lie down for few minutes and try not to think. In fact, meditation is beneficial to eliminate stress.

Frequency of Enemas:

- At the beginning, and if your body is very intoxicated, one enema a day is advisable. But, if the life style does not permit, three or four times a week is suggested.

- After 20 days of treatment and cleansing up of the colon, you reduce to one enema per week, since it may also irritate the colon. You may continue for another four weeks and stop.

Types of Enemas:

Coffee enema – this type of enema increases the intensity of elimination of residues and toxins. Take a liter of boiled water, at 98.6°, add a cup of pure, strong coffee. Or else, boil a liter of water with two spoons of ground coffee and let boil for a few minutes. Cool to body temperature then strain through a piece of pure cotton.

Castor oil enema – this type of enema was already in use by Dr. Max Gerson for his cancer patients. Castor oil is derived from the seed of the castor plant and acts as a stimulant laxative. It stimulates the walls of both the small and large intestine and empties both.

Castor oil enema recipe:

2 oz. castor oil
2 qts. warm water at 103º Fahrenheit

After making a castor oil enema you may need to take an enema with Castile Soap; otherwise, you could leak oil for hours. For more information see: http://www.health-information-fitness.com/caster-oil-enema.htm

Clay enema – used to detoxify, heal, and disinfect.

Use 1 to 2 tablespoons of powdered clay per l liter of water. Dilute the clay in half of the water, heating the other half, and then add the clay water in order to obtain the desired temperature. Pour into the application container and proceed as you would do with other enemas.

The clay enema is used above all in cases of colitis and colon inflammation. 2 tablespoons of liquid chlorophyll may be added to the mixture as it contains highly antiseptic and anti-inflammatory properties. People who have a strong odor or perspire a lot obtain excellent results from this kind of detoxification. In cases of chronic constipation, the clay enema is not advisable as it can accentuate the problem.

We can also substitute the water with a concoction of chamomile or mallow in cases of gastroenteritis or chronic inflammations of the colon.

Retention enema

Must be done at night before bed and after the intestines are clean. There are many mixtures according to the problem (see chapter on treatment).

Example:
1 small cup of carrot juice
Add 1 small cup of linseed extract
1 cup of distilled water

(This is for people with constipation and inflammation of the colon)

Apply in the same way as a normal enema. There will be no elimination. Try to keep it in as long as possible, lying down after the application. Normally, during this kind of treatment, a rubber pump is used which can be purchased from a drug store. An irrigation pump is also used in cases of treatment with substances, such as shark cartilage.

The mixtures must not be eliminated but retained in the intestines to reduce inflammation and for the process of repair.

Any person can use this method in their own home, according to these rules, and avoiding enemas or cleanses during digestion, or critical periods. For colon hydrotherapy treatments, particular care needs to be taken and it is essential to get advice from a doctor experienced in this special technique.

Changing Eating Habits

"Everything that produces a major change in the actual current state of man can be considered as a remedy. We can provoke change by modifying our food habits."
—*Hippocrates*

During my professional life, I have treated the same patients or same families for over thirty years, even some patients today for nearly forty-five years, including those with cancer, as well as educating and helping my patients to change their eating habits and lifestyle. This lengthy work was positive and allowed me to suggest some basic rules for a healthy life and healthy food diet to thousands of people of all ages and social standing.

As a result of this long work over several decades, I have been rewarded by knowing that many patients have changed their lives. Some patients have moved to countryside, starting their own organic gardens, others will search only for organic food, yet many at advanced age feel more healthy than ever. Even the younger ones that I started to treat some twenty years ago now have their own families and are all in good, healthy condition. Many adult patients that I have treated for thirty years or more, per the example given above, are now over eighty years of age and are feeling very healthy and strong.

This is something that you cannot achieve with prescription drugs. Today elderly people are literally bombarded with pharmaceutical drugs, just to try to keep them alive but left for mostly half dead, many in wheelchairs and we call it "medical progress." I have seen on TV a program about the "Centenary" from Okinawa Island in Japan. Most of the residents are over one hundred years old, they still work in in their gardens, growing their own organic vegetables, eating salads and fruits, with a large daily variety. For these Okinawans, blood pressure is in the range of 120 x 80, incredible and all without the so-called progress of medicine and having a pharmacy at home.

"Modern Medicine" is here to mainly to prescribe drugs, but it does not change our life style and keeps us ignorant of what acutely, we need to do for our health. We have a brain given to us to use, especially for thinking about what could be beneficial to keep us healthy and away from disease. One of my patients, a woman that I treated along with her husband and two daughters when they were school girls (now mothers), told me that she visited her medical doctors for a routine checkup, necessary in today's society. The doctor, a woman also was surprised since, at her age, she was without any complaint or other problems. "Strange," she said, "your cholesterol is normal, but it is best to be preventative and I am going to prescribe for you a statin drug. Of course," she said, "it may induce liver damage, but we will control it." In meantime food that prevents cholesterol, a good diet, or healthy food seems to be totally ignored by this doctor, who probably was paid to prescribe statin drugs even with toxic side effects such as blindness, as she mentioned. We call this modern medical science?

The other day I had a young couple, not even yet thirty but already with high cholesterol levels, especially the wife. What do you think happened when they consulted doctor and what was done about their condition? Statins of course, as the only solution for both, even being young, he says, "You have to take Statins for the rest of your life." Incredible!

Today modern science is in a position to present scientific data about the value of many types of foods that may prevent disease and keep us healthy. But for many people it is always difficult to change, let alone to accept this concept. Data about the value of many types of foods and dietary compounds that may prevent disease and/or treat diseases such as cancer, and keep us healthy are not made readily available or simply denied by doctors, when patients ask questions

What diet and vitamins can be taken to prevent cancer or what about a nutritional support during a course of chemotherapy? Professor Dominique Belpomme, a French oncologist wrote in his book *Healing from Cancer and Being Protected* (2005), that the so-called nutritional mechanism, including special diet is a pseudo-scientific theory and useless in the treatment of cancer. This is clearly coming from a so-called scientific person involved in cancer and that has a negative influence on other doctors.

Resveratrol, curcumin, índole-3-carbinol, green tea, polyphenols, and vegetables such as cauliflower, broccoli, tomatoes, and pomegranate are some examples of foods and dietary agents that target apoptosis that can profoundly alter gene expression to prevent cancer or to regulate oncogenes during cancer treatment. We can also mention whole rice, oats, bulgur, avocado, and almonds.

But for many people, scientific fact is not always the click that will drive them to change their habits. Usually for a radical change to occur in our dietary style we need some motivation, and because there is reason, some understanding or some circumstances beyond our control, that pushes someone to change their way of life. I remember a young lady with a severe problem of rheumatoid arthritis, without much hope of changing her state of health. Following my advice one day she became aware of the fact that it was necessary to completely revise her diet and do everything possible to establish a remission of the disease that would sooner or later leave her paralyzed. She decided to stay at home, leaving her job temporarily in order to reap the benefit from her diet, and the complete program I created for her.

On the other hand, we have a thirty-three-year-old lady with advanced diabetes, whose toes had been amputated from her left foot. She had many problems, her kidneys were functioning poorly, and she ran the risk of an amputation of her entire foot. I had seen this case eight years earlier and had made her aware of the need for a definite change in her lifestyle, both from the dietary point of view and from the hygienic point of view. But she did not understand the importance of the suggested change, or maybe she was not ready to accept it. She kept on living her more-or-less normal life and injecting herself with insulin every day.

She was not really conscious of the gravity of her case and she had recently reached a stage of facing an amputation, which she had subsequently undergone. Shortly thereafter, she died. Unfortunately, the miracle remedy has not yet been invented.

A middle aged man, mostly carnivore and not doing much for his health, changed his dietary style completely after a severe kidney stone crisis that drove him twice into the hospital. He became a vegetarian, started to learn about Indian Philosophy and yoga, taking courses on yoga, and detoxed.

While others will continue to stay on drug prescriptions, maybe undergo surgery, and remain with the same dietary style. The kidney stones were a result of a metabolic liver problem, excess of animal fats, cholesterol, and heavy crystals. After several treatments all the stones were eliminated.

We often inherit a bad education that doesn't help us in any way to discipline ourselves and be open and ready for some positive change. We have become like robots, switching human values with computers and advanced technology, but not able to live healthy and in harmony. We are our own slaves as well to the way we live.

Medicine is here to prescribe drugs, basically keeping us dependent on pharmaceutical labs for prescriptions. Doctors will usually prescribe any drug aggressively advertised by their marketing department. For example, in 1960, Richardson-Merrell Labs in the USA launched a new drug, MER/29 to decrease cholesterol levels and had recommended doctors to prescribe it to people over thirty-five years of age. The laboratory anticipated $4.25 billion per year in sales. Unfortunately, it turned into a disaster and thousands of people nearly turned themselves into crocodiles, building a formation of hard scales on their skin. The company falsified laboratory reports, showing that the product was safe, but to the contrary, they already knew about its toxicity. But unfortunately diet, anti-cholesterol, or anti-cancer food doesn't bring much profit but requires time and energy for education, but it does not change our life style either protecting us or curing us from disease. When health problems are the result of our incorrect life style, disease will constantly reappear, and then you just keep on living unhealthy, unhappy, and taking pills, feeling even worse. Today, too many people are living dependent on their doctors and prescription pills, even if they develop toxic side effects.

Most of them are absolutely conscientious about their medications, but most of the time I hear, "But it was prescribed by my doctor." An old lady with frequent headaches was prescribed several pharmaceutical drugs against epilepsy, by her doctor…to fight her headache…very strange. A list describes over fifty toxic side effects, including the idea and tentative thoughts of suicide. The poor woman was wondering if she should take this medication, or not?

> ## We Should Learn to Discipline Ourselves and to Control Dietary Errors.

The Orientals, above all the Chinese, when practicing medicine have a different view of life, putting a value on life style, spirituality, diet and even the cosmos. For example, in Chinese medicine, the cosmos (Yin and Yang) have a strong correlation to foods that are also Yin and Yang. Therefore, in this case, eating is not only a physical act but also in tune with a cosmological order, not to mention a spiritual one.

We are too materialist, and medical doctors are unable to understand about the therapeutic value of food to fight disease or to support a medical treatment or even as preventive. The majority of them do not associate disease with bad food. Most medical doctors do not even care about the vitamins and minerals contained in our food, which are not seen as important when it comes to the treatment of disease. Remember that for more than fifty years vitamins were strongly criticized, if not violently opposed. The concept of food for prevention of disease was totally denied. We are reduced to mathematics, to experimental medicine, and to infernal wars between medicine and research.

However, today we have slowly begun to acknowledge the value of whole and organic food over industrial food, along with the need for vitamin and mineral supplementation, still this is a topic wrongly criticized by medical doctors. But it is necessary to go even further into dietary traditions and break open the false ideas about some systems, such the theory of calories, which doesn't take into consideration what you eat as long as you eat your requirement in calories, whether you eat a hot dog, chili, or chicken.

In Chinese medicine the patient and his body are very important from an energy point of view. The association with the Cosmos, and Qi (or Ki) is an Oriental concept that refers to the energy that circulates within our body. Ki has its equivalent in the traditional system of Ayurveda and Prana, also known in Europe as Vitalism in our Naturopathic system. Ki-deficiency, meaning lower energy circulation in our body reflects organ function disorders such as those of the digestive system, the brain (psychic), kidney, spleen, and decline in the activity of the whole body, weakness, and fatigue. The diagnostic of Ki-deficiency is based on a score for each symptom or weakness with 10 points as a reference. A total count of more than 30 points indicates Ki-deficiency. For instance headache: 4 points – fatigue: 3 points – vertigo: 5 points – Edema: 15 points – loss of appetite: 8 points.

This Ki energy is in our body, around us, in our natural growing food, but modern life, industrial food, pollution, or stress decreases Ki production, especially for those living in big polluted cities. In this way, in order to reestablish a person's health, it is first of all important to restore the Qi energy through better food and diet, detox, relaxation, yoga, and sleeping well. Many Japanese hospitals and doctors use the QI test on patients, often along with other traditional examinations. The Japanese developed a wide range of medications from herbs called Kampo medicine, which is widely used to help restoring Ki-energy.

Once I was invited to the, "13th International Congress of Oriental Medicine", in Seoul, S. Korea, where I met Dr. Tsutomu Kamei M.D., Ph.D., who was the director of the Shimane Institute of Health Science in Tzumo, specializing in cancer treatment with Japanese herbs. He used tests and analysis from conventional medicine along with the Qi Test, the values of which in combination with good diet, who helped his patients to feel an increased sense of energy. He gave me an important document, luckily translated into English, rare for Japanese medical book called, *The Concepts of KI, Blood, Body Fluids and their Interrelation with Various Stages of Disease*. It is quite an interesting to approach patients, showing many clinical cases that go along with blood analysis, scans, and the KI score diagnostic.

In truth, today for example we begin to speak of and acknowledge the superiority of whole and organic foods and the need for supplements in the form of vitamins or minerals. But it becomes necessary to go even further into dietary traditions.

> *Medicine Must Consider the Patient, in Light of Their Dietary Style, if Not Only Half of Real Medicine is practiced. Unfortunately, this is What Happens Today.*

This is the medicine that offers thought and was developed by Hippocrates and should be the pillar for each doctor under the Hippocratic Oath. For example, I have seen patients suffering from severe liver and kidney problems, but totally unable to change their dietary style by continuing to eat red meat, white rice, black beans, and French fries. What about the duty of the doctor to do something about lifestyle and dietary concerns? Have we reached a hiatus within ourselves? Compared to Oriental Society, Western Society has lost many of its traditions, roots, and concepts. Our materialist science has cut off modern man from the old traditions and folk medicines, to become a real industry which really started back in nineteenth century in the USA, under the devilish projects of Rockefeller. Young women, nursing women, at that time were totally ignorant about the basic concepts of health and nutrition affecting both themselves and their future children.

> *We Lose Our Traditions, Roots, and Concept of Life.*

Even our ancestor's folk medicine, their herbal medicines have been slowly rejected and replaced by chemical molecules from a drug industry, that has managed to manipulate our society, having been responsible for altering our notion of health, education, and nutrition. This has resulted in today's actual situation of increased chronic and degenerative disease.

Above all, the paramount importance of food that correlates with health status or as factor to treat disease has been ignored or forgotten, and needs to be changed.

Fortunately, yet slowly but surely things are changing for the better, where we now are witnessing a reevaluation of the value of nutritional diet as a means of disease prevention. Recent published works have raised public interest in this matter. Many International and European magazines such as *Times*, *Ça m'interesse*, a reputed French magazine, and *Visão* (Vision) in Portugal, and *Der Spiegel*, in Germany have published articles and reports on the foods that heal and are also anti-cancer foods.

In 2007 one book, called *The Anti-cancer Diet* by David Servan-Schreiber, made a small revolution and was translated in twenty-four languages and most major magazines released articles about this anti-cancer diet. David Servan-Schreiber, a medical doctor in the field of research was working in USA and split his life with France, also his native country. As one can imagine, French oncologists criticized the anti-cancer diet as totally inefficient, were it up to them to help cancer disease. However, they could not stop the waves made by the book from people looking for some alternatives. Indeed it was the beginning of a change for people themselves because in truth, in each one of us there is a hidden doctor that can look out for ourselves.

We Can Heal with Foods

According to some of these articles it seems that, and I quote, "We can heal with foods," a statement that can cause a revolution in the medical field, which believes that a diet that cures must have a placebo effect. I am wondering if the placebo effect works well with dogs having a tumor?

Some years ago I was accused of using organic germanium to treat cancer, which supposedly qualified as nonsense with only placebo effects. At that time I was contacted by several people with dogs having malignant tumors, and after being treated with germanium, the dogs were tumor free. How does a dog know about what he is taking? This is not placebo but reality. In truth, many people do not understand where the real problem lies with food and above all its inherent quality.

We have fought for years to teach and explain how food can heal, but without great success. However, today, according to the articles mentioned in international magazines which proclaimed, "We can heal with foods," these words have become a statement that can now cause a revolution. Dr. Jensen, who was one of the first pioneers in this field, would be happy to know that after sixty years, science has finally come to this conclusion. In 2008 the French magazine, *Sciences et Vie* published a large article called "Food and Cancer: The conclusion of the largest International study," which really offered scientific facts on the value of food in the prevention of cancer, organ by organ. This was really a revolution.

How and why we have reached this situation, and not to exaggerate there has been repeated crimes to destroy the value of food, are interesting topics. This has been a world-wide phenomenon that comes from wrong conception, wrong education, wrong ideas, and from a total rejection of natural medicine and herbal medicine in favor of pharmaceutical drugs.

Especially coming from the idea that, "Medicine makes miracles." Modern chemistry is also very much responsible since it was through the discovery of a synthetic molecule that led to a rejection of all the natural conceptions and food in favor of industrial foods with no nutritional value.

Science Cannot Ignore Nature

There is a phenomenon that affects the entire world of nature science making us forget its laws. A void has been created between the two worlds, leading science to reject all the natural molecules from herbs or any natural compound, and substitute synthetic molecules. Today transgenic or GMO food is a good example of this rejection.

When we think about this subject from the point of view of food, especially about the question of natural food, we realize that this rift is not recent. Let's examine its origins.

In the United States, as early as 1930, research was carried out which started a war against natural foods to the benefit of the commercial food industry. The main attacks and misinformation were further implemented after 1945, becoming ever more aggressive and sometimes even laughable. Indeed, in the USA in 1949, Dr. Elmer M. Nelson was called upon to testify in a federal court to halt the comparison between quality natural foods and industrialized food products.

From this point on, a real fallacy was spread throughout the world. This doctor stated under oath, as if he were imparting "God's Word" that it was globally anti-scientific to declare a well-nourished organism is more resistant to disease than an incorrectly fed body. Even worse, in an interview with *The Washington Post Magazine*, on October 26th, 1949, he declared that, in his opinion, there is absolutely no proof that nutritional deficiencies make a body less resistant to disease. In other words, according to him, vitamins and minerals are just useless in our food consumption to activate the various physiological functions of our body. We may wonder why animals living in nature are not ill like us humans.

This is an example of the misinformation that has been spread throughout the world, through specialized magazines then taken up by the medical faculties in rejecting and denying the nutritional value of food. They were teaching the wrong conception about health and neglecting the value of natural organic food. Therefore, it's no surprise, that medical doctors coming from universities have not only a minimum of knowledge concerning nutrition, but also deny its value which makes many patients wonder about the competence of medical doctors, only to seek nutritional advice elsewhere. Of course the doctors themselves are often eating the wrong foods, and may develop disease and cancer the same as anyone, and will likely die without experimenting with other medical systems.

Facts like these make it difficult for most doctors to cross certain barriers, due to dogmatic university teaching, unless one keeps an open mind. One medical doctor, a woman of fifty-six years, came to my clinic for a consultation for her pancreatic cancer. She could not understand the necessity to undertake a special diet and preferred to follow only chemotherapy. She quickly died of course, while some of my other pancreatic cancer patients are in remission, some already with a four-year life extension.

A more rare, if not contrary example was a forty-eight-year-old woman medical doctor came to me for a breast cancer, but was very open minded, being also being married to a German medical doctor. They decided to go back to Germany to search for some other solution as an alternative to chemotherapy. She read an article about me, published in German, decided to consult with me, and undertake whatever was necessary to treat her cancer, with good results. But otherwise, things are very slow to change.

Fortunately today, there are many more publications all over on the world, as well as on the Internet that show the value of natural food intake and organic foods, to prevent the development of diseases and cancer. A simple food, such as oat cereal that I have often prescribed to my patients for over four decades, has been cited as one of the most important foods against cancer. Perhaps, as Hippocrates said, "It is a return to the past." Let me remind you of the Hippocratic Oath, which is still taken in many medical schools, "*Premium non nocere*," or "First do no harm."

Aside from having always used and advised oats above all in cases of intestinal inflammation, besides this cereal and according to each case, I used other cereals such as barley, whole rice, spelt, millet, and buckwheat, to see how the intestine reacts to these different ancient foods. I have also used them to increase energy. But for young doctors starting out and who are unaware of these foods or the way the organism accepts or rejects processed foods, it is difficult and becomes easier to just not pay any attention.

Today's young doctors coming out from university schools of medicine are just as ignorant, often only doing their job in a limited, often mechanical manner by only prescribing pharmaceutical drugs. There is reason to believe that many medical doctors have financial interest with pharmaceutical labs to over-prescribe toxic drugs, not taking into consideration the real interest of their patients, meaning they become less sick and healthier, instead of obliging them to take medications all year round. I agree that often and in case of an emergency we need medical assistance but at the same time nutrition and support with natural supplementation may be useful as well. Unfortunately it becomes easier to just ignore the issue.

They are not even passionate about their profession. They consider medication a priority to remove pain, but if in some cases pain killers or other medications are only necessary for a limited time, yet at the same time food diet is also necessary to help the body recover from disease. As I have always said, pharmaceutical drugs do not cure, but nutritional food can change your body and increase your health. The main idea is not to have the patient less sick with longer spaces between diseases, but to the contrary live without permanent relapses and more prescriptions.

It is often a fact today that they ignore dietary style, nutrition, and vitamins, plus we have reasons to believe that doctors are well paid by pharmaceutical labs to over-prescribe toxic drugs, not taking into consideration the health of their patients. They will mathematically count calories and as taught, yet nutrition and immune system support are usually forgotten. Unfortunately, it becomes easier to just ignore the issue.

Take for instance chronic fatigue syndrome (CFS), not pathology nor a localized disease, but an accumulation of several abnormal conditions including mitochondrial dysfunction. Pharmaceutical drugs are totally ineffective as a way to fight this syndrome. Here we realize that other means are necessary, that nutritional diet combined with supplementation as a mitochondria booster, vitamins, minerals, EFAs, Coenzyme Q10, NADH, and immunomodulators. Indeed, Enzyme Yeast cells preparation and Sun-Chlorella seem to be the best answer to overcome CFS. Just ask how many cases have I treated over the past decades!

Treating disease or a syndrome may take time, up to two years depending on the case, while patients start to improve little by little until full recovery. I treated a twelve-year old girl in a very bad physical and nervous condition, unable to study, even going to school. I treated her for almost two years before she became a normal girl. If you see at the end of the book the clinical cases, there are some typical examples showing what can be done using nutrition, detoxification and other natural compounds and vitamins to revitalize the entire body. Once a medical doctor called me from Johannesburg (South Africa), suffering from C.F.S. not able to drive outside of the city, feeling so tired. After taking organic germanium and Enzyme Yeast cells, for three months he could go outside of the city, however I treated him for six months. Another case was a twelve-year-old girl who had difficulties in moving more than three yards, and had been in wheelchair coming to my consultation. These are new syndromes that appear in modern society and are first above all, consequences of bad hereditary status, mitochondrial dysfunction, and the result of dietary errors. In younger people it is often a question of defective genes inherited from their parents, who are already in a bad state of health.

Recently a thirty-six-year old woman suffering from Melas Syndrome came to my clinic. Melas Syndrome is usually fatal to the patient (see clinical cases). Even though there is no treatment for this degenerative syndrome, I still decided to use my intuition to challenge the case. After three months the patient started to really improve, walk in the street, do shopping, and after six months she was a totally different person. Here, pharmaceutical drugs were totally ineffective for such progressive neuro-vegetative and muscular disease caused by mutation in the mitochondrial genome. This is what we can achieve but unfortunately we were not receiving any credit, even while this syndrome affects thousands of persons.

The Vision of the Great Pioneers

We will try and go back a hundred years, in order to show how most of the pioneers where themselves very sick, some even with little or no hope of a cure, yet healed themselves and survived because of their sense of observation and intuition using the power of nature.

The famous Abbot Kneipp, the great pioneer of Hydrotherapy had tuberculosis, which was incurable at that time (end of the nineteenth century). He cured himself by reading the book from Vincent Priessnitz, the real Father of Hydrotherapy, and started to treat himself with a water-cure and diet.

Dr. Bernard Jensen also had a severe lung disease, with no known cure at that time. "There is nothing I can do for you," he was told by doctors. The famous dietitian Gaylord Hauser was in the same situation as Dr. Krishner who introduced carrot juice. They all had severe health problems and were all seeking, observing, and adapting their own treatments. They developed methods of treatment and diets based on their own experiences.

Dr. Bernard Jensen called himself at that time a "Doctor of Natural Living." Can you imagine the reaction of people? What kind of doctor did you see, a doctor of natural living? What do you mean by natural living, if not having been taken for an eccentric or crazy guy?

I remember my landlord in Los Angeles telling me after having had a heart attack, "I don't eat your crazy food," and then eating a big steak at 6:00 a.m. on the advice of his doctor, before going back to bed. I, personally, did not follow this route and choose this profession simply by chance, but it was because of circumstances that led me to look for an alternative to what was offered to me at the time by doctors in Los Angeles where I was living, meaning pharmaceutical drugs for a nervous breakdown.

My intuition rejected the use of such chemical treatment, and after taking my own treatment with fresh organic vegetables juices such as carrot, celery, parsley, and apple that also included a diet with organic foods and a supplementation of rice bran syrup, I completely recovered.

292

This was the turning point in my life. It awakened my interest to study Naturopathic medicine which at the time was not very well known with our health community.

> ## *Fresh Vegetable Juices and Natural Foods Aroused My Interest as Healing Agents*

My interest in the study of medical care through natural process, non-toxic agents, and nutrition using organic food is still ongoing. This led me to travel the world to seek populations with better health and stronger resistance to disease civilization as compared with people of the Western world.

When I started, modern medicine reigned. Those who dedicated themselves to study and practice natural medicine were the object of laughter and mockery. This subject matter could not be freely discussed among people. What is your profession? Naturopath would silence the audience. Today it is a different story, and the maintenance of health and prevention of disease through food has once again become such an important factor, that has many progressive doctors are utilizing this in their practice.

Not long after, there was an article in a French newspaper, which read, "Our Doctors Already Cure Without Drugs" (but never follow, of course), what about the Naturopaths! We are the ones who started to cure without drugs. This was the reality we fought to see after many decades. In my opinion, this was due to great discoveries in molecular biology, immunology, nutrition, and the need to be more efficient in treating disease without harming the organism. It also highlights the importance of approaching disease from different new angles that underline the causes of disease, which can only be corrected through nutritional diet and detoxification.

Eating Habits

Each country has its own dietary style rooted in generations past. Some of them are very bad, such as in Ireland and Hungary that are consuming a higher percentage of red meat in comparison to other countries, also has the highest rate of heart disease.

Other countries, such as Italy and France, include a lot of salad and vegetables in their dietary habits. Spanish people from Spain eat too much fatty foods in their diet, especially meat and chorizo being very traditional, and in Germany the large consumption of charcuteries leads to cancer, while their excessive consumption of beer, leads to diabetes.

In Portugal we still have some balanced food habits with good fish, sardines, good virgin olive oil, cabbage, and other good vegetables. Our Mediterranean diet is one of the best in Europe.

Unfortunately, the widespread availability of processed and fast foods counteracts the consumption of good food, both here in Portugal and in all other countries. This has become tragic for the new generation, especially the young ones to come. If it takes 10-15 years to build a cancer, we are now just preparing the future with more cancer, plus there is no need to mention diabetes that has become a world epidemic, a major problem with about 382 million diabetics in the world. It is estimated that there will be 592 million diabetics worldwide by 2035.

In Japan, as explained before, but above all in South Korea, where the government worries because we see an increase in the percentage of cancer cases at the same rate as the appearance of fast foods. It is necessary to say that there is a tendency for us to get used to what is easy, to fads, to ready-made foods. And people accept the fact that their children enter this infernal cycle.

It is Necessary to Change Eating Habits

Since we know that diet can heal we must also conclude that a bad and incorrect diet leads to chronic and degenerative disease.

As we can see, the ideal situation would be to go back a century and return to the work done by the great pioneers in the field of health, disease prevention, and healing. We will learn from them and do everything possible to look for good foods. We are aware that our genome is not adapted to industrial foods, being modified only by 0.5%, over the past 2.5 million years. Therefore, it is more adapted the original food of our ancestors some 10,000 years ago. We can be grateful to these innovators who by intuition and experimentation, discovered natural food as a way to heal ourselves.

A Bad and Incorrect Diet Leads to Chronic and Degenerative Diseases

First of all, we must learn to distinguish between good and bad foods. Read the labels carefully as the food industry uses colorants, preservatives, chemicals, and artificial flavors, which although authorized by law, are not the most appropriate additives for our body that must defend itself against chemicals, often toxic. There are exhaustive lists of substances allowed in the food industry, many of which have carcinogenic effects. It is also necessary to patronize health food stores where we can find a large range of organic foods, kefir, soy milk, oats, and whole rice, as well as organic vegetables and usually, a well trained staff to advise you.

In the past few decades we have witnessed an enormous development of health food stores worldwide, even in Portugal, with the opening of large organic vegetable and fruit stores, and weekend organic markets. Even with the growing expansion of fast foods today, many people are now looking for natural food, organic foods, and seem to have more interest for better life style and health.

When I was in Montreal in 1967 there were only two stores in the whole province of Quebec. Today, there are thousands, clearly reflecting the change and the interest of the public to seek for more natural foods and vitamins, to live a healthier lifestyle.

Healing Foods

Here are some examples which are fairly simple but which show what whole foods are capable of doing. Let us consider the case of two tired people, with anemia, headaches, and vertigo. One of them is advised to do an eight day diet based on whole rice, steamed vegetables, cooked apples and a daily cocktail of vegetable juices. The other person will have a regular diet. At the end of the eight days it is surprising to see the difference between these two people.

This experiment could also be carried out for example, on middle-aged people and people who have cognitive disorders. Let us not speak of diseases or to treat a disease but only of well-being and quality of life that these people might experience.

We will divide them into groups and conduct the same experiment, but for thirty days. One of the groups will eat whole rice, and millet (rich in vitamin E, Phosphorus, magnesium, calcium, B complex vitamins, zinc and selenium) with the addition of some fish, vegetables and fresh fruit juices.

The other group will continue with white rice and white bread, meat, and all the other processed foods. Obviously, the latter will not feel any different or obtain any beneficial result as the nutritional value of these foods is low and unable to activate the cerebral neurons, balance oxidative stress, and avoid accumulation of toxins in the blood and tissues. But the group subjected to a rational diet will obviously see their cognitive capacities increase.

Unfortunately, average people are still not used to choosing the best food for their health, rushing off to the supermarket and choosing the cheapest priced food instead of quality food.

A thirty-six-year-old man came to see me after having had his fourth gout attack. During the entire time he was subject to these attacks he never altered his eating habits, sticking to drugs prescribed by the doctor, while continuing to eat spicy sausage and salty codfish. After the fourth attack pharmaceutical drugs were unable to lower the level of uric acid. Cases like this become a real vicious cycle: crisis, drug, another crisis, a stronger drug, and then other complications, which need other drugs, which are not always effective. They do not work because we do not change anything about ourselves, not for the nervous system, nor for problems of arthrosis, nor for cholesterol which is not lowered.

I wonder whether I have abused food lately? Maybe I should contact a professional Iridologist:

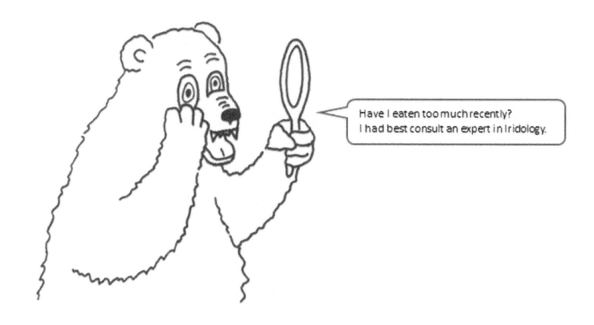

> **We suffer the consequences of an incorrect diet, of various excesses over generations.**
>
> **Our organism weakens as a result of the lifestyle and of the dietary abuses of past generations.**

Our defense and detoxification systems no longer work 100%. Our genes and the auto-regulation system that balances blood pressure, cholesterol levels, or corrects from an excess of uric acid have been altered. Today such health problems appear even more frequently at younger ages. Young men or women, 25-30 years old are already suffering from hypertension or high cholesterol. I even know boys of six, eleven, and fourteen years of age with high cholesterol and uric acid, but this seems normal to their pediatric doctors.

It is a tragedy for society, which is aging faster but does not seem to notice this decline. As soon as we realize that the drugs do not solve everything, what then? A miracle! We will then be persuaded to listen and to think about changing our eating habits. There is the case of a thirty-year-old man with 380mg cholesterol, 460 triglycerides and 180 blood pressure, or of a thirty-three-year-old woman forced to rely on drugs her entire life to prevent against a lower level of platelets.

In the first case, the patient had to constantly take pharmaceutical drugs such as statins to keep his cholesterol level and blood pressure down. When the patient asked if there was another solution, the doctor answered no and not to even think about it. Often the breach between patient and doctor comes about at this point, when he does not provide another good answer. In these two cases there is a conscientious natural denial of countering auto medication for life. Hence, we see that many people search for other solutions and means for themselves. At this point changing dietary style and favoring food that can modulate the bad cholesterol level and blood pressure is the obvious answer.

Are you already thinking about your state of health versus your eating habits? Would you be able to change your diet, detoxify yourself and help your body fight against disease? Do not wait for the onset of disease, it may be too late. A man that I knew for the past 20 years would come to our clinic (and home) to set up or repair T.V. monitors systems etc. He knew exactly what I was doing, yet he never changed his food habits. Just now he had been diagnosed with kidney failure and went immediately on dialysis (Two months later his wife was diagnosed with a colon cancer...no comment.) First begin to change your dietary style, make some corrections, and have a iridology checkup.

Soon you will see how your physical health condition and brain condition may improve. You will feel much better with a different state of mind, which is what medicine cannot do. As Dr. Bernard Jensen used to say, "A healthy spirit in a healthy body" is the key to live a better life.

Early Aging

Early aging with poor health status may also be associated with auto-intoxication and degeneration of the colon tissue, that picks up toxins more easily as well as aging characteristics. Elie Metchnikoff's (1845-1916) a Ukrainian scientist working at the Pastor Institute in Paris pioneered research in immunology but also with the bacterial life in the colon. He also is regarded as the grandfather of modern probiotics. He also asserted that some of the bacterial organisms present in the large intestine were a source of toxicants, toxic substances that contribute to illness and aging.

Normally with age the human body has less detoxification capacity resulting from decreasing kidney and liver function. Thirty years ago a Soviet Russian scientist, Dr. Popov suggested that constipation and poor elimination of toxic waste also leads toward the aging process. Dr. Norman W. Walker D. Sc. A pioneer of health and nutrition published in 1949 a book call *Become Younger* (edited and revised in 1978-1995) where he implicate the consequence of constipation and of a damaged old colon with aging. This is what I have often observed in my clinic with patients undergoing early-onset aging.

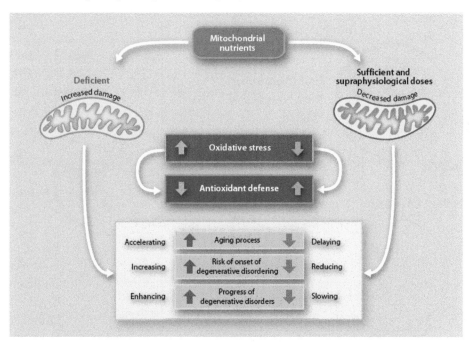

Fig. 2. Consequences of deficiency and sufficiency of mitochondrial nutrients. Deficiency can increase oxidative stress and decrease antioxidant defenses, thereby accelerating the aging process and increasing the occurrence of degenerative diseases. Conversely, sufficient mitochondrial nutrients decrease oxidative stress while fortifying antioxidant defenses, with the opposite effect.

Physical and psychological deterioration may appear, not only different from one person to another, even if they are the same age, but even before chronological age can be expected to distress middle aged individuals. I have even seen younger persons with age-related symptoms.

Aging is defined as a cumulative process of damaged body constituents, which are not repaired and renewed, further leading to a malfunctioning physiological process as well as mitochondrial dysfunction, and subsequent DNA damage dysfunction with decreasing ATP energy production. There is an accumulation and degradation of oxidized proteins, cellular membrane protein oxidation. DNA base pairs are modified mainly caused by high oxidative stress and decreasing induction of endogenous antioxidant enzymes.

However, this aging process is very much associated with our dietary style, high fat intake, a diet poor in antioxidants, an excess of cooked food, and the accumulation of toxins from colon auto-intoxication, which in turn increases the production of free radicals, poisons the tissues, which in turn disturbs the nervous system and brain function. I spent many years investigating this aspect of biological aging, but live in-person observation of early aging in patients is quite a profound experience especially when you observe their iris, and obtain overall, a better understanding of your patient. Over the years I developed a special iris chart with aging signs, presented at the New Millennium International Iridology Symposium 2000, in London. At least fourteen signs found in my iris chart directly corresponded to a "process of aging" profile.

Early aging, poor constitution, and degenerative process accompanied with chronic constipation may have other bad accompanying issues, since automatically it likely will be inherited by our children and their grandchildren, who are going to develop diseases earlier on, suffer from poor health condition, and subsequently may age even more prematurely from what we call Age Associated Memory Impairment (A.A.M.I.). According to neuroscientists this is the first disease that attacks the brain twenty to thirty years before symptoms of A.D. appear.

Aging Process in the Same Family

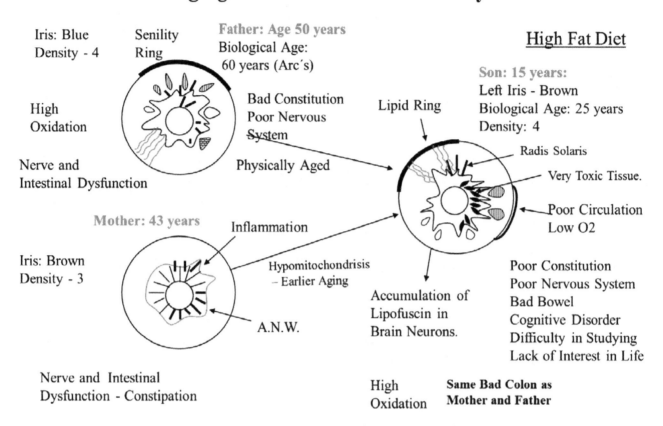

Here is a figure that I made some years ago from the iris a fifteen-year-old boy and his parents. It really shows that the boy inherited a bad constitution, a bad colon, and a bad nervous system. From what I observed the boy looked physiologically older, with a biological age of about twenty years or more. So what will be the issue when the boy grows up, gets married, and has children? What in turn, will be their health status? Soon, not only will we be old at birth, but in fact lipofuscin has been found in the brain of the dead baby during autopsy.

Lipofuscin is basically a breakdown product of peroxidized fats and proteins, like accumulated wastes in a cell's brain. It causes damage by clogging membranes so that vital nutrients cannot flow freely in the cells. Some scientists have even observed lipofuscin in fetal nerve cells. Lipofuscin accumulation in brain cells is one factor related to early aging, and from my own experience, can be interpreted according to iris observation. See my aging iris chart at www.sergejurasunas.com.

The health status, the constitution (iris density) of an offspring can be only the same or worse than the parents, and will likely determine the child's future health condition, risk of disease, or early aging during his or her lifetime.

In the upcoming chapter on clinical cases you will see iris photos and the story of a thirteen-year-old girl with a cirrhosis condition. Observing further, the iris photos of her parents, one can easily understand why the young girl inherited a bad constitution, especially a bad liver from her parents. She physically looked much older. However, from a medical standpoint, she was considered as healthy as any other child, except at nine years of age, she developed chronic hepatitis, but already carried from an embryological standpoint, a bad colon, bad liver, and a bad nervous system.

Remember that earlier, the embryonic notochord sent branches of nerve ramifications to the gut and after eight weeks, the liver budded on the colon. Therefore the iris is a real embryological indicator of our constitution and crucial to monitor children's health.

Children can also inherit from the mother's side, cells with less mitochondria, a condition called hypomitochondrisis. Adolescents with less cellular mitochondria may start an initial process of early aging and at adulthood their mitochondria may accumulate damage of the DNA components with decreasing ATP production reflected in fatigue, as well as putting on excess weight, experiencing memory loss, nerve dysfunction, heart dysfunction, and even diabetes. It can also cause DNA mutations that may drive early aging or even development of cancer.

I remember the case of a fifty-year-old man with Alzheimer 's disease, far too premature at this age, his fourteen-year-old son was already on his way, looking more like a zombie, not able to concentrate in school with no interest in life. Both the irises of the father and son were similar as far as the colon and nervous system were concerned. From the standpoint of Iridology, I had clearly determined that the condition of the central nervous system (CNS) provides the first indication of biological aging, and this together with the autonomic nervous system, which at present was under a major insult and/or badly inherited. It could be as a result of not changing his life style and dietary habits, this boy in twenty or thirty years from now, may easily suffer from Alzheimer's, being already at fourteen years of age, beset with cognitive disorders. See the upcoming case of the fourteen-year-old boy, plus other cases at www.sergejurasunas.com/index.php.aging or "Biological Aging Signs in the Iris."

In 1997 I made a study of 250 females aged from forty to fifty years (although some younger patients were later included in this study performed in my clinic with two other colleagues). We performed Iridology, Live Blood Analysis, and took readings with the Vega DFM-722.

We found the following conditions and correlations:

Poor memory 100%

Amnesia...50%

Insomnia...80%

Anxiety/sadness..................................70%

Vertigo..60%

Nerve dysfunction..............................90%

Chronic constipation...........................90%

Stress condition 70%

Low brain energy level........................80%

This clearly demonstrates first, the correlation between bad food intake and poor health status, and second, the value of Iridology as an early-warning diagnostic system for early-aging. More iris photos are included in my online paper (www.sergejurasunas.com)

Natural Foods for Improving Health

In the beginning of the last century mankind consumed a diet of 75% natural food, but unfortunately, today 75% of foods bought in supermarkets are industrially processed, that is refined, transformed, with the addition of chemical substances, colorants, and preservatives to extend food shelf life while making it more attractive for sale.

Physiologically and from a genetic standpoint we need natural food as it originated on this planet, necessary for all the body function to maintain good energy levels, since they are not transformed, manipulated and contain all the vitamins, minerals, enzymes and other natural compounds. Above and beyond all, we need natural and colored foods, with vibrations and life for the health of our organism.

The different colors such as yellow, red, and green, are not only a source of vitamins but of electrical energy concentrated from the sun with different wavelengths that are really a source of energy. Now most of the vitamins and above all enzymes are in large part, destroyed by industrial processing and more by cooking. Since natural or organic foods are a source of energy, human cells need constant energy to carry out the different functions. Ancient folk medicine practitioners, including Hippocrates, called this "the regenerating energy force." In fact, Professor E. Bouchut, referred to this energetic force in his book published in 1864 in Paris, which I mentioned previously.

Currently, we know that without energy the cells cannot communicate, neither internally nor between cells, or with one another. There is a certain similarity with the cosmos and the galaxies, which constantly produce colossal quantities of energy to balance the universe. The human cell is a fantastic world in constant turmoil, a real micro universe, functioning according to the same principles.

The cell carries out chemical and electrical processes or is simply in constant motion. A large part of the chemical work involved in activating the cells comes from the energy contained in farmed foods. These foods absorb the chemical energy from the Sun, which is used by the organism in the form of electrons. Then the electrons are used by our mitochondria that transform them into ATP energy molecules.

The sun emits radiation into space, commonly known as ultraviolet, as well as light and heat, which are essential sources of energy. Actually, light and ultraviolet rays are nothing more than the result of electromagnetic radiation, which because of its wavelength and frequency produces a usable quantity of energy. Our cells are actually a reproduction of the cosmos and of ourselves, the same as the Universe, ruled by laws, often mathematical laws. Everything has been designed to become what we are today. How our body works and how life starts on this planet and what comes as necessary for living creatures: oxygen, growing foods taken from the soil, the minerals we need, also coming from the ocean, and the sea algae, the chlorophyll which is not just a coincidence. Everything is made on purpose and not coincidence. We are very dependent on everything around us and if now scientists agree that the universe started with the Big Bang, who pulled the trigger?

To give us a better idea of this concept, consider the plants that use the energy of the sun to make their own energy. Human beings need foods that in the presence of oxygen to turn into internal fuel. It is also important to mention that natural foods grown in natural soils, in sunlight, are authentic reservoirs of solar energy used by the organism directly according to its own needs.

In truth, we are still ignorant regarding many elements such as water. Japanese scientists like Dr. Hotta, director of the Hotta Hospital in Japan, discovered that water has energy and antioxidant properties. Obviously this refers to pure Japanese spring water taken from the source. Now, vegetables alone contain 80% to 90% water. This shows how important it is for the underground water tables to remain intact and not polluted.

There is a different system to globally evaluate the vital energy of food. One of them that we have already talk about is the Bioelectronimeter of Professor J .C. Vincent that measured the PH, RH2 and Rh0 which is also now use in United States for some years for Biological Terrain Assessment. You can have the three biological measures from any food, water and see if they are living food, organic food with high redox and energy, or dead food.

Some years ago, we saw the development of the sensitive crystallography test, which provided very interesting information on the energizing quality of vegetables in relation to the way they are grown.

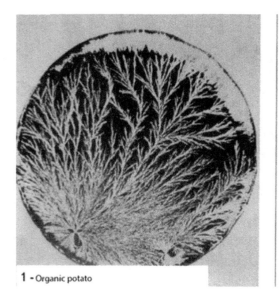 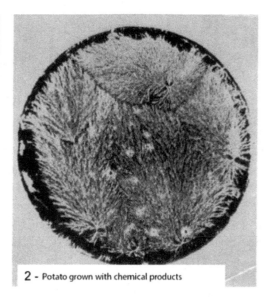

1 - Organic potato   2 - Potato grown with chemical products

1- Organic potato   2 - Potato grown with the help of chemicals

When a thin layer of copper chloride is put in a crystallized solution on a glass slide, crystal aggregates are created on the glass and are divided, more or less scattered. If we were to add small dilutions of organic extracts (plants, vegetables, etc.) to the solution before crystallization, the crystals will collect and form a particular configuration. The result is an image like the one seen in Photo 1 which is a crystallization test with organic potatoes.

Photo 2 is a test with potatoes grown with the use of chemicals and pesticides.

Another method developed by the French engineer, Andrè Simoneton, consists in capturing the electromagnetic waves corresponding to live tissues, in order to compare these same numbers in vegetables to verify their freshness and vitality. This measure is supplied in angstroms (Å) and various medical works make reference to this method.

The photographic technique using the Kirlian process is currently highly developed and allows one to photograph any object such as a fruit, vegetables or grain with an electromagnetic aura like that of the human cells. Organic fruits or seeds are photographed in order to compare their emanation of magnetic energy with that of commercially farmed fruits and seeds. The difference between them is huge and can be proven by a photo of this kind.

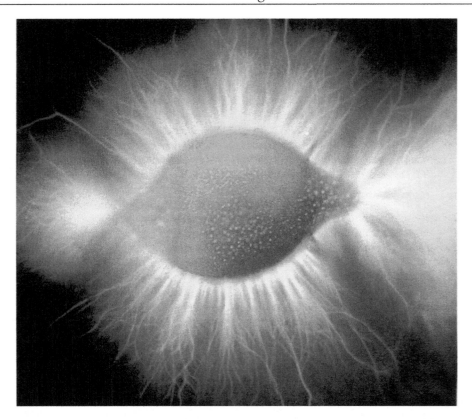

This image of Kirlian photography reveals the vitality and the fabulous energy that emanates from a freshly picked organically grown peach. We note the fantastic ramifications from the electric bundle (electrons) that emanate from this peach, which demonstrates the electromagnetic potential. This same potential is produced by the activity of healthy brain neurons.

It is easy to understand why organically farmed vegetables and fruits are superior and capable of producing beneficial, stimulating, energetic, and detoxifying effects on our organism.

Globally, the energy of each organ of the human body can be evaluated through an electronic system, using either the Voll or the Vega electromagnetic device test, which provides a whole map of every single energetic level, the organs, with a total energy value. Even electro-acupuncture devices can test this energy. This is what I am doing with all my patients in order to know their individual energy level.

In the case of disease or auto-intoxication with chronic constipation, I always notice that the energy level is always lower than average, but especially from the colon and often the brain and it always match for breast cancer patients. People with fatigue both physically or mentally also have an average lower energy level in relation to the number obtained by the test, which also represents a certain amount of intoxication in the organism.

I have already shown and proven how a poor energy level from a patient can be balanced through a diet of whole natural food, cocktails of vegetable juices, and fruit juices. The electronic tests show this clearly with increasing energy level and by additional ongoing energy testing on the patient.

Another big and current problem is that of the GMOs (genetically modified organisms) and their effects on health. At the moment this matter is creating a lot of controversy and rage as people and consumer associations as well as researchers, are unsure whether these kinds of foods are innocuous, even safe. Practically all around the world GMOs are responsible for numerous cases of allergies, sometimes very severe, causing a number of mortalities. As recent as 2010, in the United States of America, 28 million boxes of cornflakes and industrialized cereal products were withdrawn from supermarkets because of the strong allergies they caused to a high number of people.

Recently, even in England, Dr. Arpard Pusztai started a real controversy which reached the British Parliament. His research on the health of young rats fed on genetically modified potatoes for ten days clearly showed a weakening of the immune system with an abnormal development of both the liver and brain. These results were also published in the famous British medical magazine, *The Lancet*. Not with surprise, Dr. Pusztai has been strongly criticized, attacked by the food industry cartel, and lost his job. However, a few years later, in exactly September 2012, a French publication (*The New Observer – Le Novel Observateur*) published the report about a French scientific study that was like a bombshell concerning GMOs. In fact, it was first published by the U.S. magazine, *Food and Chemical Toxicology* which is a recognized reference in the field of food toxicology.

The scientific research was done in secret as not to attract the attention of Monsanto or other laboratories that have always hidden the truth to the public. The researchers fed several groups of rats during twenty-eight months with corn GMOs, either treated or not with Roundup, the Monsanto herbicide. After thirteen months, all the rats developed large tumor that often was as big as 25% of the rat's body weight and some rats developed several large tumors. At twenty-four months, meaning at the end of their life, 80% of the rats fed GMOs developed tumors against only 30% in the rats fed non-GMOs.

There are many people responsible concerning these GMOs, with the researchers of this study pointing to the sanitary agencies, the ECC commission in Brussels, Monsanto, and even governments (who may be unknowing). The consumption of GMO foods and the rate of many cancers are increasing, especially breast cancer. It could be the biggest scandal of this new century all conducted for the sake big money even if people are put at risk of cancer.

The magazine published various figures of the poor rats with large tumors and there is no way to deny how GMOs are dangerous for our health and even more so for our children. Today it becomes difficult to choose the best food, especially food which is not genetically modified, which we really have no guarantee of being of the same nutritional value compared with other food. Genetically modified foods may easily have completely unknown reactions, often dangerous, on the human body.

On the other hand, we can assist ourselves today as I explained in this book to participate in a revolution concerning the role certain beneficial foods in the prevention and treatment of disease.

As far as I am concerned, we are talking about natural, organically grown, non-manipulated food. Many new lines of research have shown that dietary components extracted from vegetables and fruits are able to inhibit tumor growth. It would be interesting to carry out the same experiments with genetically modified food, but obviously I am certain that the results will not be the same. If we remember the experience of Dr. Pusztai and the French study conducted by Gilles-Eric Seralini, professor of molecular biology, there is reason to believe that, along with the use of GMO foods, cancer risk may increase, because of further weakening of our immune system. Truthfully speaking, I don't think that GMO food is the "Food of God," not the original food that grows naturally on this planet welcoming the interaction of human kind and animals.

Science may be necessary to progress, but science can also kill us if we don't know how or learn how to use it properly. It is not always meant for the purpose of benefitting special interests from big industries.

About thirty years ago, a book was published which stunned millions of people, as it vigorously denounced polluted food and environmental pollutants. The title of this book, by Gunther Schwab, speaks for itself, *The Dance with the Devil*. Apparently, we are still dancing, but today the public is beginning to understand that this dance may end in disaster. The road to true health, and when I say "health," it is meant to be for a balanced healthy mind and body. Today, this can only be built through the intake of natural and whenever possible, organically grown foods.

Conclusions

Throughout this book I have demonstrated that the colon is the centerpiece of our body and responsible for either a good health status or an intoxication that will lead to chronic and degenerative disease. I have demonstrated that any natural treatment emphasizes detoxification, which is the first step to improve the body's function. We don't say that our treatment treats a disease but simply we are correcting some dysfunctions, which help the body to return to a normal function and health status.

We have spent time to speak about Iridology, which is a system with particular interest when it comes to know exactly about the real genetic profile of a patient, to understand exactly how each organ of their body is functioning, to know exactly about the colon, the state of intoxication, and how to treat your patient. There is no complete medical diagnosis without an Iridology checkup, and after nearly fifty years of clinical experience, I still believe that Iridology still has more to discover and may gain more and more popularity among patients and even to the new generation of young doctors.

Iridology has spread out throughout the world and is even taught in universities in countries like Russia and South Korea, while in Germany it has become a normal diagnostic tool for thousands of doctors. I have been often to Germany participating in Congresses and observed that many homeopathic doctors, Naturopaths and even medical doctors are using iridology.

In Russia there is extensive literature and an enormous database on Iridology. The irises of hundreds of workers were studied in a Russian project to determine their real state of health and the organic disorders. The results obtained were compared with conventional medical tests in order to verify the exact state of the organs and terrain. One of the objects of this project was to include the use of Iridology in hospitals, with the aim of obtaining a total diagnosis of the patient, avoiding at the same time, high-cost diagnostic methods.

Unfortunately, the general public does not have access to this information be it through television, magazines, newspapers, or other means of information. As compared to the United States, where television is open to education and public awareness of alternative methods, Europe and Portugal are far from an open democratic ideology in this field, preferring speculation and party debates, which publicly discredit these methods and use disinformation. Not long ago I was invited for a two-hour radio interview in the USA (*In Short Order*) by phone with the journalist Sue Vogan, PhD., (suevogan.net) from Tampa, Florida to speak about my professional life and topics such as cancer, detox, molecular markers, mitochondria, and what's wrong with medical doctors today. This is something impossible to do in many European countries totally controlled by pharmaceutical industries, where conventional medicine controls all the media.

304

My message has been that we cannot pretend to live healthy lives and keep our children healthy if we just limit ourselves to consulting medical doctors, run to hospitals whenever we feel sick, take pharmaceutical drugs and forget about our body and what it need. I often tell my patients you have only one body and you cannot change so be gentle with it and see what it needs.

Nutrition is an important step about which to learn and understand. First of all we should have respect for our body and give ourselves the best food possible. What value can I give to my body when I eat hot dogs and French fries? Answer: Probably, not very much.

At times we need to learn to be our own doctor and be responsible for our body, since we have only one body and cannot exchange a sick body for a healthy body. Dr. C. Kousmine said that every one of us needs to understand that he can count only on himself. He is responsible for himself, responsible for his health, where the body given to him must be highly valued as any other precious treasure. This cannot be pointed out or expressed any better, although sometimes this makes me feel as if I were talking myself.

Once again, the human body is a live unit and must be considered in its entirety. In this sense the iris is an open window into our body and personality, being a mirror between the body, nature, and the cosmos. That is, the link between the body and its environment. I am convinced that the iris was truly given to enable us to know ourselves and for self-diagnosis.

The current medical system only stresses the importance of pathology and the study of the illness forgetting about the terrain and the entire human body. Today new advances are being made in response and in justification of the theories that were resisted for so long. For example, a medical magazine recently stated that viruses are only active in an organ with a weakened immune system.

This theory is important but not new, as Naturopathy has always underlined the importance of environment, prevention, and defense of an organ. Indeed, here we see the first flaw in Pasteur's theory that proclaimed as follows, "All illnesses are caused by microbes,"

And all of a sudden, Claude Bernard's theory becomes credible, "The microbe is nothing, the environment is everything."

Through Iridology, it is now possible to reflect which are the weakest organs, as well as empirically on endocrinal dysfunction and the state of the immune defense, which has been developed by the iridologist, John Andrews, a top researcher. The bronchials, sinuses, lungs, and liver are the ideal targets for infection, colds, flu, and constipation, opening the doors to a latent virus. It is necessary to know which organ is more fragile in order to intervene effectively and reinforce the defenses of the organism. The iris is able to identify the areas in which possible health problems are likely to manifest. There's so much you can learn about your body from Iridology and I still do… its incredible!

In other chapters, I also wanted to emphasize my opinion on colon auto-intoxication and its effects on health. When the emunctory organs are deficient over a prolonged period, the progressive intoxication of the body leads to disease. Today, many Anglo-Saxon specialist magazines carry various scientific articles on intoxication. There are numerous books on this subject that provide us with valuable information and today detox is more accepted and divulged.

In truth, newly developed technology in electronics, the biomedical field, new blood and urine tests allow us to verify our organ's ability to detoxify. For example, treating the liver or kidney, which to me are very important, can give us a way to double check what you see in the iris. I think that this is a big step in line with old medical theories.

Since Hippocrates, and throughout history, the medicine of the "Entire Man," both preventative and curative, has resisted the power of allopathic or classic medicine worldwide. As a victory of the natural medical doctrine, today we are witnessing the opening of colleges of Alternative Medicine in many large American universities and a major development in some of the best Naturopathic schools.

This revolution has influenced and altered the percentage of patients who only use chemical drugs. Some years ago in a survey about CAM it showed that for the first time in United States the number of alternative medical consultations surpassed the number of consultations in conventional medicine.

This phenomenon is simply the result of a reflection, which demonstrates at first that we are now entering a new era, a real revolution in new ideas and concepts. The public and the patient are tired of being ill not to say sick of being sick. They are trying new ways and directions, looking for new solutions to their problems, diseases beyond the scope of conventional classical medicine, which does not provide answers.

Natural and organic food, previously criticized, ignored, and questioned for so long is now taking an important place in our life and has become an essential factor in health protection. Today more and more, we associate the science of nutrition, nutri-therapy, and functional foods, whatever we wish to call this, as the new medicine to treat disease. The question is really, can this be true?

About twenty-five years ago, I managed to visit a hospital in Germany run by the government. This was a special hospital where patients were treated only with natural therapeutics, no drugs, and nutritional diet from organic food. According to the director of the hospital, diets were an important means in the overall treatment. Each patient received a specific diet according to their particular case. Recently, in June of 2012, I was invited by the medical director of a German hospital to give a lecture at the 2nd International Congress of Complementary Oncology. This doctor, who set up the Congress, is also the president of the German Society of Oncology. With a group of other doctors attending the Congress, we visited the four-story hospital, which only treats cancer disease, and we not surprised that diet was an essential part of the treatment including fresh organic vegetable juices for the patient's needs. Today, in Germany there are six hospitals of this kind run by the government, two of them are specific for the treatment of cancer. Others are private hospitals.

As I said, we are assisting a true revolution, but in fact simply confirming ourselves by rediscovering the curative power of food diet as stated by Hippocrates, more than 2,500 years ago. It took so long, because during nearly a hundred years, scientists denied the powerful healing of food support by the new industry companies processing natural foods into dead food.

The same rules existed in other civilizations, such as the Oriental and Indian ones. The rules of life, hygiene, diet and spirituality were all integrated in medicine. Tibetan medicine, which became popular in the West, expounds these principles in the Wheel of Life and of the Illnesses.

Today, intoxication and detoxification are important factors in alternative medicine as they are two opposite poles, one of illness and the other of health. Unfortunately, the ratio of disease/health is today unacceptable, since health should be a dominant state and disease an occasional condition. In truth, making a human admit to a new theory or discovery is sometimes more difficult than splitting an atom. Dr. Jensen left us this interesting thought to meditate on: "Ignorance is cured with education." But ignorance is often more a fixation of the brain, which loses the sense of observation and curiosity to learn more or go further. This is often one of the reasons why official science is not interested in Iridology.

But let's analyze this example that illustrates this often holier than thou attitude of the scientists charged with considering new theories. Oxidative stress and the theory of free radicals are new advances in medicine, I would even say very recent. This shows that there is always something new to be discovered even though we may not think so.

When, by chance, the Americans, McCord and Fridovitch, discovered the enzyme superoxide dismutase (SOD) that later on led to the discovery of free radicals, some medical doctors asked McCord, "Why do you insist on discovering something that doesn't exist?" "Free radicals" were the most important medical discovery after the work of Pasteur, and who would deny today the science of oxidative stress?

We still have to keep our minds open since there is much to be discovered, to be observed, to learn and to put in practice. To have an open mind is one of the best qualities required for a researcher and for a doctor; otherwise, you are limited and make no progress. You cannot spend all your life as doctor and be limited to prescribing pills and not enjoying some good results with your patients.

Over the past decades I have practiced Naturopathic medicine, nutrition, Homeopathy, molecular medicine, complementary oncology and I am familiar with the development of non-conventional medicine around the world. But at the same time I keep one eye open to follow the work of conventional medicine which, unfortunately, has become more and more an instrument of disease repression by prescription drugs despite some significant progress. At the same time medical doctors slowly lost their link to the patient only to become increasingly computerized, the patient lost his personality and because many asked questions that for most they simply could not answer. Often they say, "This is beyond the scope of what I know."

More hospitals are being built, actual cement fortresses where patients are seen as a number, losing their personality, and often without answers to their problems. More and more interned patients die of resistant infections and viruses they catch, which is a problem that we pointed out over thirty years ago and now, here we are.

We are not speaking of course of the billions of dollars spent each year by the government for hospitals that resolve nothing, but on the contrary contribute to increased diseases. What is important today is to have in mind that people are looking to be healthier, to find a better solution for their problems, and not remain on drugs and pills all year round. Patients search for more information and explanation about their state of health and what can be done about it. Of course still many people are looking for the easy way and simply running to hospitals to get shots, antibiotics, and vaccinations even for their children with of course, no solution.

Most of them are Candidates for chronic and degenerative disease: brain stroke, heart disease, cancer, and MS, simply being not conscientious about the rules of nature and to know more about themselves.

Unfortunately, knowledge is not today a quality required in the field of conventional medicine, strictly limited to prescribing drugs or blind protocols such as in treating cancer disease. Probably they know little or none about health, about the body or about nutrition, but they are also the ones who believe in medicine and give their bodies to an over excess of drugs, chemotherapy, surgery, and radiation, where often they may die as a result.

In Europe, countries like France, England, Spain, Portugal, and probably others, TV programs rarely organize positive debates concerning alternative medicine, nutrition, or how we can be approach differently the disease of cancer, which has become a real epidemic. These are limited to real polemic critics, worthy of public market place. Often these debates turn up to ridicule our system and underline the placebo effects of most of natural medication. What about detoxification? By no means is it is activated by any placebo effect once the body has eliminated large quantities of toxic waste.

In fact, we can see the difference, before and after a diet and detox, by observing blood through the Live Blood Microscopy Analysis System, noting the shape of red blood cells, the white blood cells, and the quality of the blood free from oxidized fat, microorganisms, and heavy crystals. Definitively this is not a placebo effect but real science. I challenge conventional medicine to deny what you can actually observe in a drop of fresh blood before and after a treatment.

Under oxidative stress and radiation, damaged cells are activating DNA repair by inducing P53 gene expression leading either to cell's cycle arrest, allowing time for repair, or if not activate the apoptosis cascade and self-destruction of damaged cells. When the body is kept busy repairing, it doesn't make new proteins and tissues. This is why antioxidants, enzymes, food, or compounds containing DNA are so important since it can help in many ways. Our health status is dependent on our cells and their mitochondria. Good cells make good tissues and good organs, but medical drugs do nothing but only intoxicate the body further.

Iris observation is one important step for a doctor to have a whole view of the body from patients and especially to determine the causes of disease or symptoms. However, I insist that this practice needs to be carried out by a competent iridologist since it really requires certain knowledge beside years of experience.

According to the color of the iris, the structure of the iris fibers, the different iris markings, the observation of the main organs such as the colon, liver, and kidneys, we can define the genetic inheritance of the patient, the general health condition and his disposition towards certain illness. We can define how much intoxicated he or she is according to dietary style and environmental influence.

These must be defined, analyzed, explained to the patient with a corrective diet, detoxification program and other approaches. In fact this is the work of a Naturopath to know or discover when a patient is sick, to know about the cause of his disease or symptoms, the level or state of intoxication, provide the best treatment and most importantly educate the patient for a better way of life. This is what I usually do, it may take time, but over the years I have helped to change the lives of thousands of patients from an educational standpoint including special booklets about *How to Live a Natural Life*.

Then, in order to understand the level of intoxication in greater depth, a good, professional Naturopath may double-check the tongue (see chapter about diagnosis through the tongue), the mirror of our digestive system, the color of the skin, and the morphology of the face, which also may show what kind of food you eat and what organs may be damaged. Reflexology therapy of the foot is also a valuable diagnostic checkup for digestive organ function.

Other methods of diagnostic testing may be used along with Iridology for checkups on organic disorders, blockage of energy levels, inflammation, and intoxication that may go alone with chronic or degenerative disorders including brain function. One of the devices we use is the Vega-computerized analysis system, which performs these kinds of tests as well with energy levels, while it also permits us to exactly measure the degree of patient recovery after the treatment. In this way the patients have access to direct and immediate information which specifies the weakness of certain organs, the energy level, condition of allergy, and full condition of the digestive system.

On the other hand, if you consult a good and competent professional Naturopath, you can expect to receive full explanation about the condition of your health and disease, and the proper treatment. If you can also find a Naturopath that has a good knowledge of Iridology an examination of the irises is always valuable to profile your health and hereditary condition.

Again with Iridology, first it is very important that a competent professional carry out an Iridology examination, but this is not always the case. At first irises can define the genetic status of the patient and generally speaking the function of each organ of our anatomy and the predisposition towards certain diseases.

During my life I have observed several thousands of irises with bad colon, bad liver, bad nervous system, bad genetic status, bad constitution, and after so many years, I am really sure of what I see and I really know how to interpret what I see. You need to make the difference between a good ground and a bad ground, between a ground with a probability of cancer risk and a non-cancer ground and this is also true for rheumatism, diabetes and other diseases. The iridologist needs really to have the knowledge and experience to accurately interpret what irises show. I have an example of bad interpretation about a doctor saying there is no way for you to have a breast cancer. Then three months later, the patient was diagnosed with a breast cancer.
This is the story of a Naturopath coming from the United States seeking my help. Of course you can never be affirmative as such, best to say, according to my knowledge, I don't see any bad signs but best to check with a scan. Her irises showed me the breast cancer risk, but you may need to increase your knowledge and know how to interpret iris marks associated with inflammation, oxidative stress, how is the collarette next to the breast area, and then you can make your prognostic.

We are not practicing regular medicine but a vision of the art of healing. We need to acquire more knowledge about how the body is functioning, about how one organ can affect the other, and about what can be connected with a disease even before the disease is diagnosed. We have to see the body as a whole not only one part, this is what the irises is supposed to show. Looking into irises it is important to link what we see with what could happen or already has happened.

The iridologist needs to be the interpreter the various colors of the iris, the different spots, lacunas and other iris markings which may be detected in various tissues or on specific organs such as the liver, lung, kidney, and colon as the barometer of our health condition and by observing the iris collarette called the autonomic nervous system. This really indicates your nerve constitution and how it is associated with the good or bad function of most organs of our body. What is even more important is that irises can show the state of intoxication according to bad food style, overeating, which suggests the type of treatment and detoxification. You may have a bad liver or bad kidney function from a hereditary status and eating junk food, which overloads these two important detox organs resulting in an excess of toxins in the blood circulation. But above all, the iridologist must know about the significance of iris signs and make the correct association between one organ and another, to detect inflammatory process and how it can link with tissue inflammation and disease. Oxidative stress status is also important to profile and associate with certain dysfunction or pathology at every stage.

Looking up to the Philosophy of Naturopathy, the vision of the art of healing and upon to my own experience, a patient must be diagnosed or treated as a whole. The contrary would be a failure to attempt to treat a disease.

Our body function is also dependent on the Laws of the Universe and responds to the different seasons, moon phases, day, night, and so forth. Our physiology is also dependent on food quality. We need to rest, to breathe, to exercise, because there is no other way to balance our body. Did you know that exercises are important to keep mitochondria young and active? This is the new discovery of science.

We are subject to these rules and cannot live outside of these rules without consequences to our health status. We all are looking to be healthier, and my message is that a clean body is the first rule to protect itself against disease.

When first in consultation with a patient the time we spend is important so we can get a full profile and learn everything about the patient. By using all the diagnostic methods explained above, the patient becomes to you like an open book and you know everything about him. Indeed it is only Iridology which, from my personal experience of four decades permits me to profile the patient including the genetic status in a matter of a few minutes.

Let us not forget that our own life is an ocean of continuous observations of attempts, experiences, and fatalities. In reality practicing the true Naturopathy is not easy as medical doctors think that's because when we really follow the Hippocratic Oath it is contrary to today's practice of medicine. Practicing Naturopathy is truly an art; called the "Healing Art" that requires devotion, knowledge, reflection, observation, and experience. The Naturopath doesn't cure because this is done through nature, it's by the way nature is used that cures the patient.

This is why one must always maintain an open mind for learning. I know at least two oncologists that have changed their attitude after living through some personal bad experience with cancer that made them wonder if something different could be done, the experience having opened their minds to a new reality and vision of how cancer patients should be treated.

Were it left up to medical doctors, none of our natural medicine is proven and therefore totally rejected. What about chemical drugs with their toxic side effects, sometime dangerous, are they proven to cure? Cure the body means change something. You have to detoxify your body, reduce oxidative stress, increase nutrient supply to feed the cells, improve blood and oxygen circulation, or you make less healthy cells and healthy mitochondria. When we observe red cells through LBA microscopy with their membranes damaged by an excess of free radicals , damaged and dead white cells because of lower antioxidants defense, we can observe how they improve and regain a normal condition after a better diet and extra antioxidants in form of supplementation such as SOD, glutathione, vitamin C,E etc. This is what it means to change something and this is far from being a placebo effect.

I have accumulated enough experience and knowledge to show that our body reacts positively to selected natural compounds because it can be tested for its bioavailability, meaning the body can easily absorb the product to be used for immediate healing. Of course we can prescribe a specific product for the liver, or kidney, but it is also important to remember that the body makes a whole and cannot be separated into compartments. We have to treat the whole body. All the organs are dependent on the intestine for absorption of nutrients to feed themselves, and via reflex the colon is associated with most organs of our body. No one organ is separate from the nervous system and depends upon its quality and strength. In the observation of irises, the collarette tells us the genetic makeup of our nervous system. Some organs such as the pancreas, ovary, liver, colon, are highly dependent on a good nervous system and energy supply to function correctly. A weak nervous system can disturb or damage their function

Currently today our body has a tendency to intoxicate itself faster than ever before because of weaker detoxification and enzymatic system, poor elimination, and an excess of chemicals in the water, food, or atmosphere. That also is why more organs are affected and more people are suffering with more symptoms, more hospital and medical consultations, and more prescription drugs, resulting finally in more disease. That is why it is rare for only one organ to be affected. You have liver trouble? Look also at the colon and the nervous system and you will find correlation between the three.

Dialysis treatment is now booming in our modern society, and what is tragic now is middle age or even the youngest patients with kidney damage or atrophy. The other day I had a twenty-eight-year old young man with very weak kidney function and he had been told that soon he may need dialysis for the rest of his life. Did medicine have the ability to predict about kidney atrophy! Did we teach him about better food, to eat less meat? Probably not. He was considered as healthy, but looking into his iris, what do you think you see? He had a bad colon, bad kidney, bad nervous system, and an underlying bad food style. Too young, he was not prepared to hear about my advice to eat less red meat, one of the main problems for the kidney, and I had to spend time to explain how it is important to change one's mind about what has to be done if we could improve this situation; otherwise, he will be condemned to dialysis for the rest of his life. That give us something to think about, especially to really know what the meaning of health is and what to do to prevent such a situation or other diseases. Not being all encompassing, Iridology can still help to really define what exactly our health status is and are we subject to some health problems in the near future.

Naturopathy also includes this whole in its concept, philosophy and vision of the Art of Healing, that has been my path during the past fifty years, from what Dr. Bernard Jensen taught me, and the knowledge I learned from the great pioneers such as Dr. John Tilden and Benedict Lust. It is also important to remember that the body is a whole and each organ belongs to the whole and is not separate from each other. When we treat, it is the entire organism, since each organ communicates with the other in a mutual harmony. This is the true medicine as proclaimed by Hippocrates 2,500 years ago.

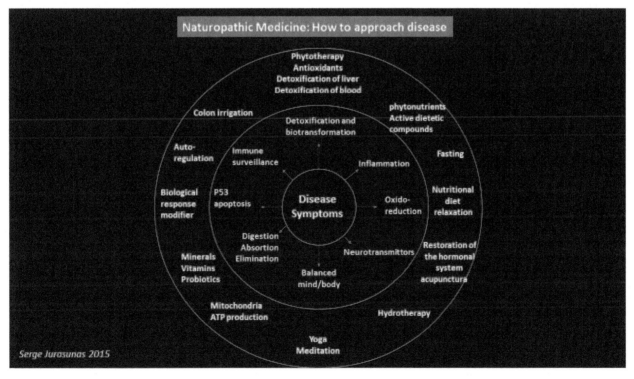

Clinical Cases

Many articles and papers have been written and published about detox, nutrition, body rejuvenation, and Naturopathic treatment, but one may ask oneself if it really works? During the past four decades, almost five, I treated all kind of diseases, of patients of all ages, cancers of all stages, including some of the worst diseases on this planet. Over 150,000 could be the approximate number of patients I treated during this time, being lucky to observe how nutrition, detox, Naturopathic treatment, and other modern approaches can be efficiently used to overcome a disease and improve health status. Treating symptoms is one thing, often chemical drugs work, but treating the whole body, improving health status is beyond the capacity of pharmaceuticals, which only serves to further intoxicate the body.

My original intention was not to include clinical cases, but some of my colleagues suggested to me that it would be important for the reader, just as book was about to be ready. I included one very bad case of a thirty-six-year-old young woman with Melas Syndrome, a progressively fatal disease, who came in my clinic in a deteriorated condition, resulting from both her physical and brain status. After six months, the patient is now able to have a normal life, to a certain extent of course, where before she could not walk even for one hour down the street.

Such admirable results could not be hidden. Therefore, I decided to include the case in this book, along with a number of other particularly interesting cases that I had treated, spanning over a thirty-five-year period where I particularly treated young children.

Case No. 1 (1984): Chronic Diarrhea

This is a little girl I wrote about in the book who had been suffering from chronic diarrhea since she was one year old. Her mother consulted three pediatric doctors and one gastrointestinal disease specialist, but without success. She was prescribed over twenty different types of antibiotics and other pharmaceutical drugs. Apparently, the only diagnosis made was an allergy to milk, but changing milk, even to soya milk, didn't resolve her problem. The little girl, Marta, continued with up to twelve and fifteen bowel movements per day and not one doctor was able to do something about her condition. We changed her diet, which her pediatric doctors did not offer to do, eventually proving they had no knowledge about her situation. I removed meat from her diet, gave her my vegetarian puree that I also mention in this book, sesame puree, cherry juice, steamed young carrots, boiled fish, and oatmeal. The supplementation I prescribed was my Apizellin formula, daily in 7.5ml ampoules, made of herbs, enzymes, biocatalyzers, glutathione, red beets, silver, potassium, and germanium, along with some bee pollen.

After two months of treatment, Marta was free from diarrhea but kept coming in for evaluation and checkups for several months to come. At the beginning we performed oxidative dried blood layer test for this little girl that showed a major inflammatory process which we slowly decreased using our Apizellin formula.

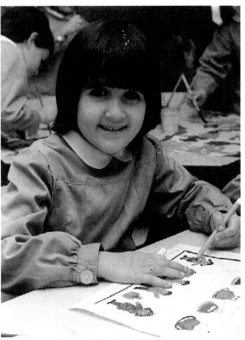

Photo nº 1

Photo No. 1 shows Marta at school, with a drawing which she gave to me inscribed with a few words on the back. She gained weight after two months of treatment.

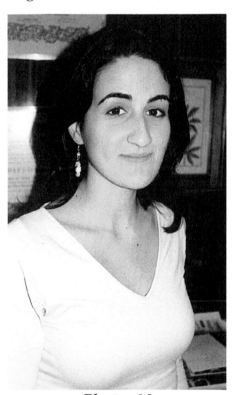

Photo nº 2

Photo No. 2 is Marta about twenty years later coming to visit me for a consultation. She never since suffered from diarrhea, due to observing a healthy diet, just as I taught to her mother.

Case No. 2 (1985): Little Girl with Organic Dysfunction

This is an extraordinary case of a little girl suffering from various organic dysfunctions. She was very nervous, had insomnia, alopecia, and no appetite, along with psychological disorders.

Her mother smoked during her pregnancy and was interned with lung emphysema. The little girl was not eating good food, or only a very small quantity. I remember that from her iris examination I diagnosed a bad liver function, toxic bowel, many nerve rings, and several dark lacunas in the lung area. Here we have a typical case of bad hereditary status and malnutrition as shown in photo No. 1.

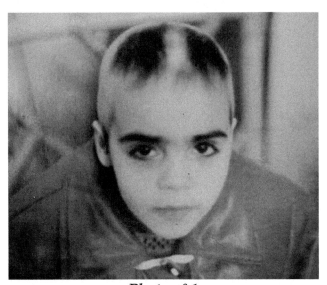

Photo nº 1

Unfortunately, this was not the photo taken at the first consultation, which we had been unable to provide, but only after thirty days of treatment and diet. What changed dramatically was a real beginning of hair growth, because at first, she was totally without hair.

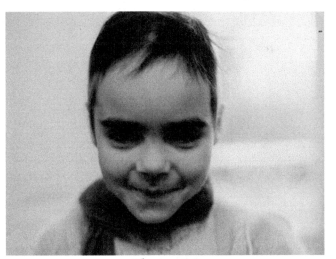

Photo nº 2

Now, photo No. 2 really shows a major change after three months of treatment. Her physical condition is remarkable, she grew and has much more hair, and looks much happier.

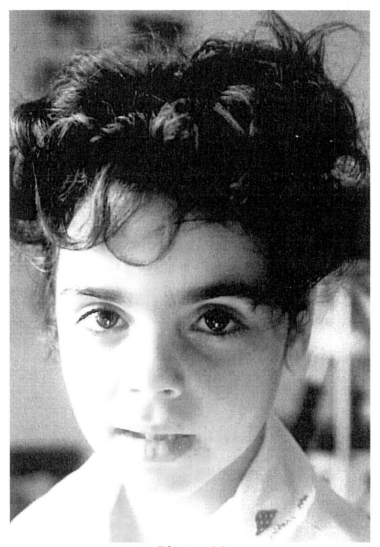

Photo nº 3

Photo No. 3, is the same girl after one year of treatment. This definitively shows what nutrition and wisely chosen food can do for our body, especially with a beautiful child. Besides the change in her diet, we helped the body to revitalize by using the supplementation, Chlorella Growth Factor, which really works at the cellular level, increasing cellular respiration.

At this level, nobody can deny the value of healthy food, organic vegetables, and juices with good supplementation in regenerating a sick body. As I repeated often in the book, pharmaceutical drugs can never make such an achievement.

Case No. 3: Seven-Year-Old Girl with Grade II Glioma

This is a seven- year-old young girl with a story of a grade II glioma who was diagnosed in September 2008, followed by chemotherapy, a two-year period of remission, and then a relapse in 2010. She was then submitted to partial surgery and chemotherapy. In 2011, she underwent a subsequent three-week period of chemotherapy, but a new scan showed no improvement.

She then was given more chemotherapy, about fifty-two sessions, but the tumor kept growing. In fact, it grew by 130%, making a strong pressure in the brain and new surgery was suggested. After the surgery, little Anoka could walk, but only with much difficulty and could only feed by using a drill (permanent surgical opening drilled into her stomach), but only with liquid food. The drill opening was also used to administer her medication. She was unable to talk for over one year and could eat only through the drill until it was possible to be removed, after which she really started to improve with our treatment and diet. She also lost the vision in her left eye, could hardly move her fingers, or raise her right arm. We are not even speaking about her psychological condition. While submitting to more chemotherapy, the mother decided to seek elsewhere for some alternative treatment, despite warning of medical doctors.

However, her mother came to me and we started to treat little Anoka with food, diet, nutritional supplementation, vegetable juices, oxy germanium in capsules, SOD capsules, glutathione i.m. and other antioxidants to be taken orally. As a result, her mother decided to stop any further chemotherapy, at least during a period, with the consent of her doctor.

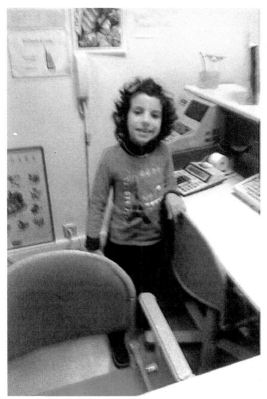

Photo nº 1

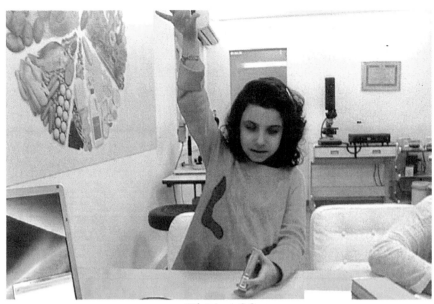

Photo nº 2

One can see for themselves in photo No. 1 at the first consultation, and how she looks in photo No. 2, about one year later, raising her arm for the first time. In photo No. 3, taken in September 2014, we can definitively observe what food, diet, and nutritional support can do in order to improve and even heal the physical body, even how this may also influence a brain tumor. This is real, not magic or a miracle, but simply the power of nature.

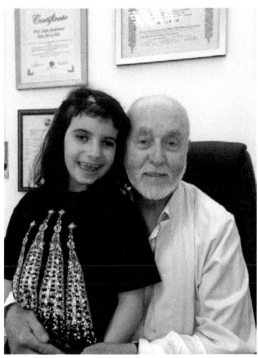

Photo nº 3

Case No. 4: Six-Year-Old Boy with Wilms Tumor

This is the story of a six-year-old boy who was diagnosed in 1983 with a Wilms tumor (7 cm) across the chest, but the mother was looking for alternative medicine, refusing surgery and chemotherapy. While this was a challenge to me, and probably a failure, I decided to treat the boy with nutrition, vegetable juices, enzymes, and other natural remedies such the organic germanium of K. Asai. After seven months of treatment, the large tumor was eliminated.

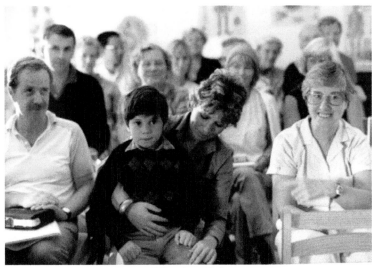

Photo nº 1

Photo No. 1 shows the boy, Tiago, seated on the knee of a doctor from a group that came from Holland to my clinic to learn my methods of treating cancer. I asked the mother to come alone with the boy and bring all the radiographs before and after to explain the case during my seminar.

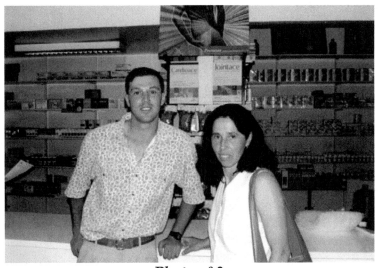

Photo nº 2

Many years later, in photo No. 2, Tiago is shown with his mother just before going to serve in the army.

Then, in photo No. 3, thirty years later, Tiago is shown with his wife and daughter. This is one of the most wonderful stories among so many others about patients that I treated during the past forty years.

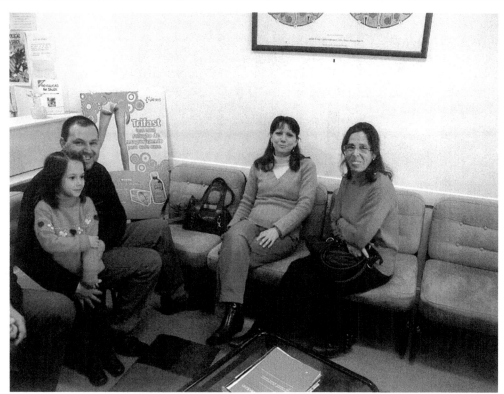

Photo nº 3

Case No. 5: Severe Allergy

Case of severe allergy – The patient is a middle-aged man with a bad diet habit, a ballooned colon, and with a busy life. The intestine functions every couple of days which increased the auto-intoxication of the colon.

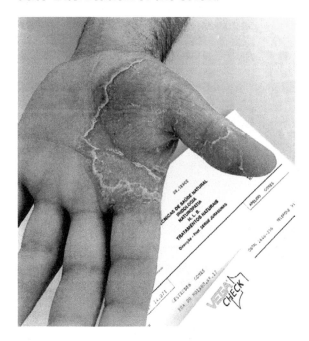
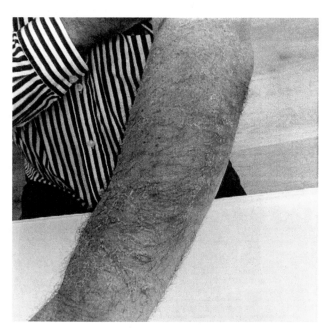

We changed the diet of the patient, suggested colonic irrigation, to have daily intake of vegetable juice such as carrot, watercress (rich in silicon), celery, parsley, and apple. Dietetic supplementation included Zell Oxygen Yeast Cells preparation, Sun Chlorella, and zinc tablets.

However, detoxification remained most important, where we can observe in the second photo that after ten days of treatment, the patient was cured from this bad allergy.

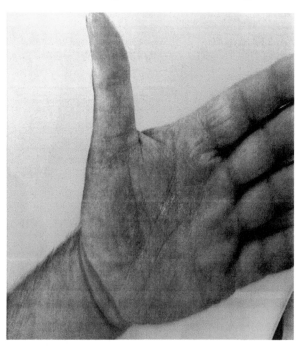
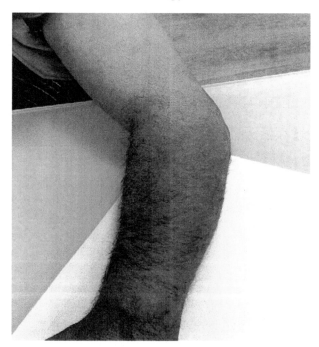

Case No. 6: Melas Syndrome Treated with Positive Results

Melas is the short definition of mitochondrial encephalomyopathy, lactic acidosis, and stroke-like episodes.

Melas is a progressive neuro-vegetative disease, a rare form of dementia caused by mutations by defects in the mitochondrial genome which is inherited purely from the female parents. MT, TH, MT, TL1, TV are the most common mutations, especially TL1, since it impairs the ability of mitochondria to make proteins, use oxygen, and produce energy. Some of the proteins normally produced are essential to synthetize enzyme complex in mitochondria that help convert oxygen, fats, and single sugars into energy. ATP is not manufactured and results in severe mitochondrial disorders. As result of this process, with disorders in the electron chain transport (E.C.T.) of mitochondria, the Melas patient builds up a large quantity of lactic acid, a waste product in the body, increasing acidity in the blood, resulting in extreme fatigue.

Melas syndrome affects many of the body's systems, but particularly the brain (encephalon) and muscles (myopathy). Repeated stroke-like episodes can progressively damage the brain, leading to vision loss, problems with movement, and dementia. Other deep symptoms include muscle weakness, extreme fatigue, headache, loss of appetite. Other damage includes hearing loss, heart and kidney problems, epilepsy, diabetes, and difficulty in walking and moving.

Prognosis

There is no known treatment for the underlying disease, which is progressive and fatal. However, some supplements have been shown to be helpful, but there have been no consistent reports of success. This includes amino acids, antioxidants, and some vitamins. COQ10 has been helpful for some Melas patients. Riboflavin has been reported to improve the function of a patient with complex 1 deficiency and the 3250 T-C- mutation. Succinate may be useful in treating uncontrolled convulsions in Melas patients, but this needs further investigation.

Clinical situation

The patient, a thirty-six-year old woman, Marta, a mother of two children, came to my clinic in January 2014 with a diagnosis of Melas Syndrome.

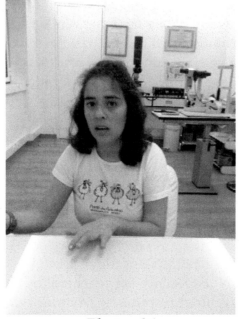

Photo nº 1

Marta was walking and moving with much difficulty, even from the waiting room to my office. She was in very bad physical condition and psychological distress. Her husband came in with her, helped her to walk and especially to have an open discussion with me. As you see in the above photo No.1, Marta also has considerable difficulty in moving her finger, difficulty in hearing, and even talking. She cannot comfortably go for a walk down the street, even slowly, for more than one hour without feeling deep fatigue. Naturally, she cannot perform normal housewife duties or take care of her two daughters. Marta is suffering from the following symptoms and dysfunctions:

- Loss of vision

- Cataracts

- Hearing loss

- Epilepsy

- Severe headache

- Diabetes

- Fatigue

Her initial treatment

Marta came to my clinic taking a number of drugs to retard some of the degenerative process and control the epileptic crisis.

What is my approach to Melas Syndrome?

While I have been deeply involved with mitochondrial dysfunction associated with cancer, I have spent decades studying the role that mitochondria plays in health and disease. I had never before had an experience with a Melas Syndrome patient, although I have experience in treating another mitochondrial disease called Amyotrophic bilateral sclerosis, fatal to patients with some relative success, but accompanied by the incapacity of the patients to pursue the treatment.

Anyhow, my experience was encouraging when Marta first faced me, being a new challenge that life offered me. In such situations, experience and intuition may drive our brain to think about what can be done, to see even if it can be done. While I have in my clinical pharmacopeia some medication and supplementation that can by-pass the blockage in the electron respiratory chain, activating the production of ATP, and decease acidosis, I asked myself: Why not attempt to regenerate the mitochondria function? Over past decades, approaching fifty years, I was confronted with so many patients with degenerative diseases, that for most of them, I resolved their diseases. I told Marta's husband, who himself investigated mitochondria in trying to help his wife. At least we could attempt to retard the progressive degeneration of her brain and muscles.

I would try one treatment over a period of 30-60 days and watch closely how she would react or not, considering my past experience treating mitochondria may help me to choose the appropriate treatment but nothing more.

My idea was to use some of the regenerative products I've used for the past twenty years, even some during the past forty years. Especially for regenerating the whole body, to improve the brain function, while activating cellular respiration. My idea was also to help promote building mitochondrial proteins, a real challenge. However, in the past and up to now, I have reversed mutated P53 and restored it to a normal wild-type function as I described in my past articles published in *Townsend Letter*; therefore, why not try this with mitochondria! So I decided to experiment with a treatment for this patient that included live cell therapy, detoxification, increasing nutritive food, cocktails of vegetables juice, and the enzyme yeast cells preparation to boost the mitochondria and Chlorella Growth Factor in liquid.

The first medication that came to my mind was the rejuvenating compound called RN13 in ampoule form, to be injected i.m. that I often used with success for over twenty years in such cases as kidney dysfunction, geriatric disorders, extreme fatigue, and to increase cellular respiration and vitality in cancer patients as explained in my article published in *Townsend Letter*, August/Sept 2012.

RN13 contains the ribonucleic acid from different organs found in the embryo, such as placenta, umbilical cord, pancreas, suprarenal, testes, etc., as well as amino acids, glutamic acid, vitamin E, B6, B12, trace elements, bio-lecithin, etc. Posology (Dosage): 3 ampoules of 5 ml i.m. 3 to 4 times per week

Enzyme Yeast cells preparation – each 10 ml dose contains 50 billion biochemically active young yeast cells containing all the vitamins, minerals, amino acids, trace elements, enzymes of the respiratory chain, coenzyme A, NADH, cytochrome and mitochondrial sequences. It is most important to mention Live Yeast Cells are high in coenzyme Q10 in a natural easy to assimilate form. The product, administered orally, reaches the small intestine, enters into the blood and releases all the substances mentioned for immediate healing.
Posology (Dosage): 20 ml mixed in a glass of apple juice or carrot/beetroot juice three times per day.

Coenzyme Q10 (100mg capsules)
Posology: 1 capsule three times per day

NADH (5 mg tablet)
Posology: 1 tablet before breakfast

Chlorella Growth Factor (liquid) contains nucleic acids and other DNA ingredients.
Posology: 10ml three times per day

The patient was also told to improve her regular diet with more vegetables and fruits, whole cereals, tofu, vegetable sprouts, rice bran, and regular intake of vegetable juices.

The Results:

After two months of treatment, Marta began to improve and move with more facility, although her husband still accompanies her on consultations.

After three months, Marta felt much better, looked healthier and can walk in the city for four hours without feeling tired, which is a major victory.

After six months, Marta is completely different comparing to the first consultation, feels healthy and especially happy, and the photo No. 2 speaks for itself.

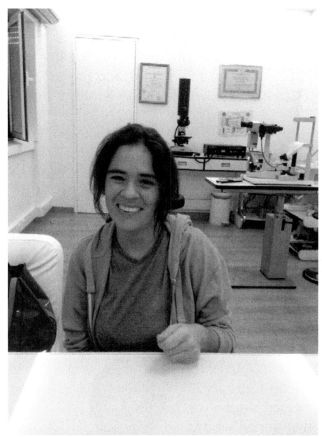

Six Months Later

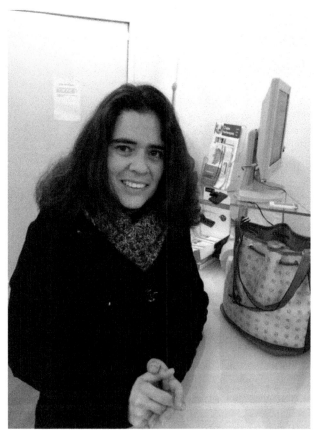

On the 7th January 2015

Conclusion:

This is more than a victory over a progressive, fatal disease that not only affects the whole body, including the brain, but leaves the patient in a distressed condition. The fact that a disease is considered incurable, doesn't mean that nothing can be done to help, and that should be the aim of an integrative doctor. Intuition is supposed to be one important quality required in the medical profession and we cannot always rely on scientific data and proof. I decided to publish this case, especially about the treatment, so doctors with similar cases may offer some better and longer lasting improvement for their patients.

While Marta is not cured, at least she can enjoy her normal life and look after her two daughters, but with precaution since tiredness overtaxes the mitochondria.

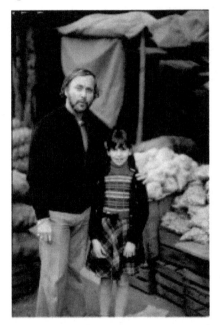

The same girl, now married with 2 children who also now are my patients.

The mother and her husband are doing regular consultation.

Here I am some 35 years ago with a young girl who at the time is my patient. She suffer from asma, constipation, physical weakness, etc...

We meet at a Agriculture exhibit in Portugal.

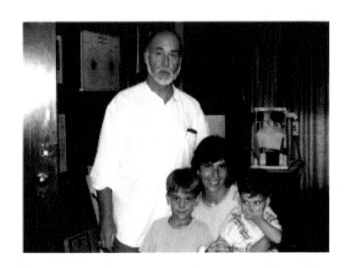

This is the most wonderful thing for a doctor treating patients to experience in one's lifetime: observing children who become adults, who still are coming to you and you even treat their own children.

Today we often receive criticisms for what we do, practicing a non-proven medicine, but we achieve results that medical doctors cannot pretend to have and are usually denied. At least one can be proud to achieve so many years of treating patients with these results, success, increasing health status, curing diseases, and changing the life style of patients. What is the satisfaction of prescribing over and over again antibiotics to children without results? Of course this book is based on colon health and detoxification, but the intestine is part of our immune system, the microbiome is one of our greatest defense systems, and we damage it with antibiotics. We have to teach this new generation about the nutritional value of food, about vitamins, minerals, about what to do to preserve the body against disease; otherwise, the predators of this new century are just ready use them as "pills-boxes" and use disease for money making. Health is probably the best thing we possess on this planet, why destroy it?

List of Cases

Clinical Cases

Bibliography

Andrews, John -- *Iris Pupillary Signs*. Publisher: Corona Books. England. John Andrews Iridology Clinic.

Baartz, Marian – Iridology Training and Research. The Iris Collarette. Collarette Changes - Collarette Structure. Lecture 28 September 2003. 7th International Iridology Symposium. London England.

Batello, Celso – Iridologia e irisdiagnose – o que os olhos podem revelar. Editora Ground. Sao Paolo, Brasil, 1990.

Bliz, F.E. – Nouvelle methode pour guerir les maladies (2000 pages). Librairie Editeur. Paris, France, 1930.

Bordeu, Theophile, Dr. – Recherces sur les maladies chronique. Imprimés chez J.A.Brosson Imprimeur Librairie. Paris, France, 1772.

Bouchut, E. Dr. Prof. – Histoire de la Médicine et des doctrines médicales. Librairies Germer Bailliéres. Paris, France, 1864.

Bouchard, Ch. Dr. - Maladie par Auto-intoxicación. Librarie F. Savy. Paris, France, 1885.

Bourget, Dr., et Dr. Rabow – Précis de Thérapeutique. Th. Sack. Librairies Editeur. Lausanne, Suisse, 1902.

Carnic, Alain, Dr. – Mèdicine Préditive – Un fantastic espoir. Èditeru Albin Michel. Paris, France, 1990.

Collings, Jollie –Principles of colonic irrigation. Thorsouse, USA, 1996.

Deledique, Alain G., Dr. – Vous ne pouvez plus ignorer la Thalassothérapie. Ed. Carmugli, Lyon, France, 1978.

Dhonden, Yeshi, DR. – Guérir ° la source. "La science et la Tradicion de la Médicine Tibétaine" (Traduit du Tibétain en Anglais). Guy Tédaniel Editeur. 2000.

Gilbert, Scot F. – *Developmental Biology*. Sixth edition. Sinauer Associates, Inc. Publisher, Massachusetts, USA. 2000

Hahnemann, Samuel –Des maladie chronique. Ed, Luois Babes. Lyon, France.1852.

Hill, Ray –Juice therapy – A story of the extraordinary healing properties of organic vegetable juice. Published by Nuhealth Books. Gloucestershire, England, 1997.

Hippocrates – Oeuvres médicales en 4 volumes. Impriemés à Toulouse, France, 1793.

Huffeland, G. – Premier médecin du roi de Prusse – Manuel de médecin pratique. Germer Bailliers. Librairie éditeur, Paris, France 1848.

Khune, Luiz – The new science of Healing (translation). Luiz Khune Edition. Leipzig, Germany 1896.

Kuhlmann, Pirk, Dr. – Die Pliz-invasion. Editeur Verlag Bio. Medoc, Germany 1991.

Kullenberg, B. – Les bienfaits du vinagre de cidre. Editions Vigo, Paris, France, 2001.

Jensen Bernard, D.C.N.D. – Iridology– The Science and Practice in the healing Art. Bernard Jensen Publisher, Escondido, California, USA, 1982.

Jensen Bernard, D.C.N.D. – Doctor-Patient Handbook, Dealing with the several processes and the healing crisis through detoxification. Bernard Jensen Publisher, Escondido, California, USA, 1976.

Jensen Bernard, D.C.N.D.- Vision of Health – what your eyes reveal about your health. Avery Publishing Group Inc. New York, USA 1988.

Jensen, Bernard + Mark Anderson – Empty Harvest – understanding the link between foods, our immunity and our planet. Avery Publishing Group Inc. New York, USA 1990.

Joseph, Deck – Principle of iris diagnosis. Published by the author. Institute for Fundamental Research in Iris Diagnosis. Etthingen, Germany , 1982.

Lo Rito, Daniele – Embryology in Iridology. Advanced Iridology Research Journal, Vol 3/4 . September, 2002.

Levy, Stuart, B. – professor of molecular biology and microbiology – The challenge of Antibiotic Resistance. Scientific American, page 32-39, 1998.

Morelle, Jean – L'oxidation des aliment et la santé. François-Xavier de Guilbert, Paris, France, 2003

Mourey, Christophe – Comment vaincre le constipation par les méthodes naturelles. Editions de Vecchi, Paris, France, 1983.

Nick, Gina L. PhD, ND – Clinical Purification. Longevity Through Prevention, Inc. USA, 2001.

Pastern, Charles A., Dr. – The Molecules within our body in health and disease. Plenum Press, New York, 1998.

Pesek, David PhD. – Holistic Iridology. Basic Course, USA.

Pithchford, Paul – Healing with whole foods Oriental Traditions and Modern Nutrition. North Atlantic Books. Berkeley, California, USA 2003.

Platen, M. Professeur – Livre d'Or de la Santé. Méthod nouvell, complet et pratique de la médecine naturelle et de l'hygiène privée. Bong Editeurs. Paris, France. 1930.

Povoa, Helion – O Cérebro Desconhecido – como o sistema digestivo afeta nossas emoções. Editora Objectiva Ltd. Rio de Janeiro, Brasil 2000

Purves, William K et al – Life the science of biology. Fifth edition.   Sinauer Associates, Inc. Publishers. Massachusetts, USA 1999.

Robert, Carola et al – Human Anatomy and Physiology. McGraw Hill Inc. USA, 1992.

Schollmann, Claudia, Dr. – Intestinal Mikroflora und Immunosytem. Forum Medzin, Deutchland, 1997.

Schneider, E., Dr. – La santé ça se mange. Edition Vie et santé. France 1985.S

Seignalet, Jean, Dr. – *L'alimentation ou la troisième médecine*. Ed. François Xavier de Guibert. Paris, France 2001.

Simnshon, Barbara – *L'ananas- miracle de la santé*. Librairie de Medicus. Entrelacs (édition française). Orsay, France 2000.

Starenkyj, Daniele – *Mon petit docteur*. Publications Orion Richmond, Quebec, Canada 1989.

Tissot, Dr., - Docteur et Professeur de médecine – *Avis ou peuple sur la santé*. Chez P. François. Didot le jeune éditeur. Paris, France 1762.

Valnet, Jean, Dr. – *Aromatherapie – traitement des maladies par les essences de plantes*. Librairie Malone, SA. Paris, France 1964.

Walker, Norman, W.D.Sc.Ph.D – *The Key to a Vibrant Life*. O'Sullivan Woodside Company. Phoenix, Arizona, USA 1979.

Wildman, Robert E.C. – *Handbook of Nutraceuticals and Functional Foods*. CRS series in Modern Nutrition. CRS press. USA 2001.

Author's Publications:

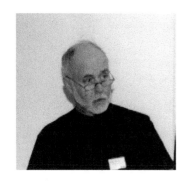

An Importancia dos Antioxidants – Natipress (2.edition 2015)

L'Iridologie – Un Diagnostic Naturel (out of print)

Le Germanium: une réponse au cancer (out of print)

Le Lapacho et le cáncer - Edition MIVA –1989 – Switzerland

Revolução Na Saúde - Natipress 1999 – Sintra, Portugal

Mitochondria DNA Mutations in Aging and Degenerative Diseases – Iridology profile and treatment.

New Millennium International Iridology Symposium, 11- 12 November 2000 – London, United Kingdom

Mitochondria DNA Mutations in Aging and ARC's Disease – Iridology Profile.

13th International Symposium "Integrative Medicine 2001" – Malta

The Therapy of Enzyme Yeast Cells in Cancer Disease, C.F.S and Aging Process. Natipress 2001 – Sintra, Portugal

"How to Interpret Iris Signs to Profile Aging," *Advanced Iridology Research Journal*

Volumes 3 + 4 – September 2002 – United Kingdom

"Biological Aging Signs in the Iris," *International Journal of Iridology*

Volume 1 n° 1 – United Stated of America

Breast Cancer Therapy and Profiling Through Iridology and Therapies (100 colored pages). 7th International Iridology Symposium, 27-28 September 2003 – London, United Kingdom

An Integrative and Naturopathic Approach to Breast Cancer. Natipress 2003 – Sintra, Portugal (Online at: www.sergejurasunas.com)

Breast Cancer Theory, Profiling Through Iridology: Therapies

7th International Symposium on Iridology– 27-28 September 2003 – London, England

For more articles, publications, and clinical cases consult: www.sergejurasunas.com

Where to Learn Iridology:

International Institute of Iridology- Dr. David
Pesek
375 Paradise Lane
Waynesville, North Carolina 28785
Email: drpesek@holisticIridology.com

John Andrews Iridology Clinic
Research Journal
www.johnandrewsiridology.net
Email:johnandrewsiridology@hotmail.com

College of Oriental Medicine
University of Health Sciences
Graduate Division
181 South Kukui Street
Suite 206
Honolulu, Hawaii

Integrated Iridology
PO Box 389
West Burleigh QLD 4219
Australia
Iridologyonline.com
Email: info@Iridologyonline.com

Institute for Applied Iridology
Harri Wolf
PO Box 301
Laguna Beach, CA 92652-0301
949-362-4959

International Iridology Practitioner Association
PO Box 1442
Solona Beach, CA 92075
www.Iridology assn.org
888-682-2208
iipacentraloffice@Iridologyassn.org

Hellenic Medical School of Iridology
2 Lidias St.
544 53 Thessaloniki
Greece
Email: irismed@otenet.gr

The Canadian Institute for Iridology
Christina Gualtieri – Program Coordinator
233 Park Lawn Rd.

Toronto – Ontario M8Y 3J3
Canada
Email: Iridologyplus@hotmail.com

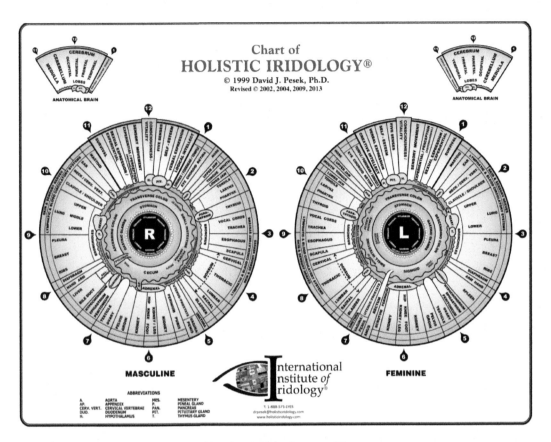

Holistic Iridology Chart

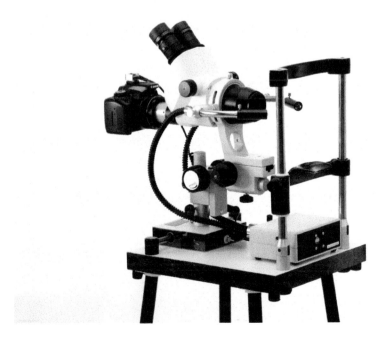

Pesek Iriscope

List of Colon Hydrotherapy Schools:

The International Association for Colon Hydrotherapy provides information and an Institute for Colon Hydrotherapy Training, along with a list of recognized schools and practitioners in the United States, Latin America/Caribbean, Canada, Australia, Asia, Israel, Japan, Hong Kong and Europe. Contact Information:

Email: homeoffice@i-act.org   Website: www.i-act.org

Phone: 210-366-2888 Fax: 210-366-2999

Special Course Just Announced for Our Readers

A complete course on colon detox and iridology, fully illustrated with colored figures will be available only for the readers of this book. This course is a must for doctors looking to further increase their knowledge after reading this book, especially for doctors working with Colon Hydrotherapy. This is a must for every practitioner looking to understand, treat, and detoxify their patients. This course was developed after nearly fifty years of clinical practice.

Readers can receive updates, new documentation, and clinical cases by sending your e-mail address to: SergeJurasunas@hotmail.com

INDEX

U

V

W

X

Z

Epigenetics: How Environment, Lifestyle and Food Modulate Our Genes

Some new lines of research now show how the environment and food can influence the expression of our genes in our present life and later on by passing them on to our children. In truth, we can modify the expression of genes to shut down or activate this mechanism leading to diabetes or cancer. A new science called epigenetics shows how we can modulate our health status, even with a family disease risk, by improving our dietary style, cutting down alcohol etc., with the genes keeping the information about what we eat, about our stress conditions; this being very important for pregnant women, transmitting this information to our children and grandchildren.

For instance, what we see now with the increasing level of juvenile and even younger diabetics is the result of an excess of consuming the wrong food by the past generation that has disturbed the pancreas. This information is then transmitted in the pancreas gene. Although Iridology is relevant to what we can observe in the irises that are associated with the pancreas, or even the liver which do not correspond as of yet to a disease, but probably in the future, as I have often observed, it will show up in iris cases concerning hepatitis, diabetics, and various types of cancer.

It is the same with the tumor suppressor genes which can be the result of environmental condition, stress shutting down by epigenetic process of the DNA methylation. For instance, the P53 tumor suppressor gene is suppressed, blocked up, or even result in P53 mutation transmitted to our descendants that are born with a deficient or mutated P53 on the way to cancer, and this is what we have seen today with juvenile or middle age cancer patients even today beginning around 26 years old including colon or stomach cancers, lymphoma, and brain cancer.

So our lifestyle and food is more important than we think, and this is not only a question of vitamins, minerals, and proteins, but it is food that modulates our genes. In fact, some years ago I wrote a document about DNA methylation and the Chlorella Growth Factors that I call a "Genomic food" since it contains nucleotides, nucleic acid, and other important nutrients such as glutathione, selenium, vitamins A,C,E, zinc, vitamin B6, and nicotinamide. Zinc is very important since it interacts with DNA-binding proteins forming what we know as "zinc fingers."

The zinc fingers act as molecular switches affecting gene expression at the level of transcription. Now DNA methylation plays an important role in gene function and requires the presence of methyl groups, and the primary donor of methyl groups in the body is S-Adenosylmethionine or SAM-e.

SAM-e requires nutrients such as methionine, choline, vitamin B12, and folate which assist in this process and are considered the primary dietary sources of methyl donors. If the body does not have enough SAM-e, cancer can arise and, as explained, can shut down tumor suppressors. Environmental toxins may also have negative effects on methylation. Of course this is only a short explanation, but I wrote a small book about it called *Liver, Detoxification of Toxins and Chemicals Using Chlorella Extract and CGF*.

The cells transmit to their descendants this configuration of tumor suppressor genes of cancer that are shut down, and in this way, cancer can arise. The epigenetic transformation can be transmitted through several generations, and with no surprise, this new generation is much more vulnerable. Empirically this is what Iridology has shown with iris examinations of the youngest, their parents and grandparents showing for most of us, the same iris signs which can be compared to information transmitted to the iris during the early development of the embryo and before the differentiation mechanism, which prove that all the information is already imprinted in the iris before the organs start to develop.

In the iris, we are not looking for disease, but how our body is being developed according to the health condition of our parents and grandparents, and the iris show many signs that can be compared to some information transmitted. In fact, it is the same as in the universe because science now agrees that what is the universe today is the result of information that pre-existed before the start of the Big Bang.

We are now approaching a new area of discovery, not only about the universe, but also our body. Another discovery is the transmission of billions of bacteria by the mother to her child to build the intestinal microbiome that we know today greatly influences our behavior, physical and psychological, and plays a key role in various body functions and immune function. But what is new is that science has now discovered that this transmission is not involuntary but really programed and essential to the good development of the newborn baby. So, as I explained, this information preexists in the embryo cells and we realize that our body has been programed since the beginning, same as the food that contains everything necessary to activate all the functions of the body and modulate our genes so that we can live healthy and avoid disease.

Industrialization of food can be seen as the worst tragedy for human kind since it has removed most of the nutrients needed for the body. Let's also mention the nervous system, which today is reaching a critical phase of deterioration from the use of denatured food, social stress, tobacco, pollution, and from generation to generation it is getting worse where psychiatric drugs seem to be the only answer offered by our medical science, which, to the contrary, makes things worse, and we end up assisting in an epidemic of suicides and crimes that are the direct result of excess usage of psychiatric drugs. Indeed, we are making things worse since these types of drugs greatly damage the mitochondria, our energy power house that is associated with all our cellular functions, differentiation, apoptosis, and cancer—not even mentioning other degenerative diseases. Now, if we all agree on the information to be transmitted to our next generation, then what are we now going to transmit if all our life we have been taking medical drugs, antibiotics without reason, anti-inflammatory medications, cortisone, wrong food, excess of food etc. What are we going to transmit to our future generations!

SERGE JURASUNAS

Readers can receive updates, new documentation, and clinical cases by sending your e-mail address to Sergejurasunas@hotmail.com

CPSIA information can be obtained
at www.ICGtesting.com
Printed in the USA
LVOW06s1224020118
561499LV00026B/438/P

9 789892 069388